COMING OF AGE

THE 75-YEAR HISTORY OF THE
AMERICAN COLLEGE OF HEALTHCARE EXECUTIVES

COMING OF AGE

THE 75-YEAR HISTORY OF THE
AMERICAN COLLEGE OF HEALTHCARE EXECUTIVES

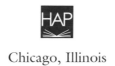

Chicago, Illinois

Your board, staff, or clients may also benefit from this book's insight. For more information on quantity discounts, contact the Health Administration Press Marketing Manager at (312) 424-9470.

12   11   10   09   08   5   4   3   2   1

Library of Congress Cataloging-in-Publication Data

American College of Healthcare Executives.
   Coming of age : the 75-year history of the American College of Healthcare Executives/ American College of Healthcare Executives.
     p. ; cm.
   Includes bibliographical references and index.
   ISBN-13: 978-1-56793-285-0 (alk. paper)
   ISBN-10: 1-56793-285-1 (alk. paper)
1. American College of Healthcare Executives. 2. Health services administration--Study and teaching--United States--History. I. Title. II. Title: 75-year history of the American College of Healthcare Executives.
   [DNLM: 1. American College of Healthcare Executives. 2. Hospital Administration--United States. 3. Hospital Administration--history--United States. 4. Health Facility Administrators--United States. 5. History, 20th Century--United States. 6. History, 21st Century--United States. 7. Societies--United States. WX 1 A5117c 2008]
   RA971.A675 2008
   362.1071'173--dc22

                                                                       2007048395

Acquisitions editor: Audrey Kaufman; Project manager: Amanda Bove; Cover designer and layout editor: Chris Underdown

Health Administration Press
A division of the Foundation
   of the American College of
   Healthcare Executives
One North Franklin Street
Suite 1700
Chicago, IL 60606
(312) 424-2800

CONTENTS

PREFACE

In celebration of ACHE's 75th anniversary, we are proud to present *Coming of Age: The 75-Year History of the American College of Healthcare Executives.* First and foremost this is a history of ACHE. In 1933, we began with a small group of select leaders in the field of healthcare administration. Since then, ACHE has grown to an international professional society of more than 30,000 members, including affiliated chapters all across the United States. Throughout this phenomenal growth, the focus of ACHE has remained constant—to advance the profession of healthcare management by providing our affiliates with the knowledge, tools, and relationships to be exceptional leaders.

The American College of Healthcare Executives represents executives who lead and manage healthcare organizations across the country. This history, therefore, not only reflects the growth of the organization but also the major changes that have occurred throughout these years in the healthcare field. For example, changes in the way healthcare is delivered have transformed the way providers are organized and managed. Such issues as safety, quality, reimbursement, and the physician workforce have all undergone change, and throughout it all, ACHE has represented its members' interests and sought to provide information and education that would enable them to lead with compassion and effectiveness.

It has been an honor for us to be part of ACHE and the healthcare field in general. We hope this book will continue to serve as both a resource for how ACHE has grown and developed over the years as well as a glimpse into the changes that have occurred in the healthcare field during that same time.

This is the fourth edition of ACHE's history. We would like to acknowledge Ira Kipnis, who started us down this road and developed the first edition, called *A Venture Forward.* We also owe a great debt to Duncan Neuhauser, who carried the history forward in the second and third editions. We would also like to thank Kathleen Vega for her editorial assistance with this edition.

Coming of Age is about the pioneers in the field, the leaders who kept the torch burning, and the many professionals who continue to work and provide leadership in this important field. We look forward to working together with you toward a future of continued growth and excellence.

Alyson Pitman Giles, FACHE, Chairman 2007–2008
Brigadier General David A. Rubenstein, FACHE, Chairman-Elect
    2007–2008
William C. Schoenhard, FACHE, Immediate Past-Chairman 2007–2008
Thomas C. Dolan, PhD, FACHE, President and Chief Executive Officer

INTRODUCTION

Corporate history can be a way of thinking about the company, a way of compre-
hending why the present is what it is, and what might be possible for the future.
*   Once managers recognize the value of the corporate past, they can enhance*
their ability to diagnose problems, reassess policy, measure performance, and
even direct change.

Smith and Steadman, 1981 [1]

The American College of Healthcare Executives (ACHE) was founded in 1933. It led to the creation of a profession out of an amorphous occupational group—those who often fell into a career of supervising hospitals by chance. The founding members of ACHE were not average administrators; they were leaders who were ahead of their time. The ideas generated by ACHE and its founders were a vanguard for the field.

Like most organizations, ACHE is a product of its environment. The changing field of healthcare delivery as well as the historical events that have occurred throughout the years have helped the organization evolve into what it is today. For example, since ACHE was founded, hospitals have become more complex with the growth of technology and greater division of labor. Formal education for hospital managers has grown so that ACHE's role has changed from primary educator to a provider of continuing education. As healthcare has evolved, ACHE members have worked for many different types of healthcare organizations, including hospitals, long-term care organizations, managed care organizations, consulting firms, and so forth. As more and more women and minorities enter the healthcare field, the membership of ACHE has become more diverse. The organization has moved from a predominantly white, male, prestige-driven organization to a diverse, inclusive organization.

The Contents of the Book

The history of ACHE cannot be understood through a narrow review of its internal organization. Such a study would ignore the close link between ACHE and the changing field of hospital administration and healthcare management. Chapters 1 and 2 provide a discussion of how healthcare organizations and their leaders have changed since ACHE was founded.

Chapter 3 provides a brief history of ACHE from the first days of J. Dewey Lutes to the present.

Coming of Age also discusses all the key functions that ACHE performs for its membership. These functions are not unlike the core functions and activities that any professional society provides for its members. These functions help serve, attract, and respond to the changing needs of healthcare leaders and include the following:

- Defining excellence through a membership recruitment and credentialing process (Chapter 4)
- Providing continuing education and becoming involved in accreditation or approval of education programs (Chapter 5)
- Producing publications (Chapter 6)
- Helping affiliates with career management (Chapter 7)
- Engaging in research (Chapter 7)
- Establishing and educating affiliates and other stakeholders on public policy (Chapter 7)
- Promoting diversity (Chapter 7)
- Maintaining the internal organization (Chapter 8)

Sidebar I-1. A Note About Terms

When ACHE was founded, it was called the American College of Hospital Administrators (ACHA) and was often referred to as "the College." In 1985, the organization changed its name to the American College of Healthcare Executives to reflect the broader definition of leaders the organization encompassed and sought to attract. More recently, the use of the term "College" has been dropped. In this 75th anniversary edition of *Coming of Age*, to prevent confusion and promote consistency, the current name of the American College of Healthcare Executives or its acronym (ACHE) is used throughout the book, except within citations, references, and direct quotations.

The Purpose of this Book

In 1980, it was written that "The history of hospitals exists primarily as introductory chapters in textbooks, while the history of hospital administration is virtually nonexistent."[2] This void began to be filled when the 50-year history of ACHE was written.[3] Since that time a lot has changed in the world, in healthcare, and at ACHE. The purpose of this edition of *Coming of Age* is to provide a brief, up-to-date history of the organization, including the internal and external forces that have molded and shaped it. The timeline in Figure I-1 offers a glimpse into the events of the world, the advances in healthcare, and the significant accomplishments of ACHE across its 75-year history. *Coming of Age* also provides some insight into the field of healthcare management and how it too has evolved over the years.

FIGURE I-1. A Timeline of Events, 1896–2007

General [4]	Healthcare [5]	ACHE [6]
1896		
	X-rays used in the United States	
1899		
	Founding of what became the American Hospital Association	
1901		
• T. Roosevelt becomes president • J. P. Morgan forms the U.S. Steel Corp.		
1903		
	New York City outbreak of typhoid fever; Typhoid Mary, a carrier, is named	
1906		
	Pure Food and Drug Act defines the pharmaceutical industry	
1909		
W. H. Taft becomes president		
1910		
	• Flexner Report • First university-based school of nursing opens in Minnesota	
1913		
• W. Wilson becomes president • Federal income tax imposed	American College of Surgeons is founded	
1914		
World War I starts		
1915		
	Number of hospitals in United States tops 5,000 (up from about 178 in 1873)	

Continued

1918		
Armistice Day (Nov. 11) ends World War I	• Worldwide influenza pandemic (estimated 500,000 deaths in United States) • American College of Surgeons starts hospital accreditation	
1919		
	Worldwide influenza pandemic ends	
1920		
Women's suffrage adopted		
1921		
W. G. Harding becomes president		
1922		
	Insulin discovered by Banting and MacLeod in Canada	
1923		
C. Coolidge becomes president		
1928		
	Penicillin discovered by Alexander Fleming in England	
1929		
• The great stock market crash • H. Hoover becomes president	Blue Cross concept starts at Baylor University	
1931		
	First randomized clinical trial in medicine	
1932		
		J. Dewey Lutes and three other administrators meet to plan association
1933		
F. D. Roosevelt becomes president		• Palmer House meeting starts American College of Hospital Administrators (ACHA) • J. Dewey Lutes appointed director general (CEO) until 1937 • First annual meeting

Continued

1934		
	University of Chicago starts first graduate degree program in hospital administration	ACHA incorporated
1935		
• Social Security Act signed by Roosevelt • Wagner Labor Relations Act	Antibacterial activity of sulfa drugs discovered	227 total affiliates
1936		
		Local committees for geographical regions appointed
1937		
		• First permanent headquarters • Gerhard Hartman, PhD, appointed executive secretary (CEO) until 1941
1938		
	Harold Cox grows typhus microbes in chick embryos, leading to development of an effective vaccine available for World War II	
1939		
Hitler invades Poland		853 total affiliates
1940		
		• First examinations conducted for entrance to ACHA • 1,016 total affiliates
1941		
Pearl Harbor invasion	• Penicillin first used on a human patient; only widely available after World War II • Effect of rubella on fetus during early pregnancy shown	*Code of Ethics* adopted
1942		
	Kaiser Permanente formed from earlier capitation plan started in 1938	Dean Conley appointed executive director (CEO) and serves until 1965
1944		
	Streptomycin discovered	1,317 total affiliates

Continued

1945		
• F. D. Roosevelt dies; H. S. Truman becomes president • V-E Day (May 7) • Hiroshima bombed • V-J Day (Sept. 2) ends World War II • United Nations formed	Fluoridation of water introduced in United States	• 1,369 total affiliates • Joint Commission on Education of ACHA and AHA begins
1946		
	• First version of Benjamin Spock's *Baby and Child Care* • Hill-Burton Program	
1947		
Taft-Hartley Act		
1948		
Transistor discovered		Joint Commission on Education of ACHA and AHA ends
1949		
		Initiation of Arthur Bachmeyer Memorial Annual Address
1950		
Korean War begins		2,486 total affiliates
1951		
	Joint Commission on the Accreditation of Hospitals formed	
1952		
	Isoniazid introduced effective chemotherapy for tuberculosis	*Hospitals Visualized* published
1953		
• Korean War ends • D. D. Eisenhower becomes president	Discovery of DNA structure by Watson and Crick	
1954		
		ACHA opens new office at 820 N. Michigan Ave., Chicago
1955		
	• Peak in number of mental patients • Salk produces polio vaccine	3,467 total affiliates

Continued

1956		
		Journal *Hospital Administration* premieres
1957		
Sputnik I launched		
1958		
		• Observance of the 25th Anniversary of ACHA • First Congress on Administration held in Chicago • Initiation of James A. Hamilton Hospital Administration Book Award
1960		
	Ultrasound used to diagnose brain damage	4,600 total affiliates
1961		
J. F. Kennedy becomes president		Initiation of Malcolm MacEachern Memorial Lecture
1962		
	The limitations of broad-spectrum antibiotics appear after 20 years of use	
1963		
J. F. Kennedy assassinated; L. B. Johnson becomes president	Government expenditures on medical research exceeds $1 billion	
1964		
L. B. Johnson begins "Great Society" legislation	New York passes first certificate-of-need law	Initiation of Gold Medal Award for Excellence in Hospital Administration
1965		
	Medicare and Medicaid legislation passed	• Richard J. Stull appointed executive vice president (CEO) and serves until 1971 • Reorganization of Council of Regents and Board of Governors • 5,276 total affiliates
1966		
	Michael DeBakey transplants first artificial heart	

Continued

1967		
	• Christian Bernard performs heart transplant • First coronary artery bypass surgery at Cleveland Clinic	• Initiation of Dean Conley Award • *Administrative Briefs* published until 1980 • The *British National Health Service Tour* (published in 1969)
1968		
• Rev. Dr. M. L. King Jr. assassinated • Senator R. F. Kennedy assassinated		
1969		
• R. M. Nixon becomes president • First moon landing		Initiation of Robert S. Hudgens Memorial Award for Young Hospital Administrators
1970		
		8,747 total affiliates*
1971		
		Richard J. Stull serves as president (CEO) until 1979
1972		
	Computerized axial tomography introduced	Computerized Membership Data Profile
1973		
Vietnam peace treaty signed	HMO Act (PL93-222)	
1974		
R. M. Nixon resigns; G. R. Ford becomes president	• Nonprofit Hospital Amendments to the National Labor Relations Act (allows unions to organize in hospitals) • Smallpox eradicated worldwide	End of special recognition of the administrative residency
1975		
	Number of patients in nursing homes exceeds patients in hospitals for the first time	9,699 total affiliates
1976		
		ACHA journal becomes *Hospital & Health Services Administration*
1977		
J. Carter becomes president		

Continued

	1979	
	Hospital Corp. of America exceeds $1 billion in revenue and total assets	Stuart A. Wesbury Jr, PhD, serves as president (CEO) until 1991
	1980	
		• Accord with AHA on public policy • 13,418 total affiliates
	1981	
R. Reagan becomes president	AIDS identified	ACHE "Programmatic Thrusts" approved
	1982	
		25th Annual Congress on Administration
	1983	
	• Medical care reaches 10% of gross national product • Creation of first artificial chromosome	• 16,433 total affiliates • 50th Anniversary • Professional Assessment Program starts • Committee on Public Policy is created
	1984	
R. Reagan elected to second term	• First successful surgery on a fetus • DRG payment method starts • 3,000 cases of AIDS reported	• Delphi Study with Arthur Anderson • Strategic plan is developed
	1985	
	HMO enrollment reaches 21 million people in 480 plans	• Name change to ACHE • 19,510 total affiliates
	1986	
Space Shuttle Challenger explodes	• FDA approves first genetically engineered vaccine (Hepatitis B) • 33 million Americans without health insurance • 19,181 cases of AIDS; 37% die	Survey of members about access to care
	1987	
		• Statement on access to healthcare • 30th Annual Congress on Administration • Statement on medical records confidentiality • Strategic plan is revised

Continued

1989		
• G. H. W. Bush becomes president • Berlin Wall comes down	Joint Comission starts Agenda for Change	Revision of Professional Assessment
1990		
• Nelson Mandela released • Lithuania declares independence • Communist Party monopoly ends in USSR • Saddam Hussein invades Kuwait • Reunion of Germany formalized		• *Code of Ethics* is amended • First study comparing the careers of men and women in healthcare management conducted • 21,048 total affiliates
1991		
Operation Desert Storm begins		• Faculty Practice Fellowship Program Guidelines • First Ethical Policy Statement • Robin Burki, MD, last founder, dies • Stuart A. Wesbury Jr., PhD, steps down; Thomas C. Dolan, PhD, becomes president (CEO)
1992		
Healthcare reform becomes a major issue	• RBRVS payment changes • Outpatient surgery exceeds inpatient surgery for first time	• *Code of Ethics* revised • 63 officially designated Healthcare Executive groups; 105 student chapters; 20 Women's Healthcare Executive Networks • Persons of color constitute 5% of active members • First study comparing career attainments of black and white healthcare executives conducted with NAHSE
1993		
• W. J. Clinton becomes president • Clinton health plan proposed		60th Anniversary
1994		
• Nelson Mandela inaugurated as president of South Africa • IRA declares cease fire in Northern Ireland	• Despite numerous proposals for healthcare reform, no such plan is approved by Congress • Over 650 hospitals are involved in mergers and acquisitions	• Creation of Healthcare Executive Career Resource Center • ACHE cofounds The Institute for Diversity in Health Management • ACHE headquarters moves to its current location at 1 N. Franklin St. in Chicago's West Loop.

Continued

1995		
• Oklahoma City bombing • Military conflict in Bosnia	Physicians' average net income increases 7.2%, one year after a 3.6% drop	• More than 10,000 healthcare executives participate in ACHE's educational programs • Health Administration Press moves from Michigan to the Chicago headquarters • Findings are released from phase two of the cross-organizational study entitled *Partnership Study: A Study of the Roles and Working Relationships of the Hospital Board Chairman, CEO, and Medical Staff President* • Mentoring program is established • Governance Task Force is formed • Second study comparing career attainments of men and women healthcare executives conducted • 30,144 total affiliates
1996		
• AIDS death toll reaches 6.4 million • A sheep named Dolly is cloned in Britain • President Clinton is reelected	President Clinton signs the Kassebaum-Kennedy bill, formally known as the Health Insurance Portability and Accountability Act, the first significant healthcare reform in years	• Creation of ACHE homepage • CEO Circle is launched • New ethical policy statement is developed regarding downsizing
1997		
• Intel microchips introduced • US space shuttle joins Russian space station	• The Joint Commission unveils plan to partially base hospital accreditation on providers' performance • Congress passes a bill cutting Medicare spending by more than $115 billion from 1998–2002	Creation of new logo and tagline for ACHE, "For leaders who care"
1998		
• Multiple severe storms are created by El Niño • US president outlines first balanced budget in 30 years	14% of 5,053 nonfederal community hospitals participate in some form of consolidation (e.g., mergers, acquisitions, joint ventures)	• Campaign launched to strengthen the value of ACHE credentials • *Hospital & Health Services Administration* is renamed *Journal of Healthcare Management*

Continued

1999		
• Kosovo War • Y2K scare • Human population of the world surpasses 6 billion • Euro is introduced • Columbine massacre	• *To Err Is Human*, IOM's report, is released, stating that 98,000 people die from medical errors in hospitals every year • Medicare payments increased $15.1 billion since 1994	• Several changes are made to the *American College of Healthcare Executives' Bylaws* (e.g., allowing Diplomates to be Regents) • Online Tutorial is introduced on ache.org for the Board of Governors Exam
2000		
• US economy achieves longest period of uninterrupted expansion • Creation of Amazon.com • G. W. Bush declared winner of presidential election over A. Gore	• The number of uninsured Americans drops by 1.7 million • Enrollments in HMOs drop for the first time since 1973 • Healthcare providers can now be subject to $10,000 in fines per false claim	• The third wave of the *Gender and Careers* study is conducted • ACHE teams up with The Society for Healthcare Strategy and Market Development of AHA to publish *Futurescan* • 27,824 total affiliates
2001		
• President Bush authorizes funding for limited research on embryonic stem cells • Terrorist attacks on the World Trade Center and the Pentagon • The start of US ground operations in Afghanistan • Letters containing anthrax spores sent through US mail	• Nursing shortage issue is brought to the forefront of the healthcare world's attention • HHS secretary Thompson launches campaign to increase organ donation	• "Leadership in Mentoring" and "CEO Focus" columns introduced to *Healthcare Executive* • Computer-based testing format is introduced for the Board of Governor's exam
2002		
• Creation of the Department of Homeland Security • Enron and Worldcom scandals • US and Russia reach landmark agreements to cut both countries' nuclear arsenals by up to 2/3 in the next 10 years	Richard Carmona named new US Surgeon General	• CEO Boot Camp is introduced at Congress • Organ donor awareness campaign is launched • Completion of three-year Kellogg-funded study of community health practices "Rekindling the Flame: Achieving Success Through Community Leadership" • The third study comparing the careers of whites with persons of color is conducted • ACHE's Board of Governors becomes "at-large," representing all affiliates instead of geographic districts

Continued

2003		
• Space shuttle Columbia disintegrates upon reentry • The start of US ground operations in Iraq • Completion of Human Genome Project • Saddam Hussein captured • SARS epidemic	• Highest one-year spike in hospital costs since 1993 • President Bush launches a plan to help 41 million uninsured people find coverage • President Bush announces Medicare reform plan that launches a year-long debate	Website improvements are made, such as online registration for the Congress on Healthcare Management and the "My ACHE" section

2004		
• First outbreak of the bird flu virus • President Bush wins reelection over J. Kerry • Tsunami hits Asia	• 45.8 million Americans are uninsured for healthcare • Lawmakers hold hearings on not-for-profit tax exemptions, executive compensation, and billing of the uninsured	• Congress on Healthcare Management achieves record attendance with nearly 4,500 attendees • *Code of Ethics* is updated • 60 independent chapters are chartered • Persons of color constitute 10% of ACHE membership

2005		
• Iraqi elections • Terry Schiavo case • Hurricane Katrina decimates New Orleans	• Healthcare spending growth decreases for the first time in seven years • President Bush proposes $2.57 trillion federal budget protecting Medicare but cutting Medicaid spending by $60 billion • IOM calls for universal evaluation of pay-for-performance plans	• *Healthcare Executive* is made available online • Number of districts is reduced from nine to six • Health Administration Press achieves record sales • 33,659 total affiliates

2006		
• NASA's Stardust mission brings dust from a comet to earth • The one billionth song is purchased from the Apple iTunes store • US Census Bureau projections for the US population reach 300 million	• Margaret Chan is elected director general of the WHO • A study shows that one in six people in the US spend more than 10% of their income on medical expenses • The first cervical cancer vaccine is approved by the FDA	• ACHE conducts fourth study comparing the careers of women and men in healthcare management • ACHE's Voluntary Giving program is launched

Continued

2007		
• Nancy Pelosi becomes the first woman Speaker of the House in the United States • A mass shooting occurs at Virginia Tech, resulting in the deaths of 32 students and faculty members • The seventh and final book in the Harry Potter series sets a record with an initial printing of 12 million copies	• Medicare board of trustees predicts exhaustion of trust fund by 2019 • Centers for Medicare & Medicaid Services unveils approach to pay hospitals in part on the quality of their care (i.e., pay for performance)	• Partnership established with the Institute for Healthcare Improvement's 5 Million Lives campaign • Credentialing reform consolidates Diplomates and Fellows into one credential: Fellow

*Begining in 1970, students are included in total affiliate number

ACHE cannot be considered as a single, distinct entity. It has been—and continues to be—composed of many extraordinary and unique leaders of the field. Their individuality is not easily expressed in the minutes of ACHE committee meetings. Above all, it can never be forgotten that ACHE is only as effective and innovative as its leadership and affiliate body. ACHE is about people. This book is a tribute to these people—a celebration of their successes, an examination of their past, and a look ahead to their future.

Endnotes

1.   Smith, G. D., and L. E. Steadman, "Present Value of Corporate History." *Harvard Business Review*, Nov.–Dec. 1981, pp. 164–165.

2.   Wren, G. R., "An Historical View of Health Administration Education." *Hospitals & Health Services Administration*, Vol. 25, No. 3, Summer 1980, p. 31.

3.   Neuhauser, D. *Coming of Age*. Chicago: Health Administration Press, 1983. This second edition includes nearly all the content of and updates the first edition.

4.   Sources for general historical events are obtained from encyclopedias, almanacs, and commonly available websites.

5.   Sources for healthcare trends include Flexner, A. *Medical Education in the United States and Canada*. New York: The Carnegie Foundation for the Advancement of Teaching, 1910; Burrow, J. G. *Organized Medicine in the Progressive Era: The Move Toward Monopoly*. Baltimore: Johns Hopkins University Press, 1977; Amberson, J. B., B. T., McMahon, and M. Pinner, "A Clinical Trial of Sanocrysin in Pulmonary Tuberculosis." *American Review of Tuberculosis*, Vol. 24, 1931, pp. 401–435; and major trade publications (e.g., *Modern Healthcare, Hospital and Health Networks*, etc.).

6.   Sources for ACHE include Kipnis, I. A. *A Venture Forward: A History of the American College of Hospital Administrators*. Chicago: ACHA, 1955; Neuhauser, D. *Coming of Age*. Chicago: Health Administration Press, 1983; Neuhauser, D.

Coming of Age: A 60-Year History of the American College of Healthcare Executives and the Profession It Serves, 1933–1993. Ann Arbor, MI: Health Administration Press, 1995; and White, E. *The History of the American College of Hospital Administrators and Public Policy.* Chicago: ACHA, 1985, p. 9.

THE EVOLUTION OF THE HOSPITAL: FROM COTTAGE ORGANIZATION TO HEALTHCARE SYSTEM

Any study of the work, responsibilities and qualifications of the present day Hospital Administrator would be quite incomplete without some introductory reference to the character of the institution with which he is associated in his daily tasks. Some knowledge of its relationships, problems, objectives, and characteristics of growth is essential to an understanding of the position of its executive officer.

ACHA, 1935[1]

The nature and character of a hospital defines what its chief executive does.[2] A hospital's relationships, problems, objectives, and characteristics can help define the role of the hospital executive. For example, a hospital that acts as a small cottage organization has a much different type of executive than a large integrated healthcare system. Because the American College of Healthcare Executives (ACHE) is made up of executives from all different types of hospitals and healthcare organizations, a look at the evolution of hospitals is valuable.

This chapter explores the changing nature of hospitals and discusses how their priorities have shifted. The evolution process, from hospital superintendency to hospital administration to healthcare management, can be separated into the following six distinctive eras since 1873. These dates do not represent sharp splits from one time to the next, but an evolution:

- The early days—1873 to 1915
- The move toward standardization—1915 to 1933
- The rise of the superintendent —1933 to 1945
- A focus on hospital management—1945 to 1965
- The birth of the healthcare system—1965 to 1992
- The modern era—1992 to the present

The following sections discuss each of these different eras, identifying the priorities and goals of each era and discussing the accomplishments realized during each one.

The Early Days (1873–1915)

And so it came to pass eventually that all mankind needed the hospital.
John A. Hornsby, MD, 1913[3]

In 1873, there were slightly more than 178 hospitals in the United States[4] (see Figure 1-1), and that number was increasing in response to new developments in the field of medicine, such as the availability of aseptic and antiseptic surgery, x-ray technology, and laboratory tests. The hospital, as an institution, became essential to the private practice of medicine; however, this explosive era of hospital growth resulted in a wide variation in quality of services.

Between 1873 and 1914, the number of hospitals grew from approximately 200 to more than 5,000. Especially in the North and East, philanthropy fueled by industrial development at the turn of the century led to the endowment and funding of voluntary hospitals. While many new hospitals were started by means of philanthropic capital, in the absence of such capital, some physicians, Catholic sisterhoods, or other religious and ethnic groups created new hospitals on a proprietary basis. The goal of these groups was to create a place to care for their patients. Later, many of these proprietary hospitals closed, while others were transformed

FIGURE 1-1
Number of
Hospitals by
Year and Era[5]

Era	Year	Number of Hospitals
The early days	1873	178+
	1903	2,500
	1914	5,047
The move toward standardization	1918	5,323
	1928	6,852
The rise of the superintendent	1938	6,166
A focus on hospital management	1946	6,125
	1950	6,788
	1960	6,876
The birth of the healthcare system	1968	7,137
	1978	7,015
	1991	6,634
The modern era	1995	6,291
	2000	5,810
	2007	6,349

into nonprofit institutions. In the South and West particularly, where philanthropy was less available, proprietary hospitals were common. As they grew, and as their original founders retired, many of these hospitals were transformed into voluntary institutions. However, even today acceptance of the proprietary hospital remains greater in the Sun Belt states than in other parts of the country.[6]

In the years 1890 to 1920, there was widespread agreement on the value of public health measures like sanitation, vaccination, pasteurization, and clean water supply.[7] These programs would ultimately result in a declining death rate from infectious disease and in the prolongation of life. However, compared with hospitals built even 30 years later, the turn of the century hospital was so simple as to be called a "boarding house for the sick."[8] Most new hospitals were very small. Often, the larger ones were built in the pavilion style of architecture, typically on one level, with long corridors between wards to control infection.[9]

In the old voluntary hospitals, philanthropy provided the power to admit patients.[10] Only at the turn of the century did trustees abandon their involvement in selecting "the deserving poor" for admission.[11] When trustees paid all the bills, their power was predominant.[12] Later, the decision to admit became the sole province of the physician. The hospital thus became an institution of medical science rather than social welfare.[13] The decline of trustee influence meant the rise of medical influence. Not until after World War II did the professionalization of hospital administration, along with the growing complexity of the hospital and the external environment, signal a rise in the administrator's influence.[14] For example, the LaCrosse Lutheran Hospital in Wisconsin, founded in 1899, had no administrator until 1921; until that time the hospital was run by a nurse-matron and a chief physician. Their first superintendent in 1924 was a general-store manager before he started work as a hospital administrator.[15]

The Move Toward Standardization (1915–1933)

With the exception of health insurance, the major building blocks of the healthcare system were in place by 1915. The hospital became universal. Between 1915 and 1945, the average hospital remained small and uncomplicated. Even in 1943, 45 percent of general hospitals had fewer than 50 beds and almost 70 percent had fewer than 100 beds.[16]

Superintendents came to their positions by chance, not through career planning. Professional "stepping-stones" included nursing, medicine, or religious administration. Superintendents were expected to know all the details of hospital work, including sterile technique, food preparation, sanitation, and medical record keeping.

The 1920s saw important advances in medical care: insulin for diabetes in 1922 and penicillin in 1928. In 1935, sulfa drugs were shown to have antibacterial effects. The effect of these changes extended over decades, and advancements greatly enhanced the role of medical care and the hospital. While penicillin was discovered in 1928, it was first used in humans in 1941 and was not widely available for the civilian population until after World War II.

The stock market crash of 1929 and the subsequent Great Depression that led to President Roosevelt's New Deal also brought changes. The Blue Cross concept began at Baylor University in 1929. The Depression encouraged the growth of this idea even more as hospitals sought to reduce their bad debt.[17] The Social Security Act of 1935 became the greatest landmark in twentieth century American social legislation, and the 1935 Wagner Act gave a boost to the union movement, laying the groundwork for negotiated healthcare benefits through collective bargaining.[18]

Between 1910 and 1933, one major development within the field of healthcare management was standardization. Standardization involves complying with a specific practice or product that is widely recognized or employed, especially because of its excellence. Standardization was a concept that came into favor during the early 1900s, and hospitals across the country embraced it.

The standardization movement was not limited to the hospital field. The National Bureau of Standards (NBS), located in the U.S. Department of Commerce, was established in 1901 for the development, construction, and maintenance of references and working standards in science, engineering, industry, and commerce. The NBS started with 14 employees, increasing to 850 by 1928.[19]

In 1910, the Hospital Bureau of Standards and Supplies was started as an independent organization. By 1938, it was performing joint purchasing for 211 member hospitals in 24 states. It standardized and tested products used by hospitals.[20] Judging by the number of articles in *Transactions* on standardization, the American Hospital Association (AHA) was actively involved in this effort from 1914 into the 1930s.[21]

Sidebar 1-1. Historical Perspective

Hospitals were ripe for standardization. For example, John R. Mannix, a founding Fellow of ACHE, remembered that 1,000 different surgical needles were available in the 1920s; 300 of these were in stock at his hospital, where only 50 different operations were performed. According to Mannix, it was finally agreed that only 17 different needles would fulfill every need—a startling example of the rewards of standardization in hospitals.[22]

Standardization in hospitals was not limited to standardizing instruments and equipment. It also applied to standardizing practices. Several healthcare organizations, including the American College of Surgeons (ACS) and The Catholic Hospital Association (CHA), developed standard practices with which hospitals had to comply to receive accreditation.

To determine whether a hospital was complying with set standards, organizations such as the ACS conducted surveys. Between 1918 and 1936, the ACS conducted more than 40,000 hospital surveys.[23] The first hospital survey in 1918 covered 692 hospitals with more than 100 beds. Only 12.9 percent of those hospitals were able to meet the ACS minimum standards, which were minimal indeed (see Figure 1-2). That so many institutions failed to meet these standards documents the negative state of most American hospitals of this time.

By 1933, in a survey of 1,603 hospitals of more than 100 beds, 93.9 percent were approved.[24] By 1936, nearly all of the largest hospitals and

1. That physicians and surgeons privileged to practice in the hospital be organized as a definite medical staff. Such organization has nothing to do with the question as to whether the hospital is "open" or "closed," nor need it affect the various existing types of medical staff organization. The word staff is here defined as the group of doctors who practice in the hospital inclusive of all groups, such as the "regular medical staff," the "visiting medical staff," and the "associate medical staff."
2. That membership upon the medical staff be restricted to physicians and surgeons who are (a) graduates of medicine of acceptable medical schools, with the degree of Doctor of Medicine, in good standing, and legally licensed to practice in their respective states or provinces; (b) competent in their respective fields; and (c) worthy in character and in matters of professional ethics; that in this latter connection the practice of the division of fees, under any guise whatsoever, be prohibited.
3. That the medical staff initiate and, with the approval of the governing board of the hospital, adopt rules, regulations, and policies governing the professional work of the hospital; that these rules, regulations, and policies specifically provide: (a) that medical staff meetings be held at least once each month; (b) that the medical staff review and analyze at regular intervals their clinical experience in the various departments of the hospital, such as medicine, surgery, obstetrics, and the other specialties; the medical records of patients, free and pay, to be the basis for such review and analysis.
4. That accurate and complete medical records be written for all patients and filed in an accessible manner in the hospital, a complete medical record being one which includes identification data; complaint; personal and family history; history of present illness; physical examination; special examinations, such as consultations, clinical laboratory, x-ray and other examination; provisional or working diagnosis; medical or surgical treatment; gross and microscopical pathological findings; progress notes; final diagnosis; condition on discharge; follow-up and, in case of death, autopsy findings.
5. That diagnostic and therapeutic facilities under competent medical supervision be available for the study, diagnosis, and treatment of patients, these to include at least (a) a clinical laboratory providing chemical, bacteriological, serological, and pathological services; (b) an x-ray department providing radiographic and fluoroscopic services.

FIGURE 1-2
ACS Minimum Standard for Hospitals[25]

Sidebar 1-2. On a Personnel Note

The growth of its survey program was so rapid that the ACS decided to find a single individual to direct it. On October 25, 1921, the Regents of the ACS authorized an agreement with Malcolm T. MacEachern, MD, to devote one-third of his time to the direction of this program. He received a total of $400 for four months a year to do this work. On June 2, 1923, he became an associate director of the ACS in charge of the program. He held this post for the next 28 years.[27, 28]

MacEachern graduated from McGill Medical School in 1910, trained in obstetrics. He became superintendent of the Montreal Maternity Hospital in 1911. In 1913, he became general superintendent of the Vancouver General Hospital. J. Dewey Lutes, one of ACHE's founders, remembers "Mac" as being known throughout the country. According to Lutes,

> Everyone loved him, and he did everything he could to help the College. I remember one meeting where MacEachern was in the back of the room asleep. (He sometimes slept during meetings.) I was speaking and I said, "I am sure you would like to hear from Dr. MacEachern." He woke up and came up front and gave a superb talk.[29]

Throughout his many years in Chicago, MacEachern regularly commuted to his home in Montreal where his wife and child resided.[30] He became an internationally recognized expert on hospital administration as a result of his work for the ACS and was one of the driving forces in ACHE.

---

many smaller ones could meet these basic standards of good organization. The hospital standardization program was a great success and eventually was transformed into The Joint Commission on the Accreditation of Hospitals (today known as The Joint Commission).

Hospital standardization and accreditation was enthusiastically adopted for several reasons, including the following:

- For the patient, accreditation was an assurance of efficient and competent care.
- For the physician, it offered the security of a proper working environment.
- For the hospital, it ensured a well-functioning operation.
- For the intern and student nurse, it guaranteed a level of organization, equipment, and personnel to ensure good education and facilitate licensure and registration.
- For the community, it resulted in pride in a hospital that was meeting universally recognized standards.[26]

Both standardization of hospitals and professional education contributed to the mobility of professional workers. A physician or nurse trained in one area of the country could quickly adapt to work in another region. This similarity of tasks, relations, and organization across thousands of independent hospitals was a remarkable social achievement.

The Rise of the Superintendent (1933–1945)

In 1935, according to the annual "Hospital Number" of the *Journal of the American Medical Association*,[31] the 6,246 registered hospitals in the United States contained 1,076,350 beds. That year, Franklin Roosevelt's Public Works Administration financed a business census of hospitals to collect information about "the financial structure of hospitals and opportunities for employment within them." This was part of a larger census of all American businesses. Nearly 6,000 hospitals responded to this government study.

The Typical Hospital

In 1935, according to the Public Works survey, the average general hospital administrator presided over a small hospital with a small number of unskilled employees (see Figure 1-3). Very likely, the hospital was running at a deficit even though expenses were very low and patients had to pay out of their own pocket. The threat of hospital closure was real. Many of these small hospitals were not unlike nursing homes of today. Although endowments and philanthropy were important, these funds were less evenly distributed across the country than were all hospital services per capita.[32]

Hospital beds per 1,000 people were maldistributed by state. Annual per capita payments (expenditures) on hospital care averaged $3.37 for the country as a whole. Per capita payments varied tenfold from the highest ranked state to the lowest. Well over half of the payments came directly from the patient paying out of pocket. Taxes supported government hospitals. For the rest, endowment income was important in areas like Massachusetts.[33]

Sidebar 1-3. Historical Perspective

Dr. Robert L. Dickinson, founding member of the American College of Surgeons,[34] presented a paper to a joint meeting of the New York Taylor Society and the Harvard Medical Society[35] that was later published in the *Bulletin of the Taylor Society* as "Hospital Organization as Shown by Charts of Personnel and Powers Functions." This was probably the first published organization chart for a hospital.[36]

Frank Gilbreth, an efficiency expert whose family was the subject of the book and movie *Cheaper by the Dozen*, presented another paper at the 16th Annual Convention of the American Hospital Association in 1914 on "Scientific Management in the Hospital."[37] His wife, Lillian, presented a paper entitled "Efficiency in the Care of the Patient" at the same St. Paul, Minnesota, meeting.[38] Lillian Gilbreth was made an Honorary Fellow of ACHE in 1961.

Sidebar 1-4. On a Personnel Note

The survey of hospitals funded by Franklin Roosevelt's Public Works Administration was directed by Elliott Pennell, Joseph Mountin, and Kay Pearson with the advice of Michael M. Davis, HFACHE, and C. Rufus Rorem.[39]

Sidebar 1-5. Historical Perspective

With the Depression came the disappearance of nearly 700 hospitals (from 6,852 in 1928 to 6,166 in 1938). Still other hospitals faded from the scene but were replaced by new ones.

FIGURE 1-3
Hospital Size
and Type,
1935[41]

Number of Beds	General and Specialty Hospitals	
Less than 25	1,287	
50–149	1,177	
150+	797	
Total	4,841	

Number of Beds	Mental Institutions	Tuberculosis Institutions
Less than 50	144	135
50–499	189	231
500+	264	140
Total	597	506

During this time, both nonprofit general and specialty hospitals were losing money. (This was the era when tuberculosis was treated by years of stay in specialized hospitals, a time before chemotherapy in the 1950s emptied these institutions.) For every dollar spent by voluntary general hospitals, only 96 cents was returned from all income sources. The smallest hospitals had the greatest deficits per bed.[40]

The income for nonprofit general and specialty hospitals came from several sources, including the following:

- Patients (70.9 percent)
- Taxes (10.3 percent)
- Endowment (6.3 percent)
- Others (12.5 percent)

On an average day, only 64 percent of all general and specialty hospital beds were occupied. For the proprietary hospitals, this number was 45 percent. Hospital expenses were payroll (48.9 percent), supplies and maintenance (47.2 percent), and other (3.9 percent).

For general and specialty hospitals, average plant assets per bed were $4,682. These assets comprised the following:

- Land (9.5 percent)
- Buildings (73.4 percent)
- Equipment (14.8 percent)
- Other (2.3 percent)

The endowment per bed was $1,090. However, 78 percent of all hospital endowments were in the northeastern quarter of the United States (north and east from—and including—Pennsylvania and Maryland).

Personal health expenditures actually fell by half a billion dollars from 1929 to 1935. Private health insurance played a negligible role prior to World War II.[42] During the war, wage freezes encouraged the growth of fringe benefits such as health insurance.

Hospital Employment 1935

Within the Public Works survey, the 5,836 reporting hospitals had 1,035,503 beds and 161,884 employees. For nonprofit general and specialty hospitals, there were 0.89 employees per bed. Of these, more than 80 percent were paid full time, 3.5 percent were paid part time, and 15.7 percent were provided maintenance (room and board) only. Workers receiving maintenance only were predominantly student nurses and resident physicians. Both of these groups provided a substantial amount of labor, particularly in the larger hospitals.

For all general and specialty hospitals, the workforce consisted of the following groups:

- Physicians (4.8 percent)
- Nurses (40.8 percent)
- Technical and other professionals (5.4 percent)
- Administrative and clerical workers (7.2 percent)
- Orderlies and other nonprofessional workers (41.8 percent)

The average monthly pay for these workers was $55.53.

Even as late as 1946, in hospitals of 200 to 299 beds (larger than average), a survey of 155 hospitals revealed that 62 had "no assistant administrator, medical director or the like"; 65 had one assistant; 23 had two assistants; and 5 had three or more assistant administrators.

Sidebar 1-6. Historical Perspective

When J. Dewey Lutes helped start ACHE in 1933, he was administrator of the 150-bed Ravenswood Hospital in Chicago. He knew every employee by name and walked through the hospital every day. "Anyone could come into my office without an appointment," he said. "There was more feeling for patients and fewer electronic things." He remembered tears in the eyes of nurses caring for dying cancer patients. Added Lutes, "That doesn't happen so much now."

Virtually every room was a patient room on the nursing floor. There were only three nonpatient rooms: one for housekeeping, a floor kitchen, and a supply room. There were no nursing stations, and hospital housekeeping was no different from that practiced in a home. At that time, Lutes's major problems were keeping the hospital in good repair and collecting bills.

The latest technology was a new EKG on rollers. "It was really something," Lutes said. The Ravenswood lab had one part-time pathologist. Technicians were trained on the job, and the whole lab was located in one little room. "We didn't know what a social worker was," said Lutes.

In 1933, there was no problem finding nurses either. The graduates of the hospital nursing schools stayed on to work in the hospital. "Nursing students really worked then," said Lutes.

The hospital's funds were in a local bank. "I took all the money out of this bank in cash and put it in a safety deposit box," Lutes reported. "Two weeks later the bank failed. The Board of Trustees gave me a pat on the back for that." While some hospitals closed during the Depression, Lutes noted of his hospital, "We all took pay cuts."[43]

Sidebar 1-7. The Miasmatic and Contagion Theories of Infection

During this time period, there were two conflicting theories about hospital infections: the miasmatic theory and contagion theory. The miasmatic theory stated that infection was caused by bad climate, bad location, or lack of fresh air. The contagion theory held that disease was spread by carriers. At the turn of the twentieth century, what is now the *New England Journal of Medicine* regularly reported the local weather conditions, thought to be related to disease. New hospitals in Boston were built on top of hills to get fresh air. The pavilion style of hospital architecture put long distances between patient wards. The Nightingale ward for inpatients had high ceilings and lots of window space. The treatment of tuberculosis was rest and fresh air, as represented by the early years of the then famous Trudeau Sanatorium (1884 to 1954).[50]

The great works of Robert Koch (tuberculosis in 1879 and cholera in 1883) and Louis Pasteur (anthrax in 1877) on the germ theory of disease eventually convinced physicians that the contagion theory of disease was the correct one. But the battle between these two ideas lasted well into the twentieth century.[51]

The Vertical Hospital

An important development in hospital architecture occurred during this era with the appearance of the vertical hospital, an alternative to the pavilion style.[44] Vertical hospitals were technically possible after the introduction of the Otis elevator in 1857[45] and the creation of the skyscraper office buildings of the Chicago school of architecture in the 1880s.[46] Growing hospital size and urbanization were also necessary preconditions. However, it was the understanding and control of hospital infections that made the vertical hospital acceptable (see Sidebar 1-7).[47]

The multistoried hospital was proposed as early as 1903 by Dr. A. J. Ochsner, yet it was only after the control of hospital infection and the disappearance of the miasmic theory of infection that the vertical hospital became a reality, according to E. H. L. Corwin, an Honorary Charter Fellow of ACHE.[48]

Building on the vertical hospital concept, S. S. Goldwater, an Honorary Fellow of ACHE, supported conveniently grouping interdependent hospital departments. This idea came from the classical school of management theory. According to Goldwater, "For the thoughtful hospital planner, the most significant contrast is not one between hospitals with vertical and horizontal lines of communication, respectively, but between hospitals in which interdependent departments are conveniently and those in which they are inconveniently grouped."[49]

A Focus on Hospital Management (1945–1965)

At the beginning of the era entitled "a focus on hospital management," the typical hospital was, by today's standards, a low-cost operation. Plant assets per bed were $4,814. Although the great majority of hospitals had x-ray equipment, not all hospitals did. For example, only 45.5 percent of hospitals in Utah had such equipment. Likewise, although the great majority of hospitals had clinical laboratories, only 62.5 percent in South Dakota did.[52]

From 1943 to 1963, hospitals became more complex.[53] Administrators no longer worked with details; instead, they recruited technically skilled workers to accomplish the work of the hospital. This era saw the growth of graduate programs in hospital administration and the creation of a separate profession chosen—and not fallen into—as a career by its members. During this time, ACHE's nondegree "Institutes" were replaced by degree programs at universities, regional meetings, and an annual Congress on Administration (see Chapter 5 for more information on ACHE's role in education).

Throughout the era, hospitals also became larger.[54] They added more staff per patient day, hired a wider range of professionally trained specialists, increased their scope of services, and became more expensive. The average general hospital of 1933, with about 50 beds and fewer than 50 employees, began to evolve, and by 1983 had an average of 200 beds and 750 employees. While the hospital of 1933 could be managed by a nurse with some on-the-job experience, the more modern hospital called for more skilled management.

After World War II, healthcare expenditures grew. For example, in 1935, there were 800,000 births in hospitals. By 1959, there were four million births in hospitals.[55] Likewise, in 1928 through 1931, the average American went to see the doctor a little less than three times in a year. By 1954 through 1959, that statistic had grown to five times a year.[56] Figure 1-4 presents a snapshot of hospitals in 1945, and Figure 1-5 shows the national health expenditures for 1935 through 2004.

The Growth of Health Insurance

By 1950, private health insurance paid 9 percent of personal health expenditures. Government expenditures rose steadily, with the largest jump occurring during the 1960s with the start of Medicare and Medicaid (for more information about the introduction of Medicare and Medicaid, see the section entitled "The Birth of the Healthcare System" later in this chapter).

Rising costs and the growing numbers of elderly and poor Americans created the need for Medicare and Medicaid, which in turn allowed costs to continue to rise. For example, total expenditures on medical research in 1949 was only $45 million. By 1963, government expenditures on medical research had grown to $1.008 billion, out

Sidebar 1-8. Significant Statistics

In 1935, 37 percent of live births occurred in hospitals. By 1953, up to 93 percent of live births were in hospitals. During this time, maternal mortality fell from 58.2 per 100,000 live births to 6.1 per 100,000. Infant mortality fell from 55.7 per 1,000 live births to 27.8. In 1935, 18 states had less than 30 percent of live births in hospitals. By 1953, 36 states had more than 90 percent of live births in hospitals.

In 1945, the average work week for untrained hospital employees was more than 48 hours. By 1954, it was down to 43 hours. In 1954, the average short-term general hospital had 102 beds, 18 bassinets, and 149 full-time-equivalent personnel.[57]

FIGURE 1-4
A Snapshot of
Hospitals in
1945[58]

Number of Beds	Total Employees	Cost per Patient Day	Personnel per Patient Day
0–49	28,904	$7.99	1.06
50–99	54,682	$8.01	1.22
100–249	158,027	$8.60	1.45
250+	188,987	$8.96	1.57

FIGURE 1-5
Personal Health
Expenditures,
1935–2005[59]

Year	Amount (billions)	Out of Pocket (%)	Private Health Insurance (%)	Government (%)	National Health Expenditures as a Percentage of Gross National Product
1935	2.7	82.4	N/A	14.7	4.0
1940	3.5	81.3	N/A	16.1	4.0
1950	10.9	65.5	9.1	22.4	4.5
1960	28	46.4	21.4	25.0	5.2
1970	63	39.6	22.3	35.3	7.2
1980	215	27.2	28.4	40.0	9.0
1990	607	22.4	33.7	38.9	12.2
2000	1,140	16.9	35.4	42.7	13.7
2001	1,239	16.1	35.6	43.7	14.4
2002	1,341	15.8	35.9	44.0	15.3
2003	1,446	15.5	35.9	44.2	15.7
2004	1,551	15.2	36.0	44.6	15.8
2005	1,661	15.0	35.9	45.0	15.9

of a total expenditure on medical research of $1.545 billion. By 1977, the government paid for $3.612 billion out of a total of $5.526 billion spent for medical research.[60] Not only did this large investment in research lead to improved medical care, but with developments including heart surgery and diagnostic devices, it also helped increase medical care costs.

Not all new treatments increased costs. Drugs to control tuberculosis emptied the once numerous tuberculosis hospitals. Effective drugs and community mental health centers led to the era of deinstitutionalization, with 1955 being the peak year for the number of mental hospital inpatients. Polio vaccines replaced the costly iron lung. As the proportion of the population over the age of 65 grew, the number of residents in nursing homes increased. By about 1975, there were, for the first time, more people in nursing homes than in hospitals.

As healthcare expenditures grew, the percent that came from direct patient payment fell from 88.4 percent in 1929 to 26.8 percent in 1980, by which time the hospital received reimbursement not only directly from patients, but also from private insurers and the government, resulting in a vastly more complex external environment. The percent of gross national product spent on health went from 3.5 percent in 1929 to 9.8 percent in 1982 and to 11.1 percent in 1988. Figure 1-6 shows the average yearly rate of change in health expenditures from 1929 through 2005.

In 1940, 12 million people had some type of health insurance. Of these, six million were covered by Blue Cross/Blue Shield plans. By 1950, 76.6 million people were covered; by 1960, 122.5 million were covered; and by 1970, 158.8 million were covered. By 1978, 166.8 million people under

Years	Average Percent Change
1929–1935	−3.5
1935–1940	6.6
1940–1950	12.2
1950–1955	6.9
1955–1960	8.7
1960–1965	8.9
1965–1970	12.2
1970–1975	12.3
1975–1980	13.6
1980–1985	11.6
1985–1990	10.2
1990–1995	7.3
1995–2000	5.9
2000–2005	8.0

FIGURE 1-6
Average Yearly Rate of Change in National Health Expenditures[61]

the age of 65 had hospital insurance protection.[62] The availability of health insurance again fueled the rise in national health expenditures. It also helped concentrate medical care in the hospital.

Health Services Employment

In 1940, a million people were employed in health services. By 1979, this number had grown to 4.93 million, with 3.84 million people working in hospitals. Not only did the total number of hospital-based employees increase; the number of hospital employees per 100 patients also increased from 226 full-time equivalents (FTEs) in 1960 to 302 FTEs in 1970, and 388 FTEs in 1979[63] (see Figure 1-7).

The Birth of the Healthcare System (1965–1992)

During the 1960s and 1970s, the nature of the average hospital was again changing. Organizations were becoming more complex and beginning to cooperate with each other to form multihospital systems. No precise date hails the era of the multi-institutional hospital system, but 1979 was the first year that the Hospital Corporation of American (HCA) exceeded a billion dollars both in revenue and assets.[64]

The introduction of Medicare and Medicaid in 1966 paralleled rising costs and government regulation. More of the hospital manager's time was occupied with external affairs, particularly with regulatory agencies. With increasing hospital size and the attractiveness of hospital management as a career, a longer portion of the manager's career was spent in middle management.

Year	Total	In Hospitals	In Nursing Homes
1940	1.0	N/A	N/A
1950	1.5	1.0	N/A
1960	2.5	1.5	N/A
1970	4.25	2.69	0.51
1980	7.34	4.04	1.2
1990	9.45	4.69	1.54
2000	13.7	5.20	1.59
2005	14.2	5.72	1.85

FIGURE 1-7
Health Services Employment (in millions of employees) [70]

Medicare and Medicaid also fostered the introduction of other organizations like neighborhood health centers, planning agencies, consultants, and large third-party payers—such as health maintenance organizations (HMOs) and preferred provider organizations (PPOs)—that all required health managers. Consequently, specialized healthcare management grew in importance.

According to Goldsmith:

> With the exception of a few large municipal hospital systems, such as that of New York City, most (nonfederal general) hospitals have developed in isolation from one another both clinically and managerially. But in the decade of the 1970s this fragmentation gave way to increasing interinstitutional cooperation as we enter the 1980s. The completely freestanding hospital is rapidly becoming a thing of the past.[68]

The 1970s saw the growth of multihospital systems and alliances. Most Catholic hospitals had been associated with a particular order of sisters but were highly decentralized in their management. A number of these congregations developed larger corporate headquarters and central management. The chief executive officer (CEO) became increasingly concerned with marketing, competition, corporate reorganization, and financing.

In 1975, an estimated 24 percent of community hospitals were in multihospital systems (see Figure 1-8). A 1978 AHA survey of 5,740 community hospitals showed the following:[69]

- 65 percent of hospitals shared purchasing services, up from 38 percent in 1975.
- 34 percent shared electronic data processing, up from 21 percent in 1975.
- 27 percent shared laboratory services, up from 17.4 percent in 1957.
- Nearly 19 percent shared biomedical engineering services, up from 7.7 percent in 1955.

Type of Ownership	Total Hospitals	Hospitals in System	In Hospital Systems	
			(% of hospitals)	(% of beds)
Voluntary				
1975	3,355	940	28	32
2006	2,990	1,567	56	63
Investor-owned				
1975	755	309	40	51
2006	723	602	83	90
State and local government				
1975	1,745	156	8	22
2006	1,112	283	25	33
Total				
1975	5,875	1,405	24	32
2006	4,625	2,452	53	61

Another measure of the hospital's increasing complexity was the growth of outpatient and emergency visits to short-term, nonfederal hospitals. In 1944, outpatient visits totaled 23.7 million; in 1953, 42 million; in 1965, 92.6 million; in 1970, 124 million; and in 1979, 203.9 million. Emergency visits went from 9.4 million in 1954, to 76.6 million in 1979.[71] In the 1980s, hospitals grew still larger and more complex. They confronted third-party payers, both government and private, in a sea of regulatory constraints fostered by a concern for rising costs. This complex environment, both internal and external, resulted in hospitals creating linkages in the interests of survival.

By 1982, several large multihospital systems were thriving with significant operating revenues. The following are a few of those systems and their 1982 operating revenues and number of hospitals:

- The HCA, with $3.5 billion in operating revenues and 349 hospitals
- Kaiser Permanente, with $2 billion in operating revenues and 30 hospitals

	Nonfederal Multi-hospital by Ownership			Number of Hospitals			Number of Beds		
	1981	*1992*	*2006*	*1981*	*1992*	*2006*	*1981*	*1992*	*2006*
Investor-owned	31	50	69	746	1,101	1,258	97,478	134,006	146,854
Catholic	113	67	43	516	503	558	137,501	118,527	108,841
Other religious	19	14	13	150	95	108	21,771	18,563	21,441
Voluntary/state and local government	93	164	249	465	799	1,217	94,658	180,649	267,090
Total	256	295	374	1,877	2,498	3,141	351,408	451,745	549,226

FIGURE 1-9
Multihospital Systems, 1981, 1992, 2006[75]

- Humana, with $1.92 billion in operating revenues and 91 hospitals
- American Medical International, with $1.41 billion in operating revenue and 70 hospitals[73]

Such large systems had political "clout" and easier access to capital markets, and attracted skilled managers looking for larger responsibilities. Figure 1-9 categorizes the multihospital systems by ownership in 1981, 1992, and 2006.

During this time, hospitals began taking on new roles, including the following:

- Hospice programs
- Nursing homes
- Emergency centers
- Wellness programs
- Mental health crisis-intervention programs
- Family planning
- Rehabilitation centers
- Congregate housing
- Industry-related programs[74]

Both vertical and horizontal integration of health services occurred. Hospitals were both evolving into community health centers (vertical integration) and joining together in new and creative relationships (horizontal integration).

The rising tide of regulation began to recede with the presidency of Ronald Reagan. Local health planning agencies disappeared in some locations; in others, their role was reduced. The key to hospital construction was less the regulatory certificate of need and more the hospital's bond rating.

Sidebar 1-11. Historical Perspective

At ACHE's 50th Anniversary Congress on Administration in March 1983, attendees could, in a seminar on "Health Provider Advertising: How to Do It Ethically and Legally," learn how to

- Lawfully combat a competing health provider's deceptive (and competitively damaging) advertising; and
- Change, as violations of the First Amendment or the federal antitrust laws, those state laws or ethical rules that unreasonably prevented a health provider from running truthful advertising.

In another session that year entitled "Creative Alternatives for Hospital Capital Formation and Financing," participants could become informed on the existence and nature of certain creative and unconventional methods of raising and utilizing hospital capital, including private capital reorganizations and private sale/leaseback reorganizations.

In the seminar on "Competition in Health Care," executives might learn to incorporate financial planning with strategic planning, especially when viewing mergers, acquisitions, restructuring, or capital expansion programs.

When John R. Mannix, a founding Fellow of ACHE, saw the announcement of these seminars, he said that most of these topics would be appropriate for the executive of any business. "We didn't concern ourselves with those things in 1933," he said.[76]

The hospitals that did well in the investment arena were those that generated sufficient revenue to repay the bonds. In such an environment, the multi-institutional systems often had more capital for expansion than isolated small community hospitals.

As previously mentioned, the hospital's complex external environment from the 1970s forward led managers to spend more time on external affairs. This encouraged the shift to the corporate form of hospital organization with a CEO often focused on external affairs, long-range planning, and governance, and a chief operating officer (COO) managing the internal organization.

In an era of multi-institutional systems, fewer managers reported directly to boards of trustees. Instead, they worked in organizations that included tens—and even hundreds—of hospitals under one corporate umbrella. Most institutions had several assistant executives, vice presidents, and middle managers.

In this evolution, the skills acquired in previous eras were not abandoned. Hospital administration still required knowledge of architecture, operations, and human resources, as well as concern for the external environment and quality improvement.

The Modern Era (1992 to the Present)

The time period from 1992 to the present has again brought tremendous changes to the healthcare field. While organizations have continued to focus on improving the quality of care provided to patients, a more focused look at medical errors and their prevention has started a movement across the country to focus on system-based improvements, open communication, patient involvement in care, and so forth. The nature of health insurance has also changed, with an initial popularity of HMOs that has given way to insurance that offers more patient control and

Sidebar 1-12. Historical Perspective

During this time, hospitals across the country were redefining themselves as medical centers. In addition, nonhospital healthcare providers, including home care organizations, hospice providers, ambulatory surgery centers, and urgent care centers, were all growing. The diversity of healthcare provider organizations was reflected in the change in employing organizations of ACHE affiliates from 1985 to 1991. Hospital employment in 1991 included 74 percent of the membership, while it included 85 percent in 1985. By 2007, hospital employment included 56 percent of the membership.

Percent of Active ACHE Members by Employing Organization

	1985	*1991*	*2007*
Hospital	84.8%	73.9%	55.6%
Corporate headquarters	N/A	N/A	10.0
Other direct providers	3.3	11.0	8.7
(including HMO, long-term care, ambulatory care, medical group practice)			
Health association/agency	4.1	2.1	3.6
Education	6.0	1.7	3.2
Consulting	N/A	5.9	9.0
Industry and insurance	1.2	1.0	3.9
Other	0.7	4.4	6.0
	100%	100%	100%
Total active ACHE members	13,782	16,667	24,880

choice. The Health Insurance Portability and Accountability Act (HIPAA) ushered in an era where patient privacy became paramount, and healthcare organizations needed to restructure the way they communicated with and about patients. The following sections discuss in greater detail some of these new and emerging trends.

The Growth in Healthcare Expenditures

As with other eras discussed in this chapter, healthcare expenditures have increased throughout the modern era, as can be seen by the growing proportion of the gross domestic product devoted to healthcare (Figure 1-10). This trend has occurred for many reasons, including the following:

- General inflation
- Medical price inflation
- The availability of health insurance and the resulting loss of individual accountability
- Population growth
- The increased number of elderly in the population, who require more health services
- Technology and the increased intensity of services provided per capita
- Growth in national and personal incomes that permits individuals to spend more on health services
- The increased complexity of administering a multipayer system
- Fraud and abuse
- Defensive medicine (which may included potentially ineffective care)
- Malpractice
- The growth of government health programs
- The system's emphasis on curative rather than preventive health services
- Fee-for-service payment systems
- Market failure[77]

Sidebar 1-13. The Decrease in Health Insurance Coverage

Rising costs and a changing economy starting in the 1980s increased the number of Americans without health insurance. By 1989, almost 16 percent of Americans were without coverage.

Percentage of People Without Health Insurance Coverage[78]

Year	Population Total (millions)	Uninsured (millions)	Uninsured (percent)	Under 65 and Uninsured
1987	241.2	31.0	12.9	13.7
1990	248.9	34.7	13.9	14.9
1998	271.7	44.3	16.3	17.0
2000	297.5	39.8	14.2	16.1
2004	291.2	43.5	14.9	16.9
2005	293.8	44.8	15.3	17.2

The Changes in Health Insurance

In the mid to late 1990s, healthcare executives were attempting to cope with the enormous growth and popularity of HMOs. However, since that time, HMOs have decreased in both the number of plans and enrollees. Now, more consumer choice is being offered through PPOs, which allow patients more latitude in deciding who will provide their care.

As shown in Figure 1-11, the number of Americans both with and without insurance has increased considerably since the 1980s. Individuals lacking coverage should not be regarded as destitute, however. Instead, 81

	National Health Expenditure (billions)	Health Expenditures as Percentage of Gross Domestic Product	Amount per Capita
1990	$ 717.3	12.4%	$ 2,821
2000	1,358.5	13.8	4,729
2005	1,987.7	16.0	6,697

FIGURE 1-10
National Healthcare Expenditures, 1990–2004

	1990	2000	2005
Enrollment in HMOs (millions)	33.0	80.9	74.0
Number of HMOs	572	568	546
Sources of insurance coverage (millions)			
Total non-elderly population	220.6	245.1	257.4
Total with private health insurance	164.7	179.9	177.3
Employer coverage	149.6	163.8	159.5
Other private coverage	15.1	16.1	17.8
Total with public health insurance	32.2	35.8	45.5
Medicare	3.5	5.4	6.5
Medicaid	22.7	26.2	34.7
Tricare/CHAMPVA	7.9	6.8	7.7
Uninsured (millions)	32.9	39.6	46.1

FIGURE 1-11
Insurance Statistics[79]

Sidebar 1-14. The Leapfrog Group

Many employers felt that HMOs failed to engage healthcare organizations in constructively improving quality; therefore, in 2000, a coalition of large employers, including more than 160 private and public sector purchasers, formed the Leapfrog Group. The Leapfrog Group works to accomplish the following tasks:

- Work with medical experts to identify problems and propose solutions that will improve hospital systems that could break down and harm patients
- Reduce preventable medical mistakes by mobilizing employer purchasing power
- Influence improvements in the safety of healthcare
- Give consumers information to make more informed hospital choices[83]

Ultimately, the Leapfrog Group works to obtain a free flow of information about providers and encourages an environment where consumers choose their care based on quality. In addition, the Leapfrog Group supports a payment system that rewards physicians and hospitals for superior quality and efficiency using evidence-based measures.[84] These purchasers buy benefits for more than 34 million Americans.

percent of the uninsured come from working families whose employers may not offer healthcare benefits or who may be part-time employees or not qualify for benefits. These individuals also may not be able to afford their portion of their health insurance premiums and thus do not enroll in company benefit programs.[80]

Most recently, "consumer driven" health plans are growing because the plans hold out the promise of employer savings and employee empowerment at the same time. Such plans include a deductible of $1,000 or more and are tied with a health savings account or health reimbursement arrangement. They can be set up so that employees have a financial incentive to spend less on healthcare, and the employees often reap the savings themselves. Employees are thus involved in the process of trying to economize on healthcare expenditures. As evidence of their increased popularity, in 2006 in the Chicago area, 23 percent of employers offered consumer-driven health plans and another 29 percent were considering adding one in 2007.[81]

The Health Insurance Portability and Accountability Act of 1996

In 1996, a fairly significant piece of legislation regarding health insurance was passed. HIPAA provides for protection of workers' insurance coverage when they change or lose jobs. It also provides administrative simplification—where all providers and payers who collect and submit electronic health information must do so using a common format. This allows providers to check for status of claims electronically, reduce or eliminate manual or paper-based activities, accelerate the receipt of payment for claims and the payment cycle, and reduce claim errors and write-offs.[82] The HIPAA legislation had significant financial and operational impact on hospitals, because most healthcare organizations were collecting only 50 percent of the more than 300 data elements required in the new claim format.

In addition, HIPAA requires organizations to safeguard clients' rights to privacy. The requirements of HIPAA demanded specific policies relating to patient privacy and education that took time, money, and staff resources to implement.

Another significant piece of legislation regarding insurance was the 1997 Balanced Budget Act (BBA). This legislation reduced payments for Medicare patients and affected both hospitals' and physicians' incomes. It represented an effort by the federal government to balance the budget by the year 2002. The BBA initiated huge Medicare cuts amounting to $116.4 billion over five years. Graduate medical education funding also experienced a decline, and incentives were provided to reduce the number of residents educated. Urban hospitals experienced a one percent annual reduction in Medicare Disproportionate Share Hospital (DSH) payments, which are payments designed to offset the increased costs of treating low-income and indigent patients.[85] From this legislation, the critical access hospital designation was also created (see Sidebar 1-15).

Balanced Budget Act of 1997

Sidebar 1-15. The Critical Access Hospital

Over the past 15 years, many community hospitals located in rural areas have experienced the challenge of trying to provide effective high-quality care with limited resources. In some cases, depending on their location, demographics, and economic climate, communities were forced to close a hospital, which resulted in the loss of physicians and other healthcare personnel from the community. In turn, the loss of skilled healthcare professionals limited the community's access to basic primary, urgent, and emergency care services.[86]

To minimize the wholesale closing of small rural healthcare facilities, the BBA authorized the creation of the Critical Access Hospital (CAH) program. This legislation allows for enhanced Medicare reimbursement for facilities located in rural areas that meet certain characteristics. By creating the CAH program, the government ensured that rural communities could still have easy access to quality healthcare, without having to produce the capital outlay necessary for a brand new general hospital.[87]

CAHs receive cost-based reimbursement from Medicare. To receive CAH designation, an organization must meet certain criteria. It must

- have no more than 25 acute beds;
- have an average annual length of stay of no more than 96 hours; and
- be located more than 35 miles from another hospital; within 15 miles from another hospital in mountainous terrain or in areas with only secondary roads; or receive state certification that the facility is a necessary provider of healthcare services to residents in that area.

If an organization receives CAH designation, it receives 101 percent of Medicare reimbursement.[88] In 2006, there were 1,283 such hospitals; they represented 56 percent of all rural hospitals.[89]

The Dawn of Evidence-Based Medicine

The total quality management and continuous quality improvement movements have played a critical role in improving the quality of healthcare provided in the United States. These two movements have been adopted by most healthcare organizations. Within the last several years, organizations are taking these two movements a step further and measuring outcomes of care. Based on these measurements, several societies—including the American Cancer Society, the American College of Physicians, and the Council of Medical Specialty Societies—and the government (through the Agency for Healthcare Research and Quality) are publishing practice guidelines relative to treating specific diseases and conditions. These guidelines are designed to help practitioners improve patient outcomes and quality of care. This evidence-based-medicine approach has been put forward as a way not only to improve the quality of healthcare but also to reduce medical errors by reducing clinical practice variation. "Ideally evidence-based medicine strikes at the heart of the poor health outcome end of the spectrum by reducing some of this variation."[90] Regrettably, the guidelines have been criticized as "cookbook medicine," and studies show that few guidelines lead to consistent changes in provider behavior. More collaboration among providers in the future may overcome this.

Another quality-oriented movement that has taken hold since 1992 is the Malcolm Baldrige Award. The Baldrige Award was created by Congress in 1987 to enhance U.S. competitiveness. The award program promotes quality awareness, recognizes quality achievements of U.S. companies, and provides a vehicle for sharing successful strategies. The Baldrige Award criteria focus on results and continuous improvement. They provide a framework for designing, implementing, and assessing a process for managing all business operations. Three awards may be given annually in each of these categories: manufacturing, service, small business, and, since 1999, education and healthcare. The award is given because a company has shown it has an outstanding system for managing its products, services, human resources, and customer relationships. As part of the evaluation, a company is asked to describe its system for ensuring the quality of its goods and services. It also must supply information on quality improvement and customer satisfaction efforts and results.[91]

A Focus on Patient Safety

In 1999, the Institute of Medicine (IOM) released its report, *To Err Is Human*, which suggested that as many as 98,000 people in American hospitals die each year as a result of preventable errors. The root causes of preventable errors are deeply embedded in a hospital's culture, and healthcare professionals are often resistant to standardizing safe practices and using mandatory checklists. These practices are commonplace in other industries such as the airline industry or the chemical industry where life and death outcomes are affected.[92]

As a result of that IOM report and its subsequent two reports, many organizations have initiated efforts to help hospitals improve patient safety. For example, the Institute for Healthcare Improvement (IHI) began and successfully concluded a 100,000 Lives Campaign designed to encourage organizations to implement specific systems to help save a potential 100,000 lives. This campaign was so successful it led to another campaign to protect patients from five million incidents of medical harm. ACHE joined with IHI in this effort.

To help further focus organizations on proactive risk identification and reduction, several accrediting organizations, including The Joint Commission (which inspects healthcare organizations for safety) are turning their focus away from document and credential reviews and shifting to a focus on improved patient care.[93] Report cards are being published that indicate how hospitals (and physicians) fare using risk-adjusted methods for various conditions. Public reporting of hospital performance has been shown to improve the clinical areas reported on.[94]

Patients now are asked to evaluate the quality of their care. A 2002 survey of ACHE-affiliated hospital CEOs showed that 79 percent measure patient satisfaction through questionnaires sent to discharged patients and another 57 percent conduct telephone interviews with those discharged.[95]

While this chapter has taken a close look at the changing nature of the healthcare organization, an equally important

Sidebar 1-16. A Changing Design for Healthcare Facilities

A groundbreaking study conducted in San Francisco in the mid-1980s called the Planetree Model Hospital Project has had an abiding influence on healthcare delivery. While including various elements of patient care, one of its key concerns was creating healing environments and using architecture and design conducive to health. Some of the main findings of this project included the importance of providing a clear way to move patients from each point of entry to all main destinations; using sunlight to improve the mood of patients; using noise-reducing ceiling materials; using colors and textures that lift the spirit; and using artwork, nature, and music to help divert patients from focusing on their problems. Just as the move to the vertical hospital in the early 1900s caused a change in the way facilities were designed and constructed, the Planetree approach may have long-lasting effects on the design and construction of modern day healthcare faculties.

Sidebar 1-17. The Increased Specialization of Physicians

As a result of the increased focus on patient safety and quality, a new type of physician is emerging that can help improve efficiency and quality of care. Today, specialist physicians outnumber primary care physicians by two to one and that trend is not abating. This continued reliance on specialists has created the opportunity for new specialists that specifically benefit hospitalized patients: hospitalists and intensivists. These hospital-based physician caregivers allow primary care physicians time to focus on their non-hospitalized patients. Hospitalists have been shown to improve patient safety and satisfaction.

aspect of healthcare delivery in the United States is the people who manage and direct these organizations. The healthcare executive of the early twentieth century is vastly different from the executive of the twenty-first century. Chapter 2 provides some insight into these changes.

Endnotes

1. ACHA, "The Hospital Administrator: An Analysis of His Duties, Responsibilities, Relationships, and Obligations," by the 1934–1935 Study Committee of the ACHA, 1935, F. G. Carter, MD, chairman, p. 3.

2. Conners, E. J., "Future of the Hospital Administrator," in *The Changing Role of the Hospital.* Chicago: American Hospital Association, 1980, p. 17.

3. Hornsby, J. A., "Standardization of Hospitals." *Transactions of the American Hospital Association*, Vol. 15, 1913, p. 176.

4. Toner, J. M., "Statistics of the Regular Medical Associations and Hospitals of the United States." *Transactions of the American Hospital Association*, Vol. 24, 1873. This census was not complete. For example, in Cleveland, Lakeside and St. Vincent's Charity Hospitals were not included. See also John R. Mannix interview, 1983.

5. Sources: Steinwald, B., and D. Neuhauser, "The Role of the Proprietary Hospital." *Journal of Law and Contemporary Problems*, Vol. 35, No. 4, Autumn 1970; Corwin, E. H. L. *The American Hospital.* New York: Commonwealth Fund, 1946, pp. 6–7; American Hospital Association. *Hospital Statistics.* Chicago: AHA, 1982, 1992–1993, 2007; Bureau of the Census, U.S. Department of Commerce. *Historical Statistics of the United States.* 2 vols. Washington, DC: U.S. Government Printing Office, 1975, Part 1, p. 78.

6. Steinwald, B., and D. Neuhauser, "The Role of the Proprietary Hospital." *Journal of Law and Contemporary Problems*, Vol. 35, No. 4, Autumn 1970.

7. Dowling, H. F. *Fighting Infection.* Cambridge, MA: Harvard University Press, 1977.

8. ACHA, "The Hospital Administrator: An Analysis of His Duties, Responsibilities, Relationships, and Obligations," by the 1934–1935 Study Committee of the ACHA, 1935, F. G. Carter, MD, chairman, p. 4.

9. Thompson, J. D., and G. Goldin. *The Hospital: A Social and Architectural History.* New Haven, CT: Yale University Press, 1975.

10. Starr, P. *The Social Transformation of American Medicine.* New York: Basic Books, 1982, p. 153; Abel-Smith, B. *The Hospitals 1800–1848.* London: Heinemann, 1964.

11. Starr, P. *The Social Transformation of American Medicine.* New York: Basic Books, 1982, p. 161.

12. Even at the turn of the century, voluntary hospitals received financial support from local and state government. Stevens, R., "'A Poor Sort of Memory':

Voluntary Hospitals and Government Before the Depression." *Millbank Memorial Fund Quarterly*, Vol. 60, No. 4, Fall 1982, pp. 551–584.

13. Starr, P. *The Social Transformation of American Medicine*. New York: Basic Books, 1982, p. 147.

14. Perrow, C. "Goals and Power Structures: A Historical Case Study," in Freidson, E. (editor), *The Hospital in Modern Society*. Glencoe, IL: Free Press, 1963, pp. 112–146.

15. Sims, S. L. *LaCrosse Lutheran Hospital: A History 1899–1979*. LaCrosse, WI: Lutheran Hospital Foundation, 1981.

16. The Commission on Hospital Care. *Hospital Care in the United States*. Cambridge, MA: Harvard University Press, 1957, p. 312.

17. Anderson, O. W. *Blue Cross Since 1929*. Cambridge, MA: Ballinger, 1975.

18. Wilson, F., and D. Neuhauser. *Health Services in the United States*. 2nd ed. Cambridge, MA: Ballinger, 1982.

19. "Standards" and "National Bureau of Standardization." *Encyclopaedia Britannica*. London: Encyclopaedia Britannica, 1939, Vol. 21, pp. 305, 310, 311.

20. J. R. Mannix interview, 1983; Hayes, J. H., "A History of the Hospital Bureau of Standards and Supplies." *Hospitals*, Vol. 12, No. 2, Aug. 1938, p. 48; Forbes, W. J., "Standardization and Purchase Agreements: Through a Central Hospital Bureau." *Transactions of the American Hospital Association*, Vol. 13, 1911, pp. 288–300.

21. "Report of the Committee on Simplification and Standardization of Furnishings, Supplies and Equipment." *Transactions of the American Hospital Association*, 1928, pp. 45–53, 1937, pp. 190–195; Ochsner, A. J., "Hospitals Are Standardizing Themselves." *Modern Hospital*, Vol. 3, No. 1, July 1914; Ochsner, A. J., "Hospitals of the U.S. to Be Standardized." *Modern Hospital*, Vol. 9, No. 6, Dec. 1917; Hornsby, J. A., "Standardization of Hospitals." *Transactions of the American Hospital Association*, Vol. 15, 1913; Drew, C. A., "The Standardization of Hospitals." *Modern Hospital*, Vol. II, No. 1, July 1918; Dickinson, R., "Standardization of Surgery: An Attack on the Problem." *Journal of the American Medical Association*, Vol. 63, No. 9, August 1914; Foote, A. E., "Simplification and Standardization." *Transactions of the American Hospital Association*, 1926.

22. J. R. Mannix interview, Mar. 1983.

23. American College of Surgeons. *Manual of Hospital Standardization*. Chicago: ACS, 1938, p. 8.

24. Ibid.

25. Ibid., p. 6.

26. Kalisch, P., and B. Kalisch. *The Advance of American Nursing*. Boston: Little Brown, 1978, p. 10.

27. Davis, L. *Fellowship of Surgeons*. Springfield, IL: Charles C. Thomas, 1960; Stephenson, G. W. *American College of Surgeons at 75*. Chicago: ACS, 1990;

American College of Surgeons Archives on MacEachern and Codman, Jan. 1993.

28.   See "Dr. Malcolm T. MacEachern Dies at 74." *Hospitals*, Vol. 30, Feb. 16, 1956, p. 88; *Hospital Management*, Vol. 80, Aug. 1955, p. 80, Vol. 82, Aug. 1956, p. 82; Prestori, C. B., 1956; Wolverton, C. A., "Dr. Malcolm T. MacEachern Honored by Hospital Administrators." Remarks in the House of Representatives, Aug. 11, 1954; *Congressional Record*. Appendix, Aug. 16, 1954, p. A6048. The *Congressional Record* records the declaration of August 16 as Malcolm MacEachern Day; "Health Care Hall of Fame." *Modern Healthcare*, Sept. 9, 1988, p. 48; "Management in Health, The MacEachern Legacy: The Next 100 Years." Program in memory of Malcolm T. MacEachern, MD (1881–1956), founder of the Program in Hospital and Health Services Management, Northwestern University, Apr. 30–May 1, 1981; Four-page printed brochure, "Malcolm Thomas MacEachern," listing his life accomplishments, no date; American College of Surgeons archives.

29.   J. D. Lutes interview, Apr. 20, 1982.

30.   D. Conley interview, Apr. 1983.

31.   "Hospital Number." *Journal of the American Medical Association*, Vol. 106, No. 10, March 7, 1935, cited by Pennell, E., J. W. Mountin, and K. Pearson. *Business Census of Hospitals 1935 General Report.* Supplement No. 154 to the Public Health Reports, U.S. Public Health Service, Washington, DC: U.S. Government Printing Office, 1939.

32.   The hospitals of this era were racially segregated with separate wards for black patients. There were over 118 black hospitals in 1931. Of these, 2 were federal, 10 state, 3 county, and 7 city-owned; 38 were proprietary, 40 independent-voluntary, and 9 church-owned. In addition, 9 were owned by fraternal organizations. Of the 118 hospitals, 95 were under the control of blacks.

33.   Pennell, E., J. W. Mountin, and K. Pearson. *Business Census of Hospitals 1935 General Report.* Supplement No. 154 to the Public Health Reports, U.S. Public Health Service, Washington, DC: U.S. Government Printing Office, 1939.

34.   Davis, L. *Fellowship of Surgeons.* Springfield, IL: Charles C. Thomas, 1960, p. 478.

35.   Rosner, D. *A Once Charitable Enterprise: Hospitals and Health Care in Brooklyn and New York 1885–1915.* Cambridge, England: Cambridge University Press, 1982, p. 61.

36.   Dickinson, R., "Hospital Organization as Shown by Charts of Personnel and Powers Functions." *Bulletin of the Taylor Society*, Vol. 3, Oct. 1917. A rival for the earliest organization chart can be found in Ochsner, A. J., and M. J. Sturm. *The Organization, Construction and Management of Hospitals.* Chicago: Cleveland Press, 1907, p. 43.

37.   Gilbreth, F. B., "Scientific Management in the Hospital." *Transactions of the American Hospital Association*, 1914. Also see Gilbreth's "Motion Study in

Surgery." *Canadian Journal of Medical Surgery*, Vol. 40, No. 1, July 1916, pp. 22–31.

38.   Gilbreth, L., "Efficiency in the Care of the Patient." *Transactions of the American Hospital Association*, 1914; Reverby, S., "The Search for the Hospital Yardstick: Nursing and the Rationalization of Hospital Work," in Reverby, S., and D. Rosner (editors), *Health Care in America: Essays in Social History.* Philadelphia: Temple University Press, 1979.

39.   Pennell, E., J. W. Mountin, and K. Pearson. *Business Census of Hospitals 1935 General Report.* Supplement No. 154 to the Public Health Reports, U.S. Public Health Service, Washington, DC: U.S. Government Printing Office, 1939, p. 1.

40.   Ibid.

41.   Source: "Hospital Number." *Journal of the American Medical Association*, Vol. 106, No. 10, March 7, 1935, cited by Pennell, E., J. W. Mountin, and K. Pearson. *Business Census of Hospitals 1935 General Report.* Supplement No. 154 to the Public Health Reports, U.S. Public Health Service, Washington, DC: U.S. Government Printing Office, 1939.

42.   National Center for Health Statistics. *Health, United States*, 1993. Washington, DC: U.S. Government Printing Office, 1994, p. 229, Table 128. [Online information; retrieved 10/10/07.] www.cdc.gov/nchs/data/hus/hus93.pdf.

43.   J. D. Lutes interview, April 20, 1982.

44.   "Germany erected the Friedrichshain [Freidrichsheim] Hospital in Berlin, generally acknowledged to be the first 'pavilion-style' hospital." ACHA, *Hospital Administration: A Life's Profession*, Chicago: ACHA, 1948, p. 13; See also Ochsner, A. J., and M. J. Sturm. *The Organization, Construction and Management of Hospitals.* Chicago: Cleveland Press, 1907, pp. 23–26. This hospital was built from 1868–1874 with 624 beds. The 17 buildings of this hospital were completely separate. Other hospitals had connecting covered passages, for example, Lariboisierre Hospital in Paris, 1846, p. 466. Of the 178 U.S. hospitals reported by Toner in 1873, 1 hospital had five floors, 35 had four floors, 55 had three floors, and 18 had two floors. The remainder (69) either failed to respond or had one floor. Corwin, E. H. L. *The American Hospital.* New York: Commonwealth Fund, 1946, pp. 6–7.

45.   Giedion, S. *Space, Time and Architecture.* 3rd ed. Cambridge, MA: Harvard University Press, 1956, pp. 206–209.

46.   Ibid., pp. 366–393.

47.   Dowling, H. F. *Fighting Infection.* Cambridge, MA: Harvard University Press, 1977.

48.   "In 1928 the Columbia-Presbyterian Hospital group of buildings rose to 22 stories, at a cost exceeding $25,000,000. Similar multistoried structures were built: the Harborview Hospital in Seattle, the Charity Hospital in New Orleans, and Lakeside (University Hospital) in Cleveland." ACHA, *Hospital Administration: A Life's Profession*, Chicago: ACHA, 1948, op. cit., p. 18.

49.   Goldwater, S. S. *On Hospitals.* New York: Macmillan, 1949, p. 240; Thompson, J. D., and G. Goldin. *The Hospital: A Social and Architectural History.* New Haven, CT: Yale University Press, 1975, p. 196 and Chapter 6; Corwin, E. H. L. *The American Hospital.* New York: Commonwealth Fund, 1946, p. 183. Ochsner, a Chicago surgeon, was one of the early members of the American College of Surgeons. See Ochsner, A. J., and M. J. Sturm. *The Organization, Construction and Management of Hospitals.* Chicago: Cleveland Press, 1907. The changes in hospital architecture are well documented in the three editions of Stevens, E. F. *The American Hospital of the Twentieth Century.* New York: The Architectural Record Company, 1918, 1921, 1928. The 1928 edition introduces a possible multistory hospital of about 25 floors, pp. 127–137. "With the crowded conditions of our city streets, the city hospital can no longer be a spread-out affair and we must look to the air rather than to land for accommodation," pp. 132, 137. Mount Sinai Hospital in New York is also shown as an example, p. 76. S. S. Goldwater was administrator of this hospital.

50.   McNeill, W. H. *Plagues and Peoples.* Garden City, NY: Anchor Press, Doubleday, 1976, pp. 265–291.

51.   Dowling, H. F. *Fighting Infection.* Cambridge, MA: Harvard University Press, 1977.

52.   Commission on Hospital Care. *Hospital Care of the United States.* Cambridge, MA: Harvard University Press, 1957, pp. 344–345.

53.   Wesbury, S. A.,"Toward a Broader View of Health Care," Chapter 19 in Sloane, R. M., and B. L. Sloane, *A Guide to Health Care Facilities, Personnel and Management*, 3rd ed. Chicago: Health Administration Press, 1992.

54.   Corwin, E. H. L. *The American Hospital.* New York: Commonwealth Fund, 1946, p. 21; The Duke Endowment. *The Small General Hospital Organization and Management.* Charlotte, NC: Duke Endowment, Bulletin No. 3, Feb. 1928, Jan. 1933, revised Mar. 1945; Neuhauser, D. *Coming of Age.* Chicago: Health Administration Press, 1983, p. 59.

55.   Lerner, M., and O. W. Anderson. *Health Progress in the United States 1900–1960.* Chicago: University of Chicago Press, 1963, p. 248.

56.   Ibid., p. 288.

57.   Block, L. *Hospital Trends, Hospital Topics.* Chicago: ACHA, circa 1957. Copies of this book were given to ACHA affiliates in 1958. Inside the front cover was a pasted label and small mirror, "Congratulations to the American College of Hospital Administrators on its Silver Anniversary. Here is a reflection of one of those who contributed to its progress [mirror]."

58.   Source: Commission on Hospital Care. *Hospital Care of the United States.* Cambridge, MA: Harvard University Press, 1957.

59.   Sources: National Center for Health Statistics. *Health, United States, 1990.* Washington, DC: U.S. Government Printing Office, 1990, p. 184, 193; for 1929 to 1940, private insurance included in out-of-pocket payment, p. 193; personal health expenditures equals national expenditures less research, con-

struction, health insurance administration, and government public health activities, p. 254; other private funds have been excluded from percentage distribution, p. 193; 1970 to 2005 data are from U.S. Centers for Medicare & Medicaid Services, "NHE Web Tables," Tables 1, 5. [Online information; retrieved 10/11/07.] www.cms.hhs.gov/NationalHealthExpendData/downloads/tables.pdf; data for 1990 from U.S. Centers for Medicare & Medicaid Services, "National Health Expenditures by Type of Service and Source of Funds, CY 1960–2005." [Online information; retrieved 10/11/07.] www.cms.hhs.gov/NationalHealthExpendData/02_nationalhealth accountshistorical.asp.

60. Mushkin, S. *Biomedical Research: Costs and Benefits.* Cambridge, MA: Ballinger, 1979, p. 37, citing U.S. Department of Health, Education and Welfare. *Basic Data Relating to the National Institutes of Health.* Washington, DC: U.S. Government Printing Office, 1962, 1966, 1978.

61. Sources: National Center for Health Statistics. *Health, United States.* Washington, DC: U.S. Government Printing Office, 1981, p. 201, 1999, p. 284, 2006, p. 374 [Online information; retrieved 10/11/07.] www.cdc.gov/nchs/hus.htm. Data for 2000–2005 from the Centers for Medicare & Medicaid Services, "NHE Historical and Projections, 1965–2016." [Online information; retrieved 10/11/07.] www.cms.hhs.gov/NationalHealthExpendData/03_NationalHealthAccountsProjected.asp.

62. Health Insurance Institute. *Sourcebook of Health Insurance Data, 1979–1980.* Washington, DC: Health Insurance Institute, 1980, p. 13.

63. National Center for Health Statistics. *Health, United States.* Washington, DC: U.S. Government Printing Office, 1981, 1990, p. 188.

64. Hospital Corporation of America, Annual Report 1980, Nashville, Tennessee.

65. Gabriel, J. *Through the Patient's Eyes: Hospitals, Doctors, Nurses.* Philadelphia: Lippincott, 1935, p. 91.

66. Goldwater, S. S., "The Future of Hospital Administration," reprinted from *Hospitals*, Nov. 1938.

67. Lerner, M., and O. W. Anderson. *Health Progress in the United States, 1900–1960.* Chicago: University of Chicago Press, 1963, p. 230.

68. Goldsmith, J. C. *Can Hospitals Survive?* Homewood, IL: Dow Jones-Irwin, 1981, p. 107. This book can stand as a symbol of a new era of thinking about multihospital systems in a competitive healthcare market. Hospital mergers have gone on throughout the century. Bradley, F. R., "How Affiliations Build Up a Great Medical Center, Barnes Hospital and Medical Center, St. Louis." *Hospital Management*, Vol. 76, July 1953, p. 34.

69. American Hospital Association, "Hospitals Save Millions and Shared Services Mushroom." Washington, DC: AHA, Feb. 5, 1979; Brown, M., and B. P. McCool. *Multi-Hospital Systems.* Germantown, MD: Aspen Systems, 1980, p. 479.

70. Sources: National Center for Health Statistics. *Health, United States.* Washington, DC: U.S. Government Printing Office, 1990, 1994, 2006; Lerner, M., and

O. W. Anderson. *Health Progress in the United States 1900–1960*. Chicago: University of Chicago Press, 1963, p. 220; National Center for Health Statistics. *Health, United States, 1980*. Washington, DC: U.S. Government Printing Office, 1980, pp. 186, 187. U.S. Department of Labor, Bureau of Labor Statistics, Occupational Employment Statistics Home Page. [Online information; retrieved 09/01/07.] www.bls.gov/oes/home.htm#overview.

71.   Dowling, H. F. *Fighting Infection*. Cambridge, MA: Harvard University Press, 1977, p. 164; American Hospital Association. *Hospital Statistics*. Chicago: AHA, 1980, Table 3, p. 12.

72.   Sources: Brown, M., and H. L. Lewis. *Hospital Management Systems—Multi-Unit Organization and Delivery of Health Care*. Germantown, MD: Aspen Systems, 1976, p. 32; Brown, M., and B. P. McCool. *Multi-Hospital Systems*. Germantown, MD: Aspen Systems, 1980; Vraciu, R. A., and H. S. Zuckerman, "Legal and Financial Constraints on the Development and Growth of Multiple Hospital Arrangements." *Health Care Management Review*, Vol. 4, No. 1, Winter 1979.

73.   American Hospital Association. *Data Book on Multihospital Systems 1980–1981*. Chicago: AHA, 1981; Coyne, J., and L. Young, "Multihospital Bed Transfers." *Health Care Management Review*, Vol. 8, No. 1, Winter 1983; American Hospital Association. *Hospital Statistics, 1993–1994*. Chicago: AHA, 1994; American Hospital Association. *Guide to the Health Care Field*. Chicago: AHA, 1993.

74.   American Hospital Association. *The Changing Role of the Hospital*. Chicago: AHA, 1981.

75.   Sources: American Hospital Association. *Data Book on Multihospital Systems 1980–1981*. Chicago: AHA, 1981; Coyne, J., and L. Young, "Multihospital Bed Transfers." *Health Care Management Review*, Vol. 8, No. 1, Winter 1983.

76.   J. R. Mannix interview, 1983.

77.   Barton, P. L. *Understanding the U.S. Health Services System*. 3rd ed. Chicago: Health Administration Press, 2006.

78.   Sources: DeNavas-Walt, C., B. D. Proctor, and C. H. Lee. *Income, Poverty, and Health Insurance Coverage in the United States: 2005*. U.S. Census Bureau, Current Population Reports, P60-231, Washington, DC: U.S. Government Printing Office, 2006 (all population totals and uninsured totals from 1987–2000); U.S. Census Bureau, *Current Population Survey, 2006*. Annual Social and Economic Supplement. [Online information; retrieved 10/1/07.] www.nber.org/cps/cpsmar06.pdf for uninsured totals 2004–2005; under 65 and uninsured totals 1987–1990 from Fronstin, P. *Sources of Health Insurance and Characteristics of the Uninsured: Analysis of the March 2003 Current Population Survey*. Employee Benefit Research Institute, 2003. [Online information; retrieved 10/1/07.] www.ebri.org/pdf/briefspdf/1203ib.pdf; under 65 and uninsured totals 1998–2000 from Fronstin, P. *Sources of Health Insurance and Characteristics of the Uninsured: Analysis of the March 2006 Current Population Survey*. Employee Benefit Research Institute, 2006. [Online information; retrieved 10/1/07.] www.ebri.org/pdf/briefspdf/EBRI_IB_10a-20061.pdf; under 65 and

uninsured totals 2004–2005 from Fronstin, P. *Sources of Health Insurance and Characteristics of the Uninsured: Updated Analysis of the March 2006 Current Population Survey.* Employee Benefit Research Institute, 2007. [Online information; retrieved 10/1/07.] www.ebri.org/pdf/briefspdf/EBRI_IB_05-20074.pdf.

79. Source: National Center for Health Statistics. *Health, United States, 2006.* Washington, DC: U.S. Government Printing Office, 2005; "The Competitive Edge, Part II: Managed Care Industry Report." Nashville, TN: HealthLeaders-InterStudy, 2006; Fronstin, P. *Sources of Health Insurance and Characteristics of the Uninsured: Analysis of the March 2002 Current Population Survey.* Employee Benefit Research Institute, 2002. [Online information; retrieved 10/1/07.] www.ebri.org/pdf/briefspdf/1202ib.pdf; Fronstin, P. *Sources of Health Insurance and Characteristics of the Uninsured: Analysis of the March 2006 Current Population Survey.* Employee Benefit Research Institute, 2006. [Online information; retrieved 10/1/07] www.ebri.org/pdf/briefspdf/EBRI_IB_10a-20061.pdf.

80. Culbertson, D., "Money," in Garber, K. (editor), *The U.S. Health Care Delivery System: Fundamental Facts, Definitions, and Statistics.* Chicago: Health Forum, 2006, pp. 47–55.

81. Meyer, A., "Consumer-Driven Plans Being Embraced by Smaller Employers." *Chicago Tribune*, June 5, 2006.

82. Lanser, E. G., "Capitalizing on HIPAA Compliance," *Healthcare Executive* May–June 2001, Vol. 16, No. 3, pp. 6–12.

83. Leonard M. D., A. Frankel, and T. Simmonds, *Achieving Safe and Reliable Healthcare.* Chicago: Health Administration Press, 2004.

84. Galvin, R.S., S. Delbanco, A. Milstein, and G. Belden, "Has the Leapfrog Group Had an Impact On the Health Care Market?" *Health Affairs*, 2005, Vol. 24, No. 1, pp. 228–233.

85. Schneider, A., "Overview of Medicaid Provisions in the Balanced Budget Act of 1997, P.L. 105-33." *Center on Budget and Policy Priorities.* [Online report; created 9/8/1997; retrieved 6/22/06.] www.cbpp.org/908mcaid.htm. Silversmith, J., "The Impact of the 1997 Balanced Budget Act on Medicare." Minnesota Medical Association. *MMA Publications.* [Online report; created 12/2000; retrieved 6/20/06.] www.mmaonline.net/publications/MnMed2000/December/Silversmith.html.

86. Missouri Hospital Association, "Critical Access Hospitals in Missouri." [Online article; retrieved 4/28/05.] http://web.mhanet.com/asp/About_MHA/directories/cah_hospitals.asp.

87. Joint Commission Resources. *Planning Design and Construction of Health Care Facilities.* Oakbrook Terrace, IL: The Joint Commission, 2005.

88. Unanue, E., "Serving the Underserved: New Design Guidelines for Small Primary Inpatient Care Facilities." Presented at ACHE's Annual Congress on Healthcare Management in Chicago, Mar. 9, 2005.

89.   American Hospital Association, "CAH Annual Report, 2006." [Online information; retrieved 8/22/07.] www.aha.org/aha/issues/CAH/resources.html.

80.   Iglehart, J. K., "Good Science and the Marketplace for Drugs: A Conversation with Jean-Pierre Garnier." *Health Affairs*, July–Aug. 2003, Vol. 22 No. 4, pp. 119–127.

91.   Six Sigma, "Malcolm Baldrige National Quality Award." [Online information; retrieved 10/4/07.] www.isixsigma.com/ca/baldridge.

92.   Bader, B., "Quality and Patient Safety." *Healthcare Executive*, Mar.–Apr. 2006, Vol. 21, No. 2, pp. 64–67.

93.   Robeznieks, A., "Oh My God, They're Here." *Modern Healthcare*. Apr. 24, 2006, p. 6 ff.

94.   Hibbard, J. H., J. Stockard, M. Tusler, "Hospital Performance Reports: Impact on Quality, Market Share and Reputation." *Health Affairs*, Jan.–Feb. 2005, Vol. 24, No. 4, pp. 1150–1160.

95.   "Measuring Patient Satisfaction." *Healthcare Executive*, July–Aug. 2002, p. 39.

THE EVOLVING ROLE OF THE HEALTHCARE EXECUTIVE: FROM SUPERINTENDENT TO ADMINISTRATOR TO CEO

In many ways the American College of Hospital Administrators is exceptional among professional societies. It rose before there was a profession, not after one had long been established. It was devoted to creating a profession, not merely advancing the professional interests of those already acknowledged as professionals. It had to develop a university without a campus, not simply to provide [an] opportunity for leaders to read papers at annual meetings. All these it has done, and done remarkably well. The time, energy, and money so freely contributed by its members would be impossible to calculate. Its achievements can be measured in part by the present status and ability of the hospital administrator, but in whole only by the high level of medical care available in American hospitals.

Kipnis, 1955[1]

The role of a healthcare executive has evolved since the American College of Healthcare Executives (ACHE) was formed. The responsibilities and management style of a hospital superintendent are significantly different from that of an administrator and even more different from that of a chief executive officer (CEO). During these transformations of the role of the healthcare executive, the activities, programs, and structure of ACHE have also changed.

This chapter explores the changing roles and responsibilities of the healthcare executive. The evolution of the position can be separated into distinct eras. As with Chapter 1, these dates do not represent sharp splits from one time to the next but an evolutionary process:

- The birth of the hospital administrator
- The growth of the hospital administrator position
- The current picture

The Birth of the Hospital Administrator

In 1927, Michael Davis, an Honorary Fellow of ACHE, described hospital administration as being "generally viewed as an inferior calling, offering a berth rather than an opportunity."[2] It was not a permanent berth either. In looking at the 1,230 hospitals in ten states during 1920 to 1926, Davis discovered the following[3]:

- 43 percent of these hospitals had the same superintendent throughout the timeframe
- 35 percent had one change of superintendency
- 19 percent had two changes
- 3 percent had three changes

Davis also looked at the characteristics of the senior manager in all 7,610 U.S. and Canadian hospitals and discovered the following[4]:

- 37 percent were directed by a physician
- 9 percent were directed by a "medical director with a lay superintendent"
- 20 percent were directed by nurses
- 8 percent were directed by sisters
- 10 percent were directed by laymen
- 11 percent were directed by laywomen
- 5 percent were unspecified

Health administration was an occupation with three origins: medicine for the men, nursing for the women, and a religious order for both genders, but mostly women.

The founding Fellows of ACHE were hardly representative of their occupation. Of the 102 Charter Fellows, 16 were women and 32 of the men were physicians. Many of the early founders of ACHE were men without even one of the three primary allegiances: medicine, nursing, or a religious order. These Fellows were enthusiastically committed to a career in hospital administration; none left the field when better economic times came. However, these Fellows became representative of hospital administration in the years to come. Not only did they seek collegial relationships through ACHE; they also used ACHE to encourage graduate education in health administration.

Surveying the Hospital Administrator

In 1936, ACHE conducted its first survey of hospital administrators. This study was conducted by a mailed questionnaire to the administrators of approximately 6,500 hospitals listed by

Sidebar 2-1. Historical Perspective

Prior to World War II, larger hospitals were typically directed by physicians; middle-size hospitals were directed by Protestant ministers or Catholic sisters; and a nurse directed the smallest hospital.[5] Physician administrators predominated in government hospitals and in proprietary hospitals. Typical administrators were in their forties.

the American Hospital Association (AHA). About 2,200 replies were received, even fewer responded to some specific questions. Of the respondents, 63 percent of the men and 91 percent of the women administrators were in hospitals of 100 beds or less, which accounted for 78.4 percent of the hospitals reporting.

Following are some of the results from the survey. Despite some statistical inconsistencies within the data, such as frequent nonresponses and the total responses varying from one question to another, some interesting points can be observed.

- Two-thirds of the administrators were women. Of these women, 26 percent held nursing degrees, but only 4.6 percent of the nurses were university-degree holders. Among the women, sisters were the most likely to be degree holders.
- Among the men who were administrators, over half were physicians. Nearly 70 percent had university degrees compared with 7.7 percent of the women. The physicians predominated among the university men. After the physicians, clergy predominated among the degree-holding men.
- Of all administrators, 12 percent had no education beyond high school.

In 1935, ACHE members were a small fraction of all hospital administrators. By 2007, ACHE members were more representative: more than 6,000 CEOs were ACHE members, although 45 percent of these were leading organizations other than hospitals.

The level of education achieved by ACHE members had also changed by 2007. For example, according to the Affiliate Profile on ache.org, 67 percent of ACHE members had a masters's degree, an additional 19 percent had two master's degrees or a doctorate, and 14 percent had a bachelor's degree or less. Of those with graduate degrees, 57 percent obtained them in hospital and health administration, 24 percent in business, 9 percent in clinical or allied health fields, 3 percent in public health or public administration, and 7 percent in other fields. Unlike 1935, in 2007 there was very little difference between men and women by degree status

---

Sidebar 2-2. Historical Perspective

In the introduction to ACHE's first survey of hospital administrators, Robert Neff—a founding Fellow and President of ACHE from 1934 to 1935—said,

The College recognizes its obligation to study and survey the administrative field in its efforts to promote and improve the efficiency of hospital administration. The variety and complexity of the numerous relationships of the administrator—social, financial, and professional—are such as to require abilities of unusual caliber, and the facts which have been gleaned by this study naturally become interesting to those who are concerned with the relationships of the hospital administrator as a professional individual.[6]

(though twice as many women as men took their highest degrees in clinical and allied health).

Salaries   Compared with today's standards, 1935 salaries were very low. Men received higher salaries on average than women. Well over half of the women received salaries of under $3,000 a year. These figures excluded fringe benefits, such as free room and board. This benefit cannot be underestimated given the state of the country during this time. On one occasion President Roosevelt said, "I see one-third of a nation ill-housed, ill-clad [and] ill-nourished."[7] No doubt there was comfort in holding any job at all, and if that job provided a place to stay and food to eat, then all the better. In the 1935 survey of ACHE members, 60 percent of members surveyed received room and board. This was especially true for physicians, sisters, and nurses. The higher-salaried men were more likely to receive full maintenance.

While they may have had jobs, administrators were affected by the Depression in terms of salary cutbacks. Only 25 percent of administrators received no reduction in their salary between 1929 (before the stock market crash) and 1935.

Why Did People Enter the Field of Hospital Administration?   In the 1936 survey, people indicated they entered the field of hospital administration for a variety of reasons (see Figure 2-1). Half of the respondents said they entered the field because of preference for administrative work. Thirty-five percent of the women were appointed or requested by their superiors—the case for nearly all the sisters. A large number of respondents admitted that they did not come into the field by preference but because of financial need, because of physical incapacity for other work, or to carry on the work of a husband or other relative. Seven percent of the men said they were "forced into it."

Survey respondents held a variety of jobs before entering the field. Twenty-three percent of respondents left private business to become hospital administrators, 21 percent came from public health and social work, 18 percent from medicine, 15 percent from nursing, 13 percent from school teaching, and the remaining 10 percent came from other fields. Sixty-six percent had more than six years of hospital administration experience before assuming their present positions. The majority (88 percent) of respondents planned to continue in hospital administration.

Hospital administration was a part-time job for many. Sixty-seven percent of

---

Sidebar 2-3. Historical Perspective

In the 1920s, administrators of larger hospitals got together and talked about problems of construction, convalescent wards, housing for employees, and pension systems. In the 1930s, the prevalent concerns included the training of nurses, low hospital occupancy, finances, the relationship of radiologists to hospitals, the Wagner Act as it related to labor unions, the Social Security Act, and national health insurance. During the war, the issues were war preparations, rationing, price and salary controls, and air raid precautions.[8]

FIGURE 2-1. Reasons for Entering Administration [9]

Reason for Entering Administrative Field	Men (years)								Women (years)								Grand	
	20s	30s	40s	50s	60s	70+	Total	%	20s	30s	40s	50s	60s	70+	Total	%	Total	%
Interest or preference for administrative work	3	60	107	75	36	3	284	40.6	20	88	177	89	16	2	392	51.4	676	46.2
Appointed or requested by supervisors	—	22	55	69	23	2	171	24.4	9	48	111	76	26	1	271	35.5	442	30.2
Financial remuneration	—	7	16	17	9	1	50	7.2	3	12	9	8	2	—	34	4.4	84	5.8
Physical incapacity for other work	—	2	4	8	2	—	16	2.3	—	—	1	3	1	—	5	0.6	21	1.4
Interest in helping the sick	1	11	34	35	14	1	90	13.7	—	5	21	6	4	—	36	4.7	132	9.1
Carried on work of husband or other relative	—	2	1	3	1	—	7	1.0	1	1	2	—	2	—	6	0.8	13	0.9
Not satisfied with existing conditions of hospital administration	1	2	10	11	5	—	29	4.2	—	1	9	3	—	—	13	1.7	42	2.8
Forced into it	1	11	10	17	7	—	46	6.6	2	—	1	3	1	—	7	0.9	53	3.6
Totals	6	117	237	235	97	7	699	100	35	155	331	188	52	3	764	100	1,463	100

survey respondents had other occupations or held other positions in addition to being administrators. Only 13 percent had a written contract as the basis of their appointment. Most of the rest had a verbal agreement or no agreement.

Defining the Role of Administrator

In 1934, ACHE's Study Committee[10] produced the report, *The Hospital Administrator: An Analysis of His Duties, Responsibilities, Relationships and Obligations.* This document defined the role of the administrator, given the conditions of the day:

> [T]he administrator is the executive head of the hospital, responsible to the governing board for efficient management.[11] Such being the case, he must be given complete authority in administration and he must collaborate with the medical staff in order that the patient may be restored to health as quickly, safely and pleasantly as possible.

The document recognized the concept of a hospital's "three-legged stool"—board, administrator, and medical staff—and advised administrators to involve themselves in formulating a body of rules, that is, a constitution and bylaws. Such rules should not be too detailed, the document noted. However, "they may and should be supplemented by more detailed rules for the guidance of hospital employees." The document also recommended the use of the following classic management tools[12]:

- Standing orders to coordinate and facilitate the work of the hospital.
- Organization charts to indicate division of labor and lines of authority, clarify the functions of the various departments of the hospital, and help prevent overlapping and the resulting friction that usually develops out of failure on the part of department heads to properly appreciate the limits of their respective functions.
- Organization record or book of job descriptions to supplement the organization chart and outline the duties and authority of each worker.

The document outlined every aspect of the administrator's role, including the following:

- Ensuring that patients receive the proper care.
- Selecting department heads yet maintaining ultimate responsibility.
- Establishing relationships between executives and employees—noting that in smaller hospitals these relationships would be very simple and in larger hospitals they would be more complex, thus warranting a more organized approach.

- Determining rates and fees and working with the business office to ensure that the fees were charged, entered, and collected. Prior to health insurance, less rate regulation existed. It was a simpler world. "The accounting office assists the administrator in preparation of the budget for presentation to the governing board," noted the report. This was an objective more than a fact; many hospitals did not use budgets until Medicare regulations required them to do so in the late 1960s.

Regarding the administrator's relationship with the medical staff, the document had the following comment:

Ordinarily the administrator acts as a liaison officer between the medical staff and the governing board, but in some hospitals there are joint conference committees consisting of board members and staff members, which meet with administrators to discuss and solve the purely medical problems of hospital administration. The danger in this type of organization is that the joint conference committee will overstep the bounds of propriety by enlarging the scope of its activities to include more than the purely medical phases of hospital administration. A more desirable arrangement is created through the appointment by the staff or its executive officer of a medical advisory committee of the staff to confer with the administrator on matters of staff interest.... The administrator relays the wishes of the staff as expressed through the committee to the governing board, and he may, if it seems desirable, in the case of highly technical matters ask the members of such advisory committee to assist him in his representations to the governing board. Incidentally, staff members should not be asked to assume the anomalous, dual role of board member and staff member because this arrangement is incompatible with sound principles of organization.[13]

This proposal, consistent with classic organization theory, was rejected in time. Evidence accumulated that good rapport between board and medical staff contributed to higher quality of care.

Regarding the human relations aspect of the administrator role, the documents suggested the following:

The administrator should be interested in the social activities of the personnel, particularly of those living in the institution. His interest should not be in the nature of interference but rather he should encourage social intercourse when off duty and render all assistance possible in promoting recreation and amusement when called on to do so.[14]

The document discussed the qualifications of the administrator, requiring him or her to have "infinite tact, diplomacy, patience and tolerance for the views and opinions of others," as well as firmness tempered with consideration for the weaknesses of others. It went on to suggest the following:

> He must be an organizer, a community leader, have a sense of seriousness in his work, be absolutely honorable and just, a judge of human nature, industrious, of broad education, neat and tidy appearance, an educator, a good buyer, of a mechanical turn of mind, an ability to work with others, familiarity with laws affecting the hospital, and he should constantly seek comments and constructive criticism.

Of the 18 listed qualifications, number nine stated, "He must have administrative ability, the degree varying directly with the size of the hospital. In the very large hospital he will be almost entirely an administrator but in the smaller one he will actually do much of the work with fewer subordinates on whom he will depend."[15]

With this list of qualifications, the report concluded, "This survey describes the niche into which the American College of Hospital Administrators feels that its members may or should strive to fit themselves in a general way."[16]

The Growth of the Hospital Administrator Position

As previously mentioned, in 1935 only a small percentage of administrators were members of ACHE. This had changed by 1944, when ACHE's survey of hospital administrators yielded 1,017 coded questionnaires from administrator members.[17] From these questionnaires, Dean Conley prepared "a statistical survey based on the 1944 Directory of Membership" for the Central Committee on Institutes of the College.[18] (Figure 2-2 shows results from this survey compared with 2007 membership statistics.)

Results of the survey showed that ACHE membership of 1944 reflected the transition away from nurse and physician administrators to younger lay administrators.[19] Laymen were the largest single group of members; sisters and nurses tied for second place; and physicians were third. More than two-thirds of the members were administrators, with the remainder being mostly associate and assistant administrators. The level of education of members in 1944 was higher than for the entire field in 1935.

Most of ACHE members represented hospitals with more than 200 beds, even when most hospitals had less than 100 beds. ACHE represented larger general hospitals that offered more services. Of the 1,017 hospitals represented in the 1944 study, 573 had outpatient departments; 703 had nursing schools; 531 had interns; and 381 had resident training programs.[20]

	1944 (%)	2007 (%)
Age		
Under 50	43	55
50+	57	45
Total	100%	100%
Country of Birth		
United States	87	99
Canada	10	1
Other	2	–
Total	100%*	100%
Education		
Less than bachelor's	60	**
Bachelor's degree	33	14
Graduate work	4	
Graduate degree	3	86
Total	100%	100%
Gender		
Female	51	41
Male	49	59
Total	100%	100%
Professional Status		
Doctor	15	3
Nurse	24	10
Member of religious order	26	**
None of the above	37	87
Total	100%*	100%
Position		
CEO/Administrator	68	23
Other	32	77
Total	100%	100%
ACHE Status		
Nominee	20	79
Member†/Diplomate	48	–
Fellow	32	21
Total	100%	100%

FIGURE 2-2
Membership
Characteristics,
1944 and 2007

*Percentages may not total 100 because of rounding.
**Less than 0.5%.
†In 2007, all Diplomates were converted to either Fellows or Members depending on whether they had accrued sufficient hours of continuing education and had sufficient tenure in ACHE.

Sidebar 2-4. Significant Statistics

The results from the 1944 survey showed there were slightly more women affiliates than men. However, Fellows were twice as likely to be men as women.[21] Although Fellows were older on average, male members were younger. For example, of members aged 30 to 39 years, 83 percent were men. The nurse and physician members were somewhat older on average than the lay members. There was a decrease in the number of nurses entering hospital administration.[22] The figure below shows the age and gender of members in 1944, 1991, and 2007.

Age and Gender of ACHE Members, 1944, 1991, 2007[23]

Age (years)	Men			Women		
	1944	*1991*	*2007*	*1944*	*1991*	*2007*
Under 30	3	295	788	0	328	1,140
30–39	104	3,684	3,114	21	1,580	2,053
40–49	163	6,245	4,650	137	1,358	3,244
50–59	148	2,443	5,963	198	517	3,768
60+	74	811	1,779	149	233	631
Not given	9	–	–	15	–	–
Percent of women ACHE members				51%	23%	40%

In 1935, ACHE surveyed approximately 6,500 hospital administrators on the mailing list of the American Hospital Association. After two mailings, 1,872 responses were received. Of these, 54 percent (1,007) were women and 46 percent (865) were men. These data were collected during peacetime and serve to indicate that in the 1930s and probably also in the 1940s, a majority of hospital administrators were women.[24]

The Effect of World War II

At the start of World War II, military hospitals were usually managed by physicians. However, as the war progressed and the need for such hospitals grew, an increasing number were managed by nonphysician male administrators. ACHE encouraged these administrators to join ACHE if they planned to continue in the field, and many did. Thus, the war helped change the profession of hospital administration.[25]

When Arthur C. Bachmeyer, MD, was Chairman of ACHE from 1940 to 1941, he predicted that there would be increased interest in hospital administration at the end of World War II. To estimate the size of this demand, ACHE sent questionnaires to Medical Service Corps administrators and received about 1,500 to 2,000 replies expressing interest in training and civilian careers.

According to Dean Conley, this survey added fuel to the postwar development of hospital administration courses.[26]

Since World War II, career officers in all branches of the military service have been actively involved in ACHE. Before the 1967 reorganization, Major General James McGibony represented the military on the Board of Regents. From 1994 to 1995, ACHE had its first Chairman from the military: Bill Head was a colonel in the Air Force. In 2007, the uniformed services were represented by a member of the Board of Governors, Air Force Colonel Kent R. Helwig. Army Brigadier General David A. Rubenstein was elected Chairman for 2008.

All the services recognize and encourage their healthcare executives to participate in ACHE. In some cases, credentials—such as those from ACHE—are necessary for advancement.

The Mid-Century Years

By 1948, annual salaries of hospital administrators were $7,500 a year and up, including maintenance (room and board). Some administrators of large institutions were "receiving upwards of $15,000 with the privilege of engaging in consultant work." In moderately sized institutions, starting salaries were around $5,000 plus maintenance.[27]

During this time, graduate education was proposed by ACHE as the primary entry point for a career in hospital administration, thus heralding a new era. By the 1950s, there were an estimated 10,000 hospital administration positions in American hospitals. By 1955, more than 2,500 of these positions were held by affiliates of ACHE.[28] In the 1960s, the weight of ACHE membership had shifted to master's-degree program graduates. The mid-1950s saw the proportionate decline of the physician administrator.[29]

As part of his work on The Joint Commission on Education of the ACHA and AHA in 1948, Charles E. Prall surveyed hospital administrators on the major problems they confronted[30] (see Chapter 5 for more information on the Prall Report). This started a series of similar surveys, including ones in 1963[31], 1978[32], 1990[33], and 2006. As seen in the results of these surveys,

---

Sidebar 2-5. Historical Perspective

In 1948, ACHE published *Hospital Administration: A Life's Profession* in response to frequent requests of ACHE, "principally for vocational guidance purposes and more specifically for men and women deciding on a life's work."[34] The book noted that

A sound case can be made for the professional status of the hospital administrator.... Hospital administration is a unique and highly complex activity. Involving as it does problems of finance, hospital care of the sick and injured, institutional management, interrelations of professional groups, as well as cutting across the fields of political economy, sociology, psychology, and technology, it encompasses many of the disciplines and principles of several distinct professional areas. Moreover [the administrator] must be skilled in effective human relations with an emphasis on such personal attitudes as diplomacy and sympathetic understanding. Further, the administrator must possess the somewhat abstract quality known as sound judgment.[35]

FIGURE 2-3
Top Issues
Confronting
Hospitals by
Rank Order,
1948–2006[38]

Issue	1948	1963	1978	1990	2006
Working with medical staff	1	4	4	2	2
Personnel management	2	3	3	3	4
Providing quality medical care	4	5	6	4	5
Business/financial management	5	2	3	1	1
Legal aspects and litigation	10	10	10	9	7

Sidebar 2-6. Historical Perspective

In 1968, Richard Stull said that one of the "major unsolved problems bedeviling the practice of truly effective administration in hospitals today...is our failure to secure competent supportive staff skills and to develop a middle level management of qualified and specialized individuals."[39]

Sidebar 2-7. Significant Statistics

As of December 31, 1983, ACHE had 17,499 affiliates. This number included 81 Honorary Fellows, 642 Life Fellows, 1,758 Fellows, 348 Life Members, 6,079 Members, 5,413 Nominees, and 3,178 Student Associates. This was the largest number of affiliates in ACHE's history.

In 1983, of the 12,471 active affiliates, 82 percent worked in hospitals and hospital systems; 3 percent in other direct providers; 8 percent in health agencies and associations; 5 percent in education and consulting; 1 percent in industry and insurance; and 1 percent in other settings. Of those working in hospitals, 63 percent were CEOs or chief operating officers. Of those working in other organizations, 47 percent were CEOs.

across the years, business and financial management went from fifth to first place in the list of top issues confronting hospitals. Quality of medical care held a steady middle place and legal issues remained a low concern (see Figure 2-3). In the 2006 survey, some new concerns rose to the forefront, including care for the uninsured, patient safety, patient satisfaction, and technology.

A Growth in Nonhospital Administrators

The 1970s saw the proportion of ACHE members who were employed in nonhospital settings reach 20 percent and remain at that level throughout the decade.[36] This growth reflected the diversity of healthcare organizations in this era of regulation and environmental complexity. By 1981, Stuart A. Wesbury Jr., PhD, president of ACHE at the time, estimated that only 60 percent of the graduates of masters' programs were employed in hospitals,[37] with the remaining 40 percent employed in a wide variety of other health-related organizations.

The Return of Women to Hospital Administration

In 1982, women were returning to hospital administration after a decline in the

1960s that accompanied a general decrease in the number of women in Catholic religious orders.[40] In 1981, 51 percent of students in graduate programs in health administration were women, up from 9 percent in 1969.[41] This growth in the percentage of women in graduate schools could also be found in law and medicine as well.

By 1991, the percentage of women in health administration had again increased, and by 2006 they represented nearly half of all members in ACHE (see Figure 2-4). While the largest percentage of female ACHE members were and still are

> **Sidebar 2-8. Significant Statistics**
>
> A 1983 staff study completed by James B. Gantenberg showed that in 1982, 202 physicians were identified as hospital chief executive officers compared to 813 in 1972. For registered nurses, 54 were identified as CEOs in 1982 compared to 294 in 1972. In 2007, there were 242 physicians and 156 registered nurses serving as hospital CEOs.

Year	Number of Women	Total*	Percent
1944	520	1,017	51
1956	913	3,828	24
1973	1,041	7,817	13
1982	1,410	12,821	11
1983	1,610	13,235	12
1985	1,925	13,854	14
1986	2,266	14,675	15
1987	2,409	14,715	16
1988	2,715	15,303	18
1989	3,042	15,925	19
1990	3,482	16,689	21
1991	4,140	17,746	23
1992	4,825	18,667	26
1993	5,660	19,853	29
1994	6,348	20,965	30
1995	7,046	22,093	32
1996	7,241	22,291	33
1997	7,204	21,747	33
1998	7,410	21,778	34
1999	7,433	21,589	34
2000	7,807	21,988	36
2001	8,306	22,668	37
2002	8,619	23,039	37
2003	9,472	24,427	39
2004	10,480	26,410	40
2005	11,176	27,779	40
2006	11,717	28,799	41
2007	11,684	28,762	41

FIGURE 2-4
Representation of Women in ACHE

*Includes Members, Diplomates, and Fellows only.

Sidebar 2-9. Significant Statistics

Since 1990, ACHE has compared the career outcomes of men and women affiliates, controlling for tenure in the field of healthcare management. Conducted at approximately five-year intervals, one of the positive gains observed in these comparisons was a narrowing of the gap between the gender groups in the proportion of individuals in CEO positions. For example, in 1990, 11 percent of women compared with 28 percent of men attained CEO positions. In 2006, 12 percent of women compared with 19 percent of men attained such positions. Thus, in 1990, women attained CEO positions at 39 percent of the rate of men; in 2006, women attained CEO positions at 63 percent of the rate of men.

Another positive trend is the proportion of both gender groups that are satisfied with their job security. In 1990, 77 percent of men and 71 percent of women were satisfied; in 2006, this rose to 86 percent for both men and women.

Other changes have appeared over time, such as the prevalence of affiliates that experienced sexual harassment. In 1995, 29 percent of women and 5 percent of men had experienced harassment sometime during the previous five years. By 2006, however, reporting of sexual harassment declined to 10 percent of women and 3 percent of men surveyed. When the issue of sexual harassment started to recieve attention, ACHE developed a policy statement on the issue, which may have helped foster improvement in the area.

In some areas, however, gender differences that may represent inequitable treatment of women persist. For example, the income gap between the gender groups has remained about the same. In 1990, the median income was $57,200 for women and $69,400 for men, showing an 18 percent gap. In 2006, the respective incomes were $107,800 and $131,000, an 18 percent gap again. Similarly, significantly more men than women continue to aspire to CEO positions. In 1990, 77 percent of men and 39 percent of women aspired to be a CEO in the coming 5 to 15 years. In 2006, 79 percent of men and 40 percent of women had such aspirations. By continuing to collect career attainment data over time, ACHE has served not only to mirror trends in the field, but also help effect positive change through its policy statements and recommendations (see Chapter 7 and Appendix 2 for more information on ACHE's policy statements.)

students, since 1982 more and more women have moved out of the student category and into the Member, Diplomate, and Fellow classifications. In 1982, 1991, and 2006, more women were Members than Diplomates and Fellows; however, as the years progressed, a greater percentage of women chose to pursue credentialed status.

ACHE, in collaboration with the AHA, studied hospital CEO turnover from 1981 to 1990[42] (see Figure 2-5). Adjusted turnover rose in the middle 1980s to more than 18 percent and then declined. Based on surveys in 1989 and 1990, 65 percent of turnover was voluntary (career moves at 31 percent; personal events like retirement at 15 percent; job dissatisfaction at 13 percent; and other at 4 percent). The 35 percent involuntary turnover was because of disagreements (14 percent) and reorganization (11 percent), with 10 percent of unknown cause.

High-turnover hospitals were more likely to be small, part of multi-hospital systems, investor-owned, located in the South or West, located in

Year	Adjusted CEO Turnovers*
1981	14.0%
1986	17.0
1991	17.0
1996	16.0
2001	15.0
2006	15.0

FIGURE 2-5
Hospital CEO
Turnover,
1981–2006[44]

* Short-term general medical and surgical nonfederal hospitals. Based on a sample survey of 150 hospitals, the total turnover rate is reduced by 18.8% due to incorrect reporting of retained CEOs or to the appointment of interim or acting CEOs.

large cities, nonteaching, have low occupancy, and have low operating margins.[43] In recent years, CEO turnover has generally stabilized and affects 14 to 16 percent of hospitals annually.

The Current Picture

The 2007 survey of ACHE affiliates reveals a different picture of the healthcare executive than that of previous eras. The profession is much more diverse, and the background of entrants to the profession is more varied. Women now represent more than 40 percent of ACHE members, and the proportion of minority members is also increasing. As with the rest of the population, the average age of the healthcare executive is also increasing, as is reflected by the fact that nearly 65 percent of ACHE affiliates are between 40 and 60 years old.

As previously mentioned, a greater percentage of affiliates are earning higher degrees than in previous eras, however, this education is not necessarily in hospital or health services administration. For example, although 86.4 percent of affiliates held a master's degree or higher in 2007, almost a quarter of those degrees were in business, not health administration. Since 1992, there has also been a growing trend for physicians and nurses to seek roles in healthcare management. Clinicians want to play a bigger role in controlling the healthcare delivery environment and effecting patient safety.[45]

A Focus on Safety
In recent years, the healthcare field has come under significant scrutiny from the public, the media, the government, and several watchdog groups. While effective healthcare executives watch the bottom line, they must also advocate on behalf of patients and families to achieve a level of

care that is safe, effective, and appropriate. As mentioned in Chapter 1, the 1999 Institute of Medicine's *To Err Is Human* report cast a harsh light on the number of medical errors occurring in the United States and placed the responsibility for addressing this pandemic squarely at the feet of healthcare executives.[46] In the years since the report, healthcare leaders have been expected to be transparent about errors occurring in their organization, proactive in addressing issues that could lead to errors, and accountable for the safety of patients and the quality of care provided in their healthcare organizations. The days of rationalizing error as a part of the complexity of healthcare delivery are over. Organizations such as the Leapfrog Group, the Institute for Healthcare Improvement, the National Quality Forum, and The Joint Commission are expecting, and often requiring, organization leadership to shift their culture to one of open communication, transparency, proactive risk reduction, safety, and quality.

The Need for Business Skills

In recent years, the demand for business skills has become paramount for effective healthcare management. Because of a variety of factors—including the advent of expensive technology, staffing shortages, and reduced reimbursement from the government and third-party payers—healthcare executives are asked to do more with less. Those individuals who have training and experience in business and financial management in addition to their health administration training have an advantage over those without such training.

In the coming years, continuous constrained reimbursement and increasing bad debt as a result of the increasing number of uninsured patients seeking treatment at healthcare organizations will require most healthcare executives to raise funds to meet financial obligations. The ability to effectively raise funds is becoming more important and could be a critical skill in the coming years.

The Importance of Strong Interpersonal Skills

In addition to business skills, an individual's interpersonal skills play as important a role today as ever before. The healthcare executive in the twenty-first century is required to balance the wants and needs of the patient and family, the medical staff, the community, and the healthcare organization's board of directors. This delicate dance requires effective communication, teamwork, conflict management, and negotiation skills. Because the healthcare executive is beholden to a variety of diverse stakeholders, the ability to manage stress has also become paramount for effective healthcare leadership.

One particular dynamic that has grown in importance in recent years is the relationship between physicians and hospitals. As third-party payers and the government rein in reimbursements, physicians are seeing their incomes decline. Consequently, physicians are looking for new ways to expand their earning potential, sometimes by investing in enterprises that directly compete with the revenue sources of the hospital. Healthcare executives must be able to negotiate win-win collaborations with physicians and partner with them to provide safe and high-quality care.

A Focus on Technology

The technological advances that have occurred since 1991 are staggering. Computerized physician-order entry systems, automated medication dispensing systems, sophisticated imaging equipment, as well as ever-changing information management systems have created an environment where a technologically savvy healthcare executive can make the difference between an efficient and innovative facility and one that is stuck in the past. Experience with, understanding of, and support of both clinical and information technology systems are critical if the healthcare executive hopes to effectively manage not only the technology in his or her facility but also the technology's impact on the healthcare organization.

The past two chapters have painted a picture of the healthcare environment—both the nature of healthcare delivery in the United States and also the nature of the individuals who lead healthcare organizations. Chapter 3 discusses how ACHE evolved within this environment. It traces the creation of the organization, its growth, and its current state.

Endnotes

1. Kipnis, I. A. *A Venture Forward: A History of the American College of Hospital Administrators.* Chicago: ACHA, 1955, p. 123.

2. Davis, M. M. *Hospitals and Health Centers.* New York: Harper & Brothers, 1927, p. 27.

3. Ibid., pp. 17–18. Based on data from American Medical Association hospital directories for these years.

4. Ibid., p. 27. Titles as listed in the 1927 *AMA Directory.*

5. J. R. Mannix interview, 1982.

6. ACHA, "A Survey of the Hospital Administrator," 1936. (Robert Neff, "General Statement.")

7. Morris, R. B. (editor). *Encyclopedia of American History.* New York: Harper & Brothers, 1953, p. 355.

8. Society of Medical Administrators. *A History of the Society of Medical Administrators and the Medical Superintendents Club.* Society of Medical Administrators, 1920–1955, 1956–1966, 1967.

9. Source: ACHA, "A Survey of the Hospital Administrator." Chicago: ACHA, 1936, p. 27.

10.   This committee consisted of Fred G. Carter, MD, chairman, Sister M. Patricia, and Asa S. Bacon. Carter was President of the ACHA from 1935 to 1936. Asa Bacon was a Charter Fellow.

11.   "The male pronoun is used throughout this study as an editorial convenience only." ACHA, *The Hospital Administrator: An Analysis of His Duties, Responsibilities, Relationships, and Obligations*, 1935, p. 3, footnote.

12.   ACHA, *The Hospital Administrator: An Analysis of His Duties, Responsibilities, Relationships, and Obligations*, 1935. Carter was President of the ACHA in 1935–1936, p. 7–8.

13.   Ibid., p. 13. The quote continues, "The preservation of the liaison characteristics of the administrator's position will be found to be highly desirable at all times. Deviations from this conception of the administrator's place in the organization lead to trouble sooner or later. The organization of the proprietary hospital represents a somewhat different problem which need not enter into present considerations."

14.   Ibid., p. 9.

15.   Ibid., pp. 19–20.

16.   Ibid., p. 24.

17.   ACHA, "A Statistical Survey Based on the 1944 Directory of Membership," Aug. 1944.

18.   The analysis was carried out by transcribing the questionnaire data onto punch cards. A statistical tabulating service was used to do the analysis that the "already overloaded headquarters staff" of ACHE was unable to complete. The result—methodologically speaking—was a major improvement over the 1935 survey.

19.   ACHA, "A Statistical Survey Based on the 1944 Directory of Membership," Aug. 1944, Part IV, Table 8.

20.   Ibid., Part III, Table 3.

21.   The number of female affiliates of ACHE increased in part because of the number of nuns who joined after Father Schwitilla lifted "the bans" on ACHE interaction. Father Schwitilla opposed ACHE at its onset. G. Hartman personal communication, 1983. Kipnis, I. A. *A Venture Forward: A History of the American College of Hospital Administrators.* Chicago: ACHA, 1955, pp. 65–66. The number of female affiliates fell during the 1960s because of the declining number of women in Catholic religious orders and the substitution of administrators who were nuns with lay male administrators. W. R. Kirk interview, 1983.

22.   ACHA *Minute Book*, Vol. 1, Aug. 19, 1944.

23.   Source: ACHA, "A Statistical Survey Based on the 1944 Directory of Membership," Aug. 1944, Part II, Table 1.

24.   ACHA, "A Survey of the Hospital Administrator," Neff, R. E. (compiler), 1936.

25.   O. Weissman and R. Griggs personal communication, 1983. ACHE continued to welcome military hospital administrators. "The Value to Medical Service

Corps Officers of Affiliation with the American College of Hospital Administrators," *U.S. Airforce Medical Service Digest*, Feb. 1959, Vol. 10, p. 27.

26.   D. Conley interview, Apr. 21, 1983.

27.   ACHA, "Hospital Administration: A Lifes Profession," 1948, p. 51.

28.   Kipnis, I. A. *A Venture Forward: A History of the American College of Hospital Administrators*. Chicago: ACHA, 1955, pp. 121, 129. There were an additional 42 ACHE members working outside of the United States and Canada as of January 1, 1955.

29.   Katzive, J. A., "The Vanishing Medical Hospital Administrator." *Hospital Topics*, Vol. 43, Feb. 1965, p. 41. This was a topic of discussion at the Society of Medical Administrators (Society of Medical Administrators. *A History of the Society of Medical Administrators and the Medical Superintendents Club*. Society of Medical Administrators, 1920–1955, 1956–1966, 1967) at their 1953, 1954, and 1956 meetings. The 1960s saw the near disappearance of the physician chairmen of the AHA and ACHA.

30.   Prall, C. E. *Problems of Hospital Administration*. Chicago: Physicians Record Company, 1948, p. 43.

31.   Dolson, M. T., "How Administrators Rate Different Tasks." *The Modern Hospital*, Vol. 104, No. 6, 1965.

32.   Carper, W. B., "A Longitudinal Analysis of the Problems of Hospital Administrators." *Hospitals and Health Services Administration*, Vol. 27, No. 3, 1982, pp. 82–95.

33.   Agho, A., and S. T. Cyphert, "Problem Areas Faced by Hospital Administrators." *Hospital & Health Services Administration*, Vol. 37, No. 1, Spring 1992 (22.6 percent response rate).

34.   Conley, D., "Foreword," in ACHA, "Hospital Administration. A Life's Profession." Chicago: ACHA, 1948. This work relies heavily on Rappleye, W. C. (*Principles of Hospital Administration and the Training of Hospital Executives*. Report of the Rockefeller Committee on the Training for Hospital Executives, 1922); Davis, M. M., (*Hospital Administration: A Career*. New York: Privately published, 1929); and the ACHA reports of 1934–35 (chaired by Dr. Fred Carter) and 1937 (chaired by Dr. Alphonse Schwitalla), and it gives thanks to Drs. Arthur C. Bachmeyer, Malcolm MacEachern, Claude Munger, Charles Prall, and John Gorrell. In the same year ACHE also published a more popular document *At the Helm of the Hospital: The Story of a New Profession*, 1948, as part of a fundraising project for ACHE.

35.   ACHA, "Hospital Administration: A Life's Profession," 1948, pp. 41–42.

36.   Wesbury, S. A., "Background Information Concerning the Proposal to Change the Name and objects of the American College of Hospital Administrators," April 1981.

37.   Ibid., p. 5.

38.   Sources: Prall, C. E. *Problems of Hospital Administration*. Chicago: Physicians Record Company, 1948, p. 43; Dolson, M. T., "How Administrators Rate

Different Tasks." *The Modern Hospital*, Vol. 104, No. 6, 1965; Carper, W. B., "A Longitudinal Analysis of the Problems of Hospital Administrators." *Hospitals and Health Services Administration*, Vol. 27, No. 3, 1982, pp. 82–95; Agho, A., and S. T. Cyphert, "Problem Areas Faced by Hospital Administrators." *Hospital & Health Services Administration*, Vol. 37, No. 1, Spring 1992; Evans, M., "CEOs Focus on Finances, Docs," *Modern Healthcare*, Vol. 37, No. 1., January 2007, pp. 8–9.

39.   Stull, R., "Management of the American Hospital," in Hague, J. E., *The American Hospital System*. Papers presented at the dedication program of the Baptist Memorial Hospital, Union East Unit, Memphis, Tennesee, Feb. 19, 1968. Pensacola, FL: Hospital Research and Development Institute Inc., 1968.

40.   W. R. Kirk interview, Mar. 14, 1983.

41.   S. Shortell personal communication, 1983.

42.   ACHE, "Hospital Chief Executive Officer Turnover 1981–1990," (with AHA, Heidrick and Struggles, Inc.), 1991.

43.   Ibid., p. 8.

44.   Source: ACHE, "Hospital CEO Turnover," 2005.

45.   T. C. Dolan interview, Sept. 15, 2006.

46.   Institute of Medicine. *To Err Is Human: Building a Safer Health System*. L. T. Kohn, J. M. Corrigan, and M. S. Donaldson (editors). Washington, DC: National Academies Press, 1999.

THE EVOLUTION OF ACHE: FROM BIRTH TO PRESENT DAY

There were five objectives when the ACHA was founded in 1933:
1. *To elevate the standards of hospital administration*
2. *To establish standards of competency for hospital administrators*
3. *To develop and promote standards of education and training for hospital administrators*
4. *To educate hospital trustees and the public to understand that the practice of hospital administration calls for special training and experience*
5. *To provide a method of conferring Fellowships in Hospital Administration on those who have rendered or are rendering noteworthy service in the field of hospital administration*

Carter, 1936[1]

As discussed in Chapters 1 and 2, the American College of Healthcare Executives (ACHE) is a product of the changing healthcare field—an evolving organization that has been and will continue to be shaped by historic events. While the previous two chapters have painted a picture of the healthcare landscape and its changing dynamics throughout the years, the focus of this chapter is on ACHE itself and how it was impacted by and reacted to historic events and eras. The chapter follows ACHE from its infancy through to the modern era. It provides an overview of how ACHE was created and how it morphed, adapted, and changed throughout the years. Chapters 4 through 7 will take a closer look at specific functions of ACHE, including those related to membership, education, publications, and other important services.

The Idea of a College: Building on the Work of Others

ACHE was not the first professional healthcare organization, by any means. The idea of a college of healthcare providers existed several hundred years prior in Britain, when King Henry VIII chartered the Royal College of Physicians in London in 1518[2] (see Sidebar 3-1). The Royal College of Surgeons was created as an offshoot of the college of physicians, and the American College of Surgeons (ACS), founded in May 1913, was modeled directly on its British counterpart.

Sidebar 3-1. Historical Perspective

The following list shows the founding dates of selected professional colleges and other organizations:

1518	Royal College of Physicians (of London)
1540	The Company of Barber-Surgeons
1745	The Company of Surgeons
1800	Royal College of Surgeons
1847	American Medical Association
1872	American Public Health Association
1899	The Association of Hospital Superintendents (to become the American Hospital Association)[3]
1913	American College of Surgeons (the first of the American medical specialty colleges)
1915	American College of Physicians
1915	Catholic Hospital Association[4]
1917	American Board of Ophthalmology (the first of the medical specialty boards)
1919	American Protestant Hospital Association[5]
1920	Society of Medical Administrators[6]
1926	Medical Group Management Association[7]
1929	Royal College of Physicians and Surgeons of Canada[8]
1931	Canadian Hospital Council
1933	American College of Healthcare Executives
1946	Hospital Financial Management (now the Healthcare Financial Management Association)[9]
1948	Association of University Programs in Health Administration[10]
1948	American Association of Healthcare Consultants
1951	The Joint Commission on Accreditation of Hospitals (now The Joint Commission)[11]
1956	American College of Medical Practice Executives (affiliated with the Medical Group Management Association)[12]
1957	The American Academy of Medical Administrators[13]
1961	Health Information and Management Systems Society[14]
1962	American College of Nursing Home Administrators (now the American College of Health Care Administrators)[15]
1966	Federation of American Hospitals[16]
1967	American Organization of Nurse Executives
1968	National Association of Health Services Executives[17]
1968	ACHESA (now the Commission on Accreditation of Healthcare Management Education)[18]
1970	Canadian College of Health Service Executives[19]
1978	The American College of Physician Executives (merged with the American Academy of Medical Directors on January 1, 1989)[20]
2005	National Forum for Latino Healthcare Executives
2006	Alliance for Pan Asian Healthcare Leaders (in the process of incorporating in 2007)

The ACS had three initial concerns:

1. To demonstrate to the public through fellowship designation the distinction between well-qualified surgical specialists and other physicians who perform some surgery as part of a general practice
2. To eliminate fee splitting between surgeon and referring physician
3. To improve hospital services through a program of hospital standardization

In addition to the previously mentioned concerns, ACS was also concerned with improving hospital management. According to the report of Arthur C. Bachmeyer, MD, to the American Hospital Association (AHA):

> During the meeting of the American College of Surgeons of October, 1917, ...at which time the campaign for improving the efficiency of hospitals was launched, the question of establishing a course of instruction for hospital executives was discussed. Many prominent men, both hospital administrators and surgeons, participated in the discussion. Dr. A. J. Ochsner of Chicago finally introduced a resolution which provided that a committee be appointed to report...in the fullest practical detail on the organization of a school for the training of hospital superintendents.... The resolution was unanimously adopted but the appointment of the committee was deferred [indefinitely].[21]

From its inception, ACHE had the American College of Surgeons to look to as a prototype organization. Dr. Malcolm T. MacEachern (see Chapter 1) was a bridge between both colleges.[22] In its own time, ACHE became a prototype for other organizations of health management specialists.

The first published prospectus of ACHE said the following:

> There is no field which requires the recognized specialist more than hospital administration. It is to this end that the American College of Hospital Administrators is proposed.
>
> So that hospital administration may be improved and eventually fully established and recognized as a profession, the American College of Hospital Administrators is proposed. The organization would bear a relationship to the American Hospital Association as the American College of Physicians bears to the American Medical Association.[23]

How ACHE Was Created

In September 1932, Paul H. Fesler, superintendent of the Wesley Memorial Hospital in Chicago[24] and president of the AHA, had the following to say at the AHA's Detroit convention:

It is deplorable to notice that some of the best hospitals in this country are administered by men with no experience or training in hospital administration. It seems that it would be for the benefit of our patients if a college of hospital administration could be created to train hospital executives. These trained executives would be known as fellows of hospital administration. A board of regents should be created, and admission to the college should be on a similar basis as fellowship in the American College of Surgeons. A candidate to be accepted should have at least five years' experience in a private and acceptable hospital and should be admitted by examination on the basis of a thesis. It is ridiculous to think that men without any training whatsoever are permitted to head institutions responsible for the saving of lives and representing millions of dollars. This would not be possible in any business organization.[25]

That same year, Matthew O. Foley, editor of *Hospital Management* and an advocate of improving the education and qualifications of administrators, approached J. Dewey Lutes—a prominent and skilled hospital administrator from Chicago—about creating an association of hospital administrators. "Foley and Lutes envisioned an organization which would define the qualifications of hospital administrators, recognize those who qualified by admitting them to membership, educate hospital governing boards to the need for qualified administrators, and elevate the practice of hospital administration to the status of a profession."[26] Lutes, in turn, approached Dr. MacEachern, who gave the project his immediate support.

On October 7, 1932, Lutes invited the following four Chicago administrators to lunch at the Hotel Sherman to discuss criteria for establishing an American Institute of Hospital Administrators: Maurice Dubin, superintendent, Mount Sinai Hospital; Ernest I. Erickson, superintendent, Augustana Hospital; L. C. Vonder Heidt, West Suburban Hospital; and Charles A. Wordell, St. Luke's Hospital (Wordell was unable to attend).[27]

These four administrators would ultimately become Charter Fellows of ACHE. The group agreed to create an organization of hospital administrators, where great care would be taken in the selection of members. The organization was to be nonpolitical and nonsectarian, open to men and women, and open to lay and religious administrators—if they could meet the qualifications.[28] Lutes proposed three classes of members:

1. Members
2. Senior Members (Members of three years, plus evidence of ability)
3. Fellows (open to Senior Members after three years)

There were also to be Honorary Members. Policy for the organization was to be determined by a Council of Regents, which was to be elected by the Fellows and Senior Members.

A month after the initial meeting at the Hotel Sherman, Lutes invited the group to dinner at Ravenswood Hospital. They selected 48 administrators to be invited to start the organization.[29] These administrators included 42 men from 20 states and 6 men from Canada. Twelve of the 48 men were physicians.

The ACS also selected its founding group in this same way, and this method produced a prolonged hostile reaction from many physicians who practiced some surgery and who objected to an elitist organization that would put some surgeons ahead of others.[30] However, ACHE presented no such economic threat. The institution met with very little hostility except from some physician administrators of larger Eastern hospitals who felt that ACHE was trying to preempt hospital administration for nonphysician managers.

On February 2, 1933, MacEachern, Lutes, Erickson, Wordell, and Fesler met at the Chicago office of the ACS. Responses of the 48 selected administrators were reviewed. It was decided to call a meeting to officially create the organization. Wordell was appointed chairman of the organizing committee.[31]

On February 13, 1933, 18 administrators, including MacEachern, Matthew Foley (*Hospital Management*) and John McNamara (*Modern Hospitals*), attended the meeting that created ACHE at the Palmer House Hotel in Chicago. This meeting was held during the meeting of the Council on Medical Education and Hospitals of the American Medical Association (AMA).[32]

MacEachern "gave many reasons why we should have an organization to elevate the standards of hospital administration," and a motion to form such an organization was unanimously adopted. The name of American College of Hospital Administrators was chosen by a large majority, and the slate of officers was unanimously elected (see Sidebar 3-2).

In the first annual report of the director general in 1934, J. Dewey Lutes reported that during the September 1933 meeting of ACHE in Milwaukee, 70 names were approved for Charter Fellowship and 11 for Charter Honorary Fellowship. By the date of the first anniversary of ACHE, this number had risen to 103 Charter Fellows and 17 Charter Honorary Fellows.[33] Lutes reports:

Sidebar 3-2. Slate of Officers at Founding of ACHE[34]

President	Charles A. Wordell
First Vice President	Robert E. Neff
Second Vice President	Joseph G. Norby
Director General	J. Dewey Lutes
Executive Committee	Rev. Herman Fritschel, Maurice Dubin, and John Smith

In a few instances fear was expressed that the College should have been organized by the American Hospital Association and that we would duplicate the work of that organization. In these cases, it was clearly pointed out that the American Hospital Association could not, by virtue of its own constituency, show any distinction of standards of competency for hospital administrators and that the trustees of the AHA were agreed on this point.[35]

From the very beginning, J. Dewey Lutes and the AHA Trustees saw a clear distinction between the AHA and ACHE. The AHA would seek to represent all hospital superintendents, while ACHE would work to single out more qualified superintendents for designation as Fellows, thereby raising the standards of the profession. The relationship between ACHE and the AHA was to be a close one, as was reflected by the number of Charter Fellows who became or had been presidents of the AHA[36] (see Sidebar 3-4).

Defining the Profession

To understand the role ACHE selected for itself and its relation to other professional organizations, it is useful to consider types of organizations, as well as their relationships and functions. Within the healthcare field, there are basically five general types of organizations for each profession:

1. An inclusive organization open to all, often called an "association"
2. An exclusive organization whose fellowship is open to the qualified elite, usually called a "college"
3. A hybrid of the first two
4. An association for educators in the profession
5. A specialized organization for professionals with focused interests

In medicine, the inclusive organization welcoming all physicians is the AMA. The exclusive organizations are primarily the specialty colleges. The organization of medical educators is the Association of American Medical Colleges. Specialized organizations abound.

Sidebar 3-4. On a Personnel Note

Of the 120 Charter and Honorary Charter Fellows of ACHE, 17 became Chairman Officers (formerly called Presidents) of ACHE and 15 became chairmen of the AHA. Eight were all three. Frank J. Walter was the last ACHE Chairman to be all three. Seven additional people, although not Charter Fellows, have been chairmen of both ACHE and AHA[38]:

1. James A. Hamilton
2. Frank Bradley
3. Frank Groner
4. Ray Brown

5. Tol Terrell
6. D. Kirk Oglesby Jr.
7. Larry L. Mathis

The table below lists administrators who were Charter Fellows, Chairman Officers of ACHE, and/or chairmen of AHA and the Association of University Programs in Health Administration (AUPHA) and their dates of office.[39]

Name	Charter Fellow (CF), Honorary Charter Fellow (HCF), or Fellow (F)	ACHE Chairman (Date)	AHA Chairman (Date)	AUPHA Chairman (Date)
Charles Wordell	CF	1933–34		
Robert Neff	CF	1934–35	1938	
Fred Carter, MD*	CF	1935–36	1940	
Basil MacLean, MD*	CF	1936–37	1942	
Howard Bishop	CF	1937–38		
Robin Buerki, MD*	CF	1938–39	1936	
James A. Hamilton	F	1939–40	1943	1951–53
Arthur C. Bachmeyer, MD*	CF	1940–41	1926	1948–49
Lucias R. Wilson, MD*	CF	1941–42		
Joseph G. Norby	CF	1942–43	1949	
Claude W. Munger, MD*	CF	1944–46	1937	
Frank R. Bradley, MD*	F	1946–47	1955	1954–55
Jessie Turnbull	CF	1948–49		
Frank J. Walter	CF	1950–51	1944	
Ernest Erikson	CF	1951–52		
Merrill Steele, MD	CF	1954–55		
J. Dewey Lutes	CF	1955–56		
Arthur Swanson	CF	1956–57		
Frank S. Groner	F	1957–58	1961	
Ray Brown	F	1959–60	1956	1966–67
Melvin Sutley	CF	1960–61		
Tol Terrell	F	1961–62	1958	
Thomas Howell, MD	HCF		1914	
Asa Bacon	CF		1923	
Malcolm MacEachern, MD	HCF		1924	1949–50
G. Harvey Agnew, MD	HCF		1939	1953–54
B. W. Black, MD*	CF		1941	
Donald C. Smeltzer, MD*	CF		1945	
Peter D. Ward, MD*	CF		1946	
D. Kirk Oglesby	F	1986–87	1992	
James O. Hepner, PhD	F	1990–91		1975–76
Larry L. Mathis	F	1997–98	1993	

*Members of the Society of Medical Administrators

In hospital management, the inclusive organization is the AHA. The hybrid (or mixture of the inclusive and exclusive organization) is ACHE, which reaches beyond hospitals. The relevant association of educators is the Association of University Programs in Health Administration (AUPHA) (see Chapter 5). A number of specialty national health organizations exist; some of these are inclusive, others are exclusive, and some may be a mixture of the two.

Sidebar 3-5. Remembering the Charter Fellows

Following are some insights from John R. Mannix, a Charter Fellow of ACHE, regarding the personalities and histories of a few of the other Charter Fellows:

- George O'Hanlon, MD, of the New Jersey Medical Center in Jersey City, was loyal to Mayor Hague, who ran that city the way Richard J. Daley ran Chicago.
- Bryce Twitty, a devout Methodist, was at Baylor University Hospital when Justin Ford Kimball started prepayment there for teachers, thus precipitating Blue Cross.
- Melvin Sutley was a lawyer who taught commercial law in Japan before becoming an administrator. Most of his administrative career was at Delaware County Hospital in Drexel Hill, Pennsylvania.
- Joe Norby was administrator of the Fairview Hospital in Minneapolis. His son, Morris Norby, was associated with Blue Cross of Pittsburgh and was given the Justin Kimball Award.
- Basil MacLean, MD, was Canadian and served with the Touro Infirmary in New Orleans. Later, he became president of the National Blue Cross Association prior to Jeb Stuart, who preceded Walter McNerney.
- Arthur C. Bachmeyer was a dean and a great administrator of this century. As the father of Bob Bachmeyer, he helped form the only father and son pair who would both be Presidents of ACHE.
- E. M. Bluestone (he never used anything but "E. M.") was administrator of Montefiore Hospital in New York and trained by Dr. S. S. Goldwater. He was one of the first people interested in geriatrics.
- Albert G. Hahn, administrator of Deaconess Hospital in Evansville, Indiana, was the only blind man in the founding group. His wife, Grace, was always with him. Mannix never saw them apart and met Hahn several times before he realized he was blind. ACHE made Grace an Honorary Charter Fellow in 1953.
- Mannix remembered Asa Bacon as always remaining young at heart. "I always came away with a great deal of sound advice from him," said Mannix.
- Bob Jolly, a Texan from Houston, was a close friend of MacEachern.
- Jessie Turnbull was a nurse and a real leader of the Hospital Association of Pennsylvania.

Eighteen of the founders were Canadian, including A. J. Swanson, Muriel Anscombe, Peter Ward, George F. Stephen, and Donald Smeltzer, MD. "All of the 103 Charter Fellows were outstanding leaders," Mannix noted.[40] The last living Charter Fellow, Robin Buerki, MD, died in 1991, bringing the founding era to a close. For a complete list of Charter Fellows, see Appendix 3.

Inclusive professional organizations tend to develop a stable central leadership, reflecting the senior, elite members of the occupation. For example, with the AMA this is accomplished through the leadership of state constituencies that make up the national house of delegates. In medicine, specialization and elite organizations are combined in the specialty colleges like the ACS. In hospital administration, the hybrid organization—ACHE—came before managerial specialization. Professional educators have sufficiently distinct interests, so they created their own organizations: the Association of American Medical Colleges for physicians and the AUPHA for health administration educators. However, the practitioner organizations have a continuing interest in education and do not leave these concerns solely to the educators. There is a partial overlap between these educational and practitioner organizations.

> **Sidebar 3-6. On a Personnel Note**
>
> Of the early administrators, many held major academic positions in health administration programs during their careers:
>
> - James A. Hamilton (Minnesota)
> - Arthur Bachmeyer, MD (Chicago)
> - Ray E. Brown (Chicago, Duke, Northwestern)
> - Frank Bradley, MD (Washington University, St. Louis)
> - G. Harvey Agnew, MD (Toronto)
> - Malcolm MacEachern, MD (Northwestern)
>
> More recently, Everett Johnson, PhD (ACHE Chairman 1971–1972), and James Hepner, PhD, have directed health administration degree programs. Hepner was president of the AUPHA from 1975 to 1976 and Chairman of ACHE from 1990 to 1991.

Overwhelmingly, the field of healthcare management is defined by organizational position rather than by licensure. In the field of medicine, becoming a generalist precedes specialization. In health administration, specialization often occurs before promotion to a generalist position.

Creating a Code of Ethics

While the opportunity to renew old acquaintances, make new ones, and talk with like-minded peers is an important part of a professional society, professional societies should also be concerned with the ethical conduct of their profession.

Unlike the professions of medicine, law, dentistry, and nursing, no code of ethics exists for managers in general, and unlike graduates of medical schools who traditionally have risen to take the Hippocratic oath or its equivalent when receiving their degrees, graduates of business schools initiate their careers unrestrained by such professional standards.[41]

However, from its earliest days ACHE maintained its concern for a code of ethics for hospital administration. As early as 1934, it was noted that:

In the Fellowship Pledge of the American College of Hospital Administrators this sentiment stands out in bold relief: "Especially do I pledge myself to honest administration within my own hospital, to consider ever primary to my own welfare that of my institution." The Fellows of the College in faithfully keeping this their pledge, will make an immense contribution to hospital administration not only in their own institutions but, by their precept and example, to every hospital on this continent.[42]

In 1938, ACHE's Executive Committee appointed a special committee, chaired by Dr. G. Harvey Agnew, secretary-treasurer of the Canadian Hospital Council in Toronto, to develop a code of ethics. "The drafting proved to be long and painful."[43] "After the ACHE committee had struggled with the code for some time, it was decided that an administrator's code could not logically be separated from a code applying to all hospital workers, so a joint ACHA and AHA Committee was established," said Dr. Agnew.

Since the subject matter was ethics, the views of the various religious hospital associations were considered, and care was taken to see that major religions had influential members on the drafting committee. Initially, soliciting the views of some of the religious hospital associations was problematic because of ACHE's membership requirement that an administrator/affiliate's hospital be approved by the ACS (the forerunner of approval by The Joint Commission) and be registered with the AHA. This resulted in a controversy with the Catholic Hospital Association (CHA), because Catholic hospitals were "registered" with the CHA rather than the AHA. Rev. M. F. Griffin, vice president of the CHA, wrote to ACHE President Arthur Bachmeyer that he could not serve on the Code of Ethics Committee "because of the strained relations between our organizations due to the refusal of your board to recognize the Catholic Hospital Association." The problem was aggravated by the fact that sisters constituted a large percentage of the potential ACHE membership. ACHE revised its position and deleted the ACS and AHA requirements for candidates for admission. By 1942, sisters were 13 percent of Fellows; 29 percent of Members; and 20 percent of Associate Members. Rev. Griffin was included as a member of the Joint Committee.[44]

In June 1941, the *Code of Ethics* received final approval by both ACHE and AHA and was published, further developing the profession of hospital administration.[45]

The Evolution of the Code of Ethics

Throughout the years, the *Code of Ethics* has undergone several revisions (see Figure 3-1). As the healthcare field has changed, the *Code* has changed along with it. In the early days, the basic *Code* was summarized as: "If you can stand to have that story printed on the front page of your local paper, it's probably

1938	ACHE Executive Committee appoints a special committee chaired by Dr. G. Harvey Agnew to develop a code of ethics
1939	The Joint ACHE–AHA Committee established to develop a code of ethics
1941	*Code of Ethics* approved by both the AHA and ACHE; published by the AHA
1942	*Code of Ethics* published in ACHA *News*
1947	Joint Committee revises *Code of Ethics*; approved by AHA and ACHE
1956	New Joint Committee appointed by Dr. A. P. Merrill, chairman
1957	Revised *Code of Ethics* accepted by both organizations
1958	Revised *Code of Ethics* published
1963	New Joint Committee, chaired by Jack A. L. Hahn, revises the *Code of Ethics*; approved in June by ACHE and in November by the AHA Trustees
1964	New *Code of Ethics* published
1970	ACHE publishes its own code; adopted September 14
1973	Special Committee on Ethics of ACHE revises the *Code of Ethics*; approved by the Council of Regents on August 20
1974	The Board of Trustees of the AHA accepts its "Guidelines on Ethical Conduct and Relationships for Health Care Institutions"
1980	ACHE republishes its 1973 *Code of Ethics* and the 1974 AHA Guidelines; the AHA revises and updates its Guidelines
1985	ACHE develops Public Policy Statement on Ethics
1987	New *Code of Ethics* published; review of Grievance Procedure
1987	AHA Guidelines on Ethical Conduct for Health Care Institutions approved
1991	First Ethical Policy Statement, "Impaired Health Care Executive"
1992	Second Ethical Policy Statement, "Responsibility to Employees"
1992	*Code of Ethics* revised, as amended by the Council of Regents on July 28
1995	*Code of Ethics* revised
2000	*Code of Ethics* revised
2001	*Code of Ethics* revised
2003	*Code of Ethics* revised
2007	*Code of Ethics* revised

FIGURE 3-1
The *Code of Ethics* Chronology[46]

OK." At that time, unethical behavior included personal aggrandizement, proselytizing employees of other neighborhood hospitals, and actively seeking to displace a colleague. Teas or open houses for nurses of other hospitals as a recruitment technique were considered unethical. Administrators were criticized if they used the shotgun approach to send out large numbers of résumés.

In 1967, the AHA and ACHE codes separated. One reason for this was the unwillingness of the AHA to adjudicate ethics violations. ACHE went on to develop and publish a definitive grievance procedure.

ACHE again revised the *Code* in 1973; that version remained in effect through 1983. The 1973 *Code of Ethics* for ACHE focused specifically on the administrator: "Health services administration must meet two primary accountabilities—one as a member of ACHE, and the other in activities performed as an institutional executive."

In 1983, the ACHE Ethics Committee focused on much more critical ethical violations than nurse recruitment teas; they focused on violations such as kickbacks, theft, sexual harassment, and misappropriation of funds. This is not to imply that the ethics of hospital executives had deteriorated but that times had changed. Gone were the days, for example, when the trustees of one hospital took home five percent of hospital revenues, or when an executive in another city kept a 45-caliber revolver in his desk drawer.[47]

The 1992 *Code* allowed both cooperation and competition. It referred to "consumers" and was explicit about avoiding discrimination. The 1992 *Code* did not mention specifically the governing board or medical staff.

In 2003, a task force carefully examined the *Code* and recommended changes. The task force met with the Ethics Committee, conducted an affiliate survey on issues and use of the *Code*, analyzed and discussed the results of this survey, and used the resulting data to update the *Code*.

The primary intent of the changes was to underscore the ethical responsibilities of healthcare executives in their various roles with patients, employees, organizations, the community, and society. The importance of implementing an organizational code of ethics was articulated. Responsibilities were also added to ensure the existence of a process to resolve conflicts when the values of patients and families differ from those of employees and physicians.

Additional formatting changes served to separate the administrative aspects of grievances and the responsibilities of the Ethics Committee from the *Code*.

Since then, several other changes have been made to both the *Code* and the grievance procedures. The *Code* was changed to provide greater clarity about its scope within the area of professional activity and practice. Language was added to articulate what is more likely to be within the control of healthcare executives as they carry out their responsibilities. The most recent revision of the *Code* was approved by the Board of Governors in March 2007 and can be found in Appendix 1. At the same time, the Board approved changes to the grievance procedures. These changes serve to better align the grievance process with the current procedure for conducting investigations and provide respondents the opportunity for a hearing earlier in the process.

In addition, ACHE has developed several practical resources to help healthcare executives address ethical issues in the workplace. This has been in response to affiliates' requests that the organization do more to help with the practical side of ethics. ACHE uses a tool-kit approach to providing ethics resources and houses this tool kit on its web site. Following are some of the resources included in the tool kit:

1. An article from *Healthcare Executive* magazine that outlines the following multistep process for ethical decision making:
   * Step 1: Clarify the ethical conflict
   * Step 2: Identify all of the affected stakeholders and their values
   * Step 3: Understand the circumstances surrounding the ethical conflict
   * Step 4: Identify the ethical perspectives relevant to the conflict
   * Step 5: Identify different options for action
   * Step 6: Select among the options
   * Step 7: Share and implement the decision
   * Step 8: Review the decision to ensure it achieved the desired goal
2. An explanation of the history and purpose of the *Code of Ethics* and how it can be used in practical, every-day situations
3. Strategies for applying ACHE's specific policy statements, such as "Decisions Near the End of Life" or "Ethical Issues Related to Staff Shortages," to organizational decisions and policy development
4. Tips for getting the most out of an ethics self-audit, and how to address potential red flags that may be identified in the process

> **Sidebar 3-9. On a Personnel Note**
>
> Members of the 2002–2003 *Code of Ethics* task force included the following:
>
> * William A. Nelson, PhD (chair)
> * Paul Hofmann, DrPH, FACHE
> * Diane Howard, PhD, FACHE
> * Mark Howard, FACHE
> * CDR Patrick Malone, PhD, FACHE
> * Karen Hackett, FACHE, staff liaison

FIGURE 3-2. Active Affiliates of ACHE*

ACHE Status	1932	1937	1942	1947	1952
Fellow	34	188	301	268	386
Diplomate	0	198	577	867	1,325
Member	0	33	269	619	1,128
Subtotal	34	419	1,147	1,754	2,839
Students	0	0	0	0	0
Total	34	419	1,147	1,754	2,839

ACHE Status	1957	1962	1967	1972	1977
Fellow	681	1,134	1,388	1,601	1,519
Diplomate	1,852	2,458	2,980	3,758	4,682
Member	1,291	2,067	1,749	2,739	2,730
Subtotal	3,824	5,659	6,117	8,098	8,931
Students	0	0	480	778	2,254
Total	3,824	5,659	6,597	8,876	11,185

Continued

ACHE Status	1982*	1987*	1992*	1997	2002	2007
Fellow	1,654	1,899	2,343	2,877	3,107	5,461
Diplomate	5,781	7,206	7,240	7,188	5,762	
Member	5,395	6,396	9,291	11,690	14,195	23,341
Subtotal— Dues Paying	**12,830**	**15,501**	**18,874**	**21,755**	**23,064**	**28,802**
Students	3,201	4,297	5,460	5,913	3,213	3,306
Faculty		59	207	247	236	254
Candidate for Associate				236		
International				30	49	112
Retired				80	190	301
Life Diplomate	979	1,184	1,489	629	629	
Life Fellow				1,101	1,170	2,050
Honorary Fellow				61	57	30
Subtotal— Non-Dues Paying	**4,180**	**5,540**	**7,156**	**8,297**	**5,544**	**6,053**
Overall Total	**17,010**	**21,041**	**26,030**	**30,052**	**28,608**	**34,855**

*Note that in 1982, 1987, and 1997, the number in the Life Diplomate row represents the total number of Retired Affiliates, Life Diplomates, Life Fellows, and Honorary Fellows.

5. An article that offers strategies senior leaders can use to enhance their ethical awareness and make better ethical decisions
6. A list of books, magazine and journal articles, periodicals, and web sites that can provide additional ethics guidance

The Growth of ACHE

By 1957, ACHE had 3,824 affiliates (see Figure 3-2). ACHE began to publish the journal *Hospital Administration* in 1956, and the 25th anniversary of ACHE in 1958 saw the start of ACHE's annual Congress on Administration. (More information on these programs can be found in Chapters 5 and 6.)

As discussed in Chapters 1 and 2, a growing complexity in the healthcare environment followed this time period, yielding health maintenance organizations, neighborhood health centers, health planning agencies, nursing homes, and increasing government involvement in the regulation of health services. As a result, a higher proportion of ACHE members than ever before were managing health organizations other than hospitals.

In 1980 to 1981 ACHE developed "programmatic thrusts" (see Figure 3-3) as a guide to planning and future development. These became the blueprint for ACHE development in the 1980s. According to Stuart A. Wesbury Jr., PhD, president of ACHE at the time, they were based on "thoughts floating around."[50] The largest activity, according to Wesbury, was the self-assessment project, which allowed affiliates to assess their own skills and compare their performance to their peers. More information on the self-assessment project can be found in Chapter 4.

ACHE was also reorganized during this time. In 1980, ACHE was a 501(c)3 nonprofit organization. This type of organization does not allow for political involvement or public policy advocacy. ACHE was transformed into two corporations:

1. the Foundation of ACHE, classified as a 501(c)3; and
2. ACHE itself, which is a 501(c)6 organization.

The latter can include unrelated business income from a for-profit subsidiary, which in the case of ACHE was called Professional Society Services Incorporated (PSSI). PSSI in turn held Career Decision, Inc. (see Chapter 7). The Foundation included Health Administration Press (see Chapter 6) as well as the Division of Education (see Chapter 5).

In 1981, a proposal was put forward to change ACHE's name from the American College of Hospital Administrators to one that reflected the diversity of the executives the association served. The proposed change required a two-thirds vote of the Regents and won only 102 of 178 Regents'

FIGURE 3-3
Programmatic
Thrusts,
1980–1981

According to the 1985–1986 Annual Report, programmatic thrusts, which were later incorporated into the Strategic Plans, consisted of specific projects classified into seven special areas and designed to help affiliates in their continual challenge to enhance their administrative performance and improve their managerial competence.

A. Professional Development (Lifelong Learning)
    1. Self-Assessment (Diagnosis/Treatment)
    2. Beginning and Early Career Development
    3. Governing Body Relationships
    4. ACHE Publications and Tapes
    5. New Educational Approaches
B. Credentialing
C. Recredentialing
D. Research
E. Public Policy
F. Academic Relationships
G. Professional Organization Relationships

votes (17 short). Former Chairman Henry X. Jackson said at the time that the new name would make the ACHA the "American College of Almost Anything."[51] Another four years passed before a name change was approved.

In 1983, ACHE's 50th year, membership was at a record 17,405 affiliates, reflecting both the size of the healthcare field, which then consumed about 10 percent of the gross national product, and the continuing value of ACHE to the profession of hospital and health services administration.

When ACHE did change its name from the American College of Hospital Administrators to the American College of Healthcare Executives (effective July 29, 1985), the name reflected the change of focus to healthcare systems, where ACHE members held positions in many different organizations, and the hospital became a part of a continuum of care. Stuart A. Wesbury Jr., PhD, said, "we like to think that we made 'healthcare' one word.... Others followed our example."

By 1990, systems thinking and continuous quality improvement/total quality management brought a new vision for healthcare as reflected in The Joint Commission's "new initiative" for accreditation, ACHE's 1990 Standards of Excellence for Staff (see Figure 3-4), and the start of ACHE's own internal continuous quality improvement effort in 1992.

The Modern Era

As mentioned in Chapter 2, ACHE has become even more diverse since 1992. Members come from a greater variety of healthcare settings, including

Service:	We are committed to exceeding the expectations of our affiliates and our coworkers in a helpful and courteous manner.
Quality:	We do things right the first time.
Integrity:	We can be trusted to perform our jobs with honesty, sincerity, and respect for others.
Timeliness:	We promptly respond to affiliates because they are our highest priority; we need to meet or exceed all deadlines and help our coworkers to do the same.
Reliability:	We can be trusted to do what we say we are going to do and to follow through on tasks to successful completion.
Teamwork:	We work harmoniously with others to get the job done.
Competitiveness:	We do not stand alone in the marketplace—healthcare executives have other organizations to which they can turn for professional services. Therefore, we must always be responsive to our affiliates' needs.
Professionalism:	We consistently demonstrate behavior that is worth emulating and reflects well on the organization.
Fiscal responsibility:	We use our resources wisely and efficiently to achieve our goals.
Staff development:	We constantly work to enhance our knowledge and skills.

hospitals, group practices, managed care organizations, post acute and chronic care organizations, consulting organizations, higher education, and research organizations. ACHE is not just for executive-level leaders anymore, but has members at all stages of their career from student through early careerist, mid-careerist, and chief executive officer. The educational background of members is also diversifying, with more physicians, nurses, and individuals with advanced business degrees seeking membership.

As previously mentioned, the average age of an ACHE member is increasing, as the U.S. population as a whole is aging. Women are playing an increasing role in ACHE, as the percentage of woman affiliates has increased from 23 percent in 1990 to 40 percent in 2007. Minority representation in ACHE is also increasing as more and more African American, Latino, and Asian healthcare executives are joining ACHE. For example, in 1992, 5 percent of ACHE's affiliates were persons of color; by 2004, persons of color constituted 10 percent of the affiliate body. (More information on diversity and the role of minorities in ACHE can be found in Chapter 7.)

One of the main reasons for this increased diversification is an effort on the part of ACHE to be more accessible and inclusive. Through programs and initiatives such as the forming of local chapters (see Chapter 4), the launching of a comprehensive Web presence (see Chapter 7), strong career development support (see Chapter 7), and the elimination of the mandatory membership testing requirement (see Chapter 4), ACHE has worked diligently to provide opportunities for individuals with an interest in healthcare management to take part in the organization. Chapters 4 through 7 explore each of these programs and initiatives, as well as many others that ACHE has pursued throughout the years.

Endnotes

1.   Carter, F. G., "Award of Merit." *Hospitals*, Vol. 26, July 1936, p. 67, based on ACHE's Articles of Incorporation, March 26, 1934.

2.   Reader, W. J. *Professional Men*. London: Weidenfeld and Nicolson, 1966.

3.   Caldwell, B. W., "American Hospital Association," in *American and Canadian Hospitals*. 2nd ed. Chicago: Physicians Record Company, 1937, pp. 11–35. The AHA was founded in 1899, but the AHA symbol shows 1898. This is not correct, but the AHA has found it too expensive to change its symbol. Quoting from a letter from John Sullivan of the AHA to John R. Mannix dated October 1, 1979: "You are right of course. The founding date [of the AHA] is 1899 no doubt. The error was made half a century ago or however long ago the seal was designed. The story I have heard is that the individual designing the seal assumed that the first annual meeting occurred at the end of the first year. In any event, because the seal has been registered as a service mark for over 30 years, no one wants to correct the error. I think, too, it would be more confusing to the field than living with the error."

4.   Shanahan, R. J. *The History of the Catholic Hospital Association 1915–1965*. St. Louis, MO: The Catholic Hospital Association of the United States and Canada, 1963.

5.   *American and Canadian Hospitals*. 2nd ed. Chicago: Physicians Record Company, 1937.

6.   Society of Medical Administrators. *A History of the Society of Medical Administrators and the Medical Superintendents Club*. Society of Medical Administrators, 1920–1955, 1956–1966, 1967. This society of physician administrators met once or twice a year from its precursor in 1909 through 1966 and beyond. Up to 1966, it only had about 120 members. However, out of this group, 38 members became presidents of the AHA between 1907 and 1969, and 13 became Chairman Officers of ACHE. M. Brown, personal communication, Apr. 8, 1983. According to several people interviewed for this history, some of the members of this Society opposed the founding of ACHE, saying "the politics" were "dirty." The members of this Society were all physicians and administrators of general hospitals, typically on the East Coast. Malcolm MacEachern was not a member. "There was intrigue and warfare between MacEachern and Bachmeyer," Lewis Weeks's

interview of Gerhard Hartman, p. 10. Bachmeyer was a leading light of the Society of Medical Administrators.

7.   Medical Group Management Association, "Dedicated to Improving Medical Group Practice." Denver, CO: The Association, 1982. Stevens, E. B. *The History of the Medical Group Management Association 1926–1976.* Denver, CO: The Association, 1976. *Encyclopedia of Associations,* 1988, p. 1193.

8.   Soderstrom, L. *The Canadian Health System.* London: Croom Helm, 1978.

9.   "Healthcare Financial Management Association," *Encyclopedia of Associations,* 1988, p. 1192.

10.   Hartman, G., et al., "The Impact of Graduate Programs in *Hospital Administration.*" *Hospital Administration,* Vol. 7, Spring 1962.

11.   Joint Commission web site. [Online information; retrieved 1/15/07.] www.jointcommission.org

12.   American College of Medical Group Administrators, "So Now You're a Nominee." Denver, CO: The College, May 1981; American College of Medical Group Administrators, "Admission Advancement Criteria." Denver, CO: The College, Jan 1982; Graham, F. E., and R. J. Wright, "The American College of Medical Group Administrators: Twenty-Five Years in Brief Perspective." *Medical Group Management,* Sept.-Oct. 1981; *Encyclopedia of Associations,* 1988, p. 1192.

13.   "American Academy of Medical Administrators," *The AAMA Medical Administrative Executive,* Southfield, MI: The Academy, Vol. 19, No. 6, Aug. 1982; *Encyclopedia of Associations,* 1988, p. 1191.

14.   Health Information and Management Systems Society (HIMSS) web site. [Online information; retrieved 1/15/07.] www.himss.org

15.   Becker, C. A. *History and Handbook of the American College of Nursing Home Administrators.* ACNHA, 1982. AUPHA, 1989, pp. 331–332

16.   American Federation of Hospitals web site. [Online information; retrieved 1/15/07.] www.fahs.com

17.   See Bellin, L., and L. Weeks. *The Challenge of Administering Health Services: Career Pathways.* Washington, DC: AUPHA Press, 1981. AUPHA, 1989, p. 336.

18.   Commission on Accreditation of Healthcare Management Education web site. [Online information; retrieved 5/7/07.] www.cahme.org

19.   Canadian College of Health Service Executives, Toronto, Ontario, Canada, Feb. 1975. AUPHA, 1989, p. 334.

20.   S. Wesbury interview, Jan. 1983; *Encyclopedia of Associations,* 1988, p. 1192.

21.   Bachmeyer, A. C., "A Course in Hospital Administration." *Transitions of the American Hospital Association,* Vol. 21, 1919, pp. 279–280.

22.   J. R. Mannix interview, 1982; J. D. Lutes interview, 1982.

23.   "American College of Hospital Administrators," 1933. Signed by J. Dewey Lutes, Robert E. Neff, Joseph A. Norby, and Charles A. Wordell, "provisional committee," p. 3. Also see Lutes, J. D., "Why the College of Hospital Administrators?" *Hospital Management,* Nov. 1933.

24. Paul Fesler was formerly superintendent of the University of Minnesota Hospitals. He started Dean Conley and Ray Amberg in their careers in hospital administration, and Amberg replaced him at Minnesota. D. Conley interview, Apr. 1983.

25. ACHA *Minute Book*, Vol. 1, Oct. 7, 1932.

26. Kipnis, I. A. *A Venture Forward: A History of the American College of Hospital Administrators.* Chicago: ACHA, 1955, p. 9–10

27. ACHA *Minute Book*, Vol. 1, Oct. 7, 1932.

28. Ibid.

29. Kipnis, I. A. *A Venture Forward: A History of the American College of Hospital Administrators.* Chicago: ACHA, 1955, p. 12.

30. Davis, L. *Fellowship of Surgeons.* Springfield, IL: Charles C. Thomas, 1960.

31. Kipnis, I. A. *A Venture Forward: A History of the American College of Hospital Administrators.* Chicago: ACHA, 1955, p. 12.

32. Lutes, J. D., "To the Members of the Board of Regents," First Annual Report of the Director-General of the ACHA, in ACHA *Minute Book*, Vol. 1, 1934.

33. Lutes (1934) includes 100 Charter Fellows and 16 Charter Honorary Fellows in his report. However, he was probably not counting exactly. According to John R. Mannix, 114 administrators were elected to become active Charter Fellows. Of these, 102 accepted (32 of these were physicians) and 12 declined (of these, nine were physicians). Of the nine physicians who declined, six were later made Honorary Members: Drs. Christopher Parnall, William H. Walsh, John M. Peters, S. S. Goldwater, Frederic Washburn, and Winford Smith. Of the three lay administrators who declined, two later joined. Mrs. Albert C. Hahn was made an Honorary Charter Fellow retroactively.

34. ACHA *Minute Book*, Vol. 1, Feb. 13, 1933.

35. Lutes, J. D., "To the Members of the Board of Regents," First Annual Report of the Director-General of the ACHA, in ACHA Minute Book, Vol. 1, 1934.

36. In 1943 and 1944, there was serious consideration of merging ACHE into the AHA. A joint commission developed recommendations for merger, but they were rejected by ACHE Regents in February 1944, who voted for a continued independent existence. An agreement was made that ACHE would be concerned with continuing education for administrators and the AHA for departmental groups in the hospital. Kipnis, I. A. *A Venture Forward: A History of the American College of Hospital Administrators.* Chicago: ACHA, 1955, pp. 83–87.

37. Lutes, J. D., "To the Members of the Board of Regents," First Annual Report of the Director-General of the ACHA, in ACHA Minute Book, Vol. 1, 1934.

38. "Among the past Chairmen of the American Hospital Association, it would appear that obtaining ACHA Fellowship is almost a prerequisite to assuming this leadership role," Wesbury, S. A., "Background Information Concerning the Proposal to Change the Name and Objects of the American College of

Hospital Administrators," ACHA, April 1981, p. 6. In recent years, to become president of the AHA (like the AMA for physicians) has required years of active work at the state level, which makes becoming head of both organizations very difficult. Further, the growth in the number of hospital administrators has increased the pool of people from which to draw leadership (S. A. Wesbury interview, 1983).

39.   Sources: American Hospital Association. *Guide to the Health Care Field.* Chicago: AHA, 1982, p. B4; Kipnis, I. A. *A Venture Forward: A History of the American College of Hospital Administrators.* Chicago: ACHA, 1955; ACHA, 1981, 1992 Directory; AUPHA, "AUPHA 1948–1973: Twenty-Fifth Anniversary Dinner." AUPHA Library, 1973; Society of Medical Administrators. *A History of the Society of Medical Administrators and the Medical Superintendents Club.* Society of Medical Administrators, 1967, p. 73. Other members of the Society of Medical Administrators who became Chairman Officers of ACHE were Robert H. Bishop, MD, 1943–1944; Wilmar M. Allen, MD, 1949–1950; Fraser D. Mooney, MD, 1952–1953; Albert C. Kerlikowski, MD, 1954–1955; and Frank C. Sutton, MD, 1962–1963. M. Brown, MD, personal communication, Apr. 8, 1983.

40.   J. R. Mannix interview, Oct. 1982.

41.   Friedlander, W. J., "Oaths Given by U.S. and Canadian Medical Schools, 1977: Profession of Medical Values." *Social Science and Medicine*, Vol. 16, 1982.

42.   *Bulletin of the American College of Hospital Administrators*, Vol. 1, No. 1, 1934–1935, quoting B. W. Caldwell, MD, executive secretary of the AHA.

43.   Kipnis, I. A. *A Venture Forward: A History of the American College of Hospital Administrators.* Chicago: ACHA, 1955, p. 53.

44.   Ibid., pp. 65–66.

45.   Ibid., pp. 53–54.

46.   Sources: Kipnis, I. A. *A Venture Forward: A History of the American College of Hospital Administrators.* Chicago: ACHA, 1955, pp. 53, 65–66; AHA and ACHA. *Code of Hospital Ethics Approved and Adopted by the American Hospital Association and the American College of Hospital Administrators.* Nov. 21, 1941, revisions 1947, 1958, 1964; ACHA. *Code of Ethics.* 1970, revisions 1973, 1980, 1987, 1992; AHA. *Ethical Conduct for Health Care Institutions.* Chicago: AHA, 1981.

47.   J. Mannix personal communication, 1982.

48.   AHA and ACHA. *Code of Hospital Ethics Approved and Adopted by the American Hospital Association and the American College of Hospital Administrators.* Nov. 21, 1941. AHA. *Ethical Conduct and Relationships for Health Care Institutions.* Chicago: AHA, 1981.

49.   "AHA, ACHA Approve Revised Ethical Codes," *Hospitals JAHA*, Vol. 31, Oct. 16, 1957, pp. 124, 126, 127.

50.   S. Wesbury interview, Dec. 29, 1992. Much of what follows in this chapter comes from this interview.

51.   "Regents Rebel, Veto Name Change Proposal." *Modern Healthcare*, Oct. 1981, pp. 77, 78.

52.   In 1989, ACHE established an award honoring the memory of Alton E. Pickert, Chairman in 1983 to 1984. Each year the Pickert Award recognizes employees who have demonstrated significant service.

.

THE FUNCTIONS OF ACHE: MEMBERSHIP AND CREDENTIALING

Undoubtedly the American College of Hospital Administrators, by its empha-sis upon higher standards for administrators, will be of inestimable assis-tance in elevating the status of this field and already it has had a very appre-ciable effect.

G. Harvey Agnew, MD, 1939 Honorary Charter Fellow, ACHA[1]

An important function of any professional society is to define its boundaries. For some organizations, licensure or certification makes these boundaries rel-atively easy to define. However, as mentioned in previous chapters, entry into the field of healthcare administration is not governed by state licensure; instead, a voluntary credentialing program established by the American Col-lege of Healthcare Executives (ACHE) is one way to ensure competence. To elevate the standard of hospital administration, ACHE had to establish early on a standard of competency for hospital executives that would be reflected in the qualifications for both Membership and Fellowship in ACHE[2] and that would change with time.

This chapter discusses the standards of competency initially created and how they have changed throughout the years. It discusses both the cer-tification and recertification processes. As with other chapters in the book, this chapter follows a timeline through the history of ACHE, offering per-spectives on how the various time periods affected ACHE's position on membership and credentialing.

In the Beginning

The first qualification for membership in ACHE was the personal selection of J. Dewey Lutes and the gentlemen discussed in Chapter 3 who helped create ACHE: Maurice Dubin of Mount Sinai, Ernest Erickson of Augustana, and Charles A. Wordell of St. Luke's.[3]

At the Chicago meeting on February 13, 1933, Maurice Dubin out-lined a constitution and bylaws providing for three classes of membership: Member, Fellow, and Honorary Fellow.[4] On February 14, 1933, the offi-cers were authorized to develop temporary standards for membership.[5] The standards were designed to be based on professional evaluation, distinct from simple economic measures such as employment and salary, and distinct from the predilections of trustees who, in 1933, had to be educated as to the need for professionally qualified administrators.

In Milwaukee on September 10, 1933, in conjunction with the annual American Hospital Association (AHA) meeting, a secret Credentials Committee of five was appointed to propose names for ACHE membership. The anonymous chairman of this committee was Malcolm MacEachern.[6] "No other individual knew so many administrators personally, nor was acquainted with the actual administrative conditions of so many hospitals."[7] As mentioned in Chapter 3, the Credentials Committee approved 70 names for Charter Fellowship and 11 for Charter Honorary Fellowship. In February 1934, an additional 44 names were approved for admission as Charter Fellows and four for Charter Honorary Membership.[8] As Ira Kipnis notes in his 1955 history of ACHE, membership classifications were a bit confusing in those days.[9]

This early membership and credentialing effort created the Charter Fellows and Charter Honorary Fellows (see Appendix 3 for a list of Charter and Charter Honorary Fellows). In the second year, the first Members were elected along with other administrators who were appointed directly to Fellowship[10] and Honorary Fellowship.

The Criteria for Membership and Fellowship

Because of the tradition of the American College of Surgeons, as discussed in Chapter 3, ACHE was able to reach consensus on the criteria for Fellowship within the first two years of its existence. The criteria were based on the following categories.

Position   At the September 23, 1934, meeting of the Board of Regents, the general feeling was that membership should be limited to active hospital administrators. ACHE decided to admit associate administrators and assistant administrators, but not specialized department heads. It was also proposed that eligibility for admission be expanded from "administrators" to those "whose major interest lies in hospital administration." This proposal was defeated. Another proposal to make executive secretaries of hospital associations eligible was similarly voted down. It was felt that individuals who were active in the healthcare field, whose work merited recognition by ACHE, but who were not hospital administrators would be eligible to election as Honorary Fellows.[11] Through 1941, administrators of hospitals with less than 25 beds were also not considered eligible for membership. From the start, Fellows of ACHE would not lose their standing if they went on to manage another type of organization during a later phase of their careers.

This specific focus on the hospital administrator was a critically important decision for ACHE.[12] It set the conditions that would result in the creation of other specialized associations such as the American Association of Healthcare Consultants and the American College of Medical Practice Executives. By 1967, ACHE had changed its focus and turned away from exclusively admitting hospital administrators and began to admit non-hospital administrators as well.[13]

In the original constitution, Members were to have five years of experience in "an acceptable institution." Members in good standing for three years might advance to Fellowship by "application and qualification."[14] Age was not used as a criterion, although it was indirectly involved in the experience standard.

Experience

At the start, Members were to have "adequate academic education," although they were not required to have a college degree.[15] Elaboration of these standards would come at a later time.

Education

As previously mentioned, Malcolm MacEachern's opinion was important at the beginning of ACHE. Ethical conduct was also considered important. J. Dewey Lutes remembers the early expulsion of an ACHE member for unethical conduct.[16] By 1973, this process was to become a formalized grievance procedure.

Reputation and Recommendation

A written examination for advancement from Nomineeship to Membership began in 1951.[17]

Examination

In 1933, it was proposed that all members submit a yearly thesis on hospital administration. By 1934, this was changed from annually to periodically. By 1938, the thesis had become a one-time requirement for Fellowship, although advancement to Fellowship was possible without it until 1940.[18]

Case Reports or Thesis

In 1936, ACHE had 191 Fellows, 184 Members, and 33 Junior Members. In 1940, there were 334 Fellows, 395 Members, and 161 Associate Members (formerly Junior Members and later to be designated Nominees). By that time, some of the Fellows had concluded that Fellowship was simply too easy to achieve. They felt that the Junior Membership was diluted by "personnel directors, directors of nurses, administrative and executive assistants, chiefs of clinics, chief accountants, superintendents of surgery, purchasing agents, etc."[19] These individuals had gained admittance as Junior Members by having three years experience in responsible hospital positions and by indicating that they desired to prepare themselves for careers in hospital administration. In addition, they had been recommended by a Fellow and had passed an examination.[20] As time progressed, ACHE adjusted, and in some instances completely altered, the original membership criteria. Figure 4-1 outlines the chronology of these changes.

FIGURE 4-1

Changes in
ACHE
Credentialing
Program

1933–1934	Admission to Fellowship by invitation.
1934–1935	First admission to Membership by invitation; Membership to be limited to active hospital administrators.
1935	Admission by application begins.
1938	Junior Members (Nominees) admitted for the first time.
1940	End of direct admission to Fellowship. From now on the thesis or equivalent is required for Fellowship.
1941	Strict requirement that the administrator's hospital be accredited was dropped.
1944	Educational psychologist consultant hired for expert advice on examination, content, and evaluation.
1947	Nominee category created, replacing Junior Membership and requiring a baccalaureate degree or the equivalent.
1950	Master's degree proposed (but not mandated) as minimum requirement for membership.
	Nomineeship required plus written and oral examinations before advancement to Membership, with some exceptions for candidates with "extraordinary qualifications." Up to 1951, a written exam (short essay, true/false, and fill-in-the blank) was a typical requirement.
1951	Written objective examinations are held in 50 cities for Nominee advancement to Membership. The writing of case reports instead of a thesis became typical for advancement to Fellowship.
1965	Annual revision of written exam starts.
1966	Introduction of structured oral interview with rigorous standards.
1967	Baccalaureate degree plus three years' experience required for admission (baccalaureate equivalency no longer allowed).
1970	Admission of nonhospital health administrators allowed.
1974	In-depth review of oral examination for Membership.
1975	August 18, *Regulations Governing Admission and Advancement* approved.
1977	Change in entry level, allowing admission of lower-level administrators.
1982	New category of affiliation: Candidate for Nomineeship.
1984	Adoption of recertification program for Members and Fellows. Two additional Fellow projects approved: continuing education seminars, which were later dropped due to lack of interest, and mentorship. Development of a new Membership exam with a generic core exam and five specialty tracks.

Continued

| 1987 | First year of recertification program. Members required to recertify every 6 years and Fellows every 10 years. |

1992   Credential Task Force established to recommend changes in *Regulations Governing Admission, Advancement, and Recertification.*

1993   Nominee status is replaced by Associate status. Associates must reappoint every six years to keep their status.

Member status is replaced by Diplomate status and "CHE" (Certified Healthcare Executive) is introduced. Diplomate requirements include:

- Master's degree plus two years' healthcare management experience; or bachelor's degree plus five years' healthcare management experience (one less year); or no degree plus 12 years' experience in a healthcare leadership position

- 20 hours of continuing education—either Category I (ACHE education) or Category II (non-ACHE education)

- Five years of tenure with ACHE for advancement to Fellow

1995   Board of Governors Examination revised to include a comprehensive generic core. Specialty tracks, which had increased to 10 since 1984, were eliminated.

1999   Regular Member status replaces Associate status.

Candidate for Regular Member replaces Candidate for Associate status.

All Regular Members are given the right to vote in Regent elections (previously, only Associates with two years' tenure with ACHE could vote).

Reference requirement eliminated for Regular Members.

Reappointment requirement eliminated for Regular Members.

2000   Candidate for Regular Member status eliminated.

Regular Member changed to Member. The collective term "member" changed to "affiliate" to avoid confusion with Member status.

2002   Position requirement removed for admission to Member, as long as the candidate attests that he or she has an interest and commitment to the profession of healthcare management.

2003   Recertification requirements changed to every three years for both Diplomate and Fellow. Continuing education requirement changed to 24 hours over previous 3 years, of which 12 must be Category I credits. Recertification held in abeyance during a phase-in period until 2006. Tenure requirements for advancement to Fellow reduced from five years to three years in Diplomate

Continued

	status. Continuing education requirements reduced to 30 hours, 15 of which must be Category I.
2004	Advancement to Diplomate continuing education requirement reduced from 20 hours to 12 hours of Category I or II over the most recent two years.
	Advancement to Fellow continuing education reduced from 30 hours to 24 hours over the most recent three-year period; half must be Category I.
2007	Credentialing program combined to one credential—the FACHE. Individuals can join as Members; after two years of healthcare management experience, members can seek Fellow status by taking a written exam and supplying three references. To complete the Fellow requirements, candidates must have 40 hours of continuing education units (12 of which are Category I), three years' tenure, five years of experience, and must attest to community and civic involvement.
2008	Effective December 31, candidates with only a bachelor's degree will no longer be eligible for Fellow status.

Admission and Advancement Procedures Upgraded

In 1944, ACHE retained an educational psychologist to upgrade admission and advancement procedures.[21] She reported that it would be difficult to improve procedures without a defined criterion of competency in hospital administration. With the help of Ralph W. Tyler, dean of graduate education at the University of Chicago, proposals were developed leading to a Kellogg Foundation grant to improve educational courses and develop more effective procedures for selection and advancement of personnel in the field of hospital administration. This project was undertaken by the ACHA–AHA Joint Commission on Education, with Charles Prall serving as the Senior Staff Member.[22] More information on this can be found in Chapter 5.

In 1947, the Junior Membership category was replaced by the Nominee category. At this time, entry into ACHE required a baccalaureate degree or its equivalent. A registered nursing (RN) degree was considered equivalent to two years of college training.

By 1950, Nomineeship was the required first step to membership, with some exceptions given for candidates with extraordinary qualifications. For example, during this time, special provision was made for faculty members of approved courses in hospital administration who did not have the hospital experience required of all other candidates.[23] According to one expert,

These comparatively stringent requirements for the rank of Nominee—rank
which no longer even brought Membership in the College—indicate the
remarkable advance in qualifications
which the College had been able to
insist upon in less than twenty years.
Few professions have been able to
make such rapid progress in so short a
time.[24]

Later, two years of college were
considered to be equivalent to two years
of healthcare management experience.
For example, a candidate could join
ACHE with a master's degree and one
year of experience or a bachelor's degree
and three years' experience.

In 1951, with the aid of Dr. Lillian
Terris, Honorary Fellow, a written examination was developed. The examination was
given in 50 cities in 1951 for advancement
from Nomineeship to Membership.[26] This
examination remained in place until 1966,
when Richard Stull initiated steps to completely overhaul the exam. Figure 4-2 offers
some sample questions from the 1952 examination.

Sidebar 4-1. Historical Perspective

At the founding of ACHE, the Constitution read:

> Application for Membership or Fel-
> lowship may be made voluntarily or
> by invitation. Before the application is
> considered by the Credentials Com-
> mittee, all Members and Fellows
> within the same state as that of the
> applicant will be asked to render an
> opinion regarding his or her adminis-
> trative ability and other qualities. In
> this respect you are reminded that
> friendship should not obscure your
> vision.
> Bear in mind that Fellows and
> Members share the responsibility for
> maintaining an organization of Dig-
> nity and Quality. The Credentials
> Committee suggests that the present
> Members and Fellows survey the
> administrative field in their state and
> propose the names of those who in
> their judgment meet the require-
> ments for membership.[25]

Strengthening the Requirements for Membership

In 1966, a structured oral interview was introduced as a requirement for membership, and the written exam was revised. Prior to this time, the failure rate for
the exam was only 6 percent. With the new version, failures rose to 28 percent
and remained from 18 to 26 percent for several years thereafter. In 1967, the
last group of non–baccalaureate degree candidates entered Nomineeship. From
that time on, all affiliates were required to have an undergraduate degree; no
more baccalaureate equivalencies were accepted (except from 1993 to 1994 to
allow older, distinguished practitioners to join ACHE).

In 1969, the Council of Regents approved an additional year of
tenure as necessary for advancement to Member or Fellow. So, in 1971, no
Nominees or Members were eligible for advancement unless they had
already accumulated the required seniority.

FIGURE 4-2
American
College of
Hospital
Administrators
Examination
for Member-
ship, Sample
Questions,
1952

Part I.

(Time: One hour)

Note: Answer numbers 1 and 5 plus any other three questions.

1. You are the administrator of a 150-bed hospital which operates its own essential facilities or departments, including pharmacy, laundry, bakery, cafeteria, etc. You desire to show the lines of authority and interrelationship of the various departments of your hospital in order that your department heads may fully understand the organization plan. Draw a schematic chart outlining the various relationships from the Governing Board to each of the departmental activities in the hospital.

2. What is a Medical Audit? From an administrative standpoint, what are its chief advantages?

3. Outline the essentials of an effective Public Relations Program for the hospital.

4   Enumerate briefly the steps which should be taken by the administrator in the preparation of the hospital budget.

5. Name five evils or abuses in hospital practice against which the administrator must be constantly alert.

6. Distinguish between the responsibilities of the Hospital Administrator and the responsibilities of the Governing Body.

7. What are the basic causes for shortages of nurses (etc.)?

Part II.

[A selection of true/false questions from a total of 25 on the exam.*]

1. T/F   Education is THE principal function of a hospital.

2. T/F   The administrator is acknowledged to be the head of the hospital responsible for the physical plant and every act committed therein.

3. T/F   The legally constituted governing body has supreme authority for the administration of the hospital.

4. T/F   It is considered good policy for a member of the Active Medical Staff to be also a member of the Board of Trustees.

5. T/F   Under no circumstances may a patient leave the hospital without the consent of the attending physician.

6. T/F   All employees who handle hospital funds should be bonded.

The correct answers were Question (1) False, (2) True, (3) True, (4) False, (5) False, (6) True.

Continued

In 1970, the admission criteria were changed again to allow the acceptance of candidates holding administrative positions in health-related organizations. ACHE's annual report stated that,

Health delivery was evolving as a system of many components with varied forms of leadership, but all with a significant impact on the operations of hospitals and health institutions. It was felt that this total leadership should be incorporated under the umbrella of professionalism as represented by the College in order to expedite and facilitate communications and relationships essential for our common goals.

Part III.
(Time: 30 Minutes)
Administrative Problems (Answer both problems)
The following problems are given to elicit administrative judgment and analysis in situations which come within the purview of a hospital administrator. There is no one classic solution to either problem. You will be graded solely on the practicability of your answer. Allow yourself 15 minutes for each question.

1. You are the administrator of a hospital and have just been informed of the death of a patient from a serious over-dosage of a potent drug administered by a general duty nurse. It is alleged that the death occurred as a result of an error in the nurse's interpretation of a doctor's correctly written order for the drug. What steps would you take in the complete handling of this death case?

2. You are the administrator of a 150-bed voluntary non-profit general hospital in a Midwestern city of 25,000 population.
    Your hospital maintains a favorably known and accepted school of nursing, also an internship and residency training program, although it has no direct university or medical school affiliation. At present the pathologist and the chief of staff in internal medicine are jointly engaged in a modest research study which has been subsidized in part by a grant from a national foundation.
    Your hospital is a major beneficiary of the community chest. In connection with the annual community fund drive, you have been asked "to portray your hospital's picture" to a large mass meeting. Your audience, being a fair cross-section of the community, is quite remote from considerations of medical and nursing education and medical research.
    Someone in the audience wants to know how you justify the teaching and research program at your hospital, the expense of which is not entirely related to patient care. What would you tell the audience?

In 1974, admissions requirements were once again amended, calling for "the elimination of the residency as fulfilling the requirement for the one year of administrative experience." The genesis of this amendment was a change in the educational practice of health administration graduate programs. Many of them began offering two years of academic study without a residency, while a considerable number continued to offer one year of graduate study and one year of residency education. In a sense, ACHE's regulations, before they were amended, discriminated against the two-year programs, since students of the other programs automatically fulfilled the experience requirement.

In addition, with the waning of interest in the residency on the part of graduate programs, the experiences of the students during their residency in some cases were becoming less meaningful. It was doubtful, in fact, that the residency could validly be given consideration as a measure of expected performance, since it was so basically educational in nature.

In 1977, the admissions requirements were again modified to allow acceptance of candidates at lower administrative levels. This amendment addressed the problems encountered by the increasing number of graduates who were finding it more and more difficult to obtain health service positions at a level that met the stipulated requirements of ACHE. The growing number of graduate programs made senior-level administrative jobs more difficult to find, and graduates took more junior-level positions. At the same time, hospitals grew in size and complexity. Some of the "lower level" jobs carried more responsibility than many senior positions had in the early years of ACHE. Finally, the number of years spent in middle management by healthcare executives grew steadily. Proportionately fewer executives could become a CEO. As stated in the Annual Report,

> Certainly when one considers the number of candidates competing for a limited number of managerial posts, the diverse factors impacting on the time schedule for ascension on the career ladder to responsible administrative positions, and the desire to involve young men and women early in the affairs of the College in order to inculcate them with the attitude and spirit of professionalism, this was a realistic move.

This amendment in the regulations also had another dimension: it effected a reconsideration of Nominee status in ACHE. What emerged was the belief that the Nominee period was "a time of transition during which there is an opportunity to monitor a candidate's progress and adaptability as he or she proceeds up the job ladder. In addition this period of Nomineeship also allowed the candidate time for broader exposure to the operations of institutions." In other words, Nominee status was viewed as a period of transition and development, with the Membership examination becoming the real screening device to determine an individual's eligibility for full status in ACHE and complete identification as a professional.

In the early 1980s and 1990s, ACHE developed management tracks. In 1984, the Board of Governors Examination consisted of a generic core and five specialty tracks; five more specialty tracks were added between 1987 and 1990.

By 1992, ACHE had the following affiliation categories:

- Candidates for Nomineeship
- Nominees

- Members
- Fellows
- Life Members, Life Fellows, and Honorary Fellows
- Student Associates
- Faculty Associates

After graduation, Student Associates were encouraged to become either Candidates for Nomineeship or Nominees. Graduates who had not been Student Associates could also apply for admittance into these categories.

After three years a Nominee could advance to Membership. This required references, current work in the field, demonstrated leadership, education, and the completion of the Board of Governors Examination in Healthcare Management.

After six years, Members could apply for Fellowship. This required references, work in the field, leadership, education, and continuing education. A Fellowship project was also required and could take one of three forms:

1. A thesis of about 30 to 50 pages
2. Four case reports of 10 to 12 pages each

Sidebar 4-2. Self-Assessment Programs

In May 1979, a self-assessment project was funded by the W. K. Kellogg Foundation to provide healthcare executives with a mechanism to assess their knowledge and skills in a variety of healthcare management areas and serve as a basis for developing a personal program for continuing education and lifelong learning. The project resulted in the development of the following three health executive professional assessment programs:

1. The General Management Assessment consisted of 175 scenario-based questions designed to assess the participant's applied knowledge in 11 healthcare management areas. Participants self-scored the questions and then used the results to develop an education plan based on areas of strength or need.
2. The Ambulatory Care Assessment was developed jointly with the American College of Medical Practice Executives and consisted of a short booklet of scenario-based exercises to assess knowledge in three areas. In addition, participants completed a simulation exercise to assess problem-solving and decision-making skills in an ambulatory care/medical group management setting.
3. The Administrative Communication Techniques program was designed to assess the participant's administrative and communication skills. It consisted of an in-basket exercise and a writing skills exercise.

More than 10,000 affiliates participated in the programs from the early 1980s through 1995, when the programs reached the end of their product life cycle and were discontinued.

Sidebar 4-3. Recertification

In 1987, a recertification program was implemented for Fellows and Members. Recertification offered affiliates the opportunity to demonstrate their commitment to continuing education and lifelong learning. Fellows were required to recertify every 10 years by participating in 90 hours of continuing education (half from Category I [ACHE education] programs) or successfully completing the Board of Governors Examination in Healthcare Management. In addition, candidates were required to show evidence of participation in healthcare and community/civic activities.

Members were required to recertify every 6 years by participating in 50 hours of continuing education (half from Category I programs) or successfully completing the Board of Governors Examination in Healthcare Management. In addition, candidates were required to show evidence of participation in healthcare and community/civic activities.

Sidebar 4-4. The Board of Governors Exam

In 1992, the Board of Governors Examination had 200 general multiple-choice questions and 50 questions in seven specialty tracks. There was also an oral interview.

3. Two years of structured mentorship with quarterly reports

About 10 percent of applicants for Fellowship chose to complete the thesis, 85 percent chose the case reports, and 5 percent chose mentorship. Fellowship recertification was required after 10 years of Fellowship. Ninety hours of continuing education were required over the previous nine years in addition to participation in health and community affairs.

Membership recertification required a formal application and continuing education of 25 hours of ACHE credits and 25 added hours of ACHE or non-ACHE credits over a six-year period. Evidence of participation in healthcare affairs and community affairs was required along with 6 years' tenure as a Member.

In late 1993, major changes to the membership regulations were passed. The highlights of these changes are as follows:

- All Nominees in ACHE were called "Associates."
- All Members in ACHE were called "Diplomates."
- An individual could remain an Associate without ever advancing to Diplomate, provided reappointment requirements were met every six years.
- Healthcare executives could join ACHE as Diplomates, provided the Diplomate eligibility requirements were met, including the successful completion of the Board of Governors Examination in Healthcare Management.
- Diplomates could use the "CHE" (Certified Healthcare Executive) credential after their names.
- An individual had to be a Diplomate in good standing for at least five years to be eligible to advance to Fellow (a change from six years).
- ACHE and/or non-ACHE continuing education credits could be used to meet continuing education requirements for Diplomate status.

- Individuals could be accepted as Diplomates without a college degree, provided they had at least 12 years of experience in the field and only if they were admitted under the no-degree option, which was limited to the years 1993 and 1994.

By 1994, two additional membership categories were added: "International Associate" was added in 1993 and "Retired Status" was added in 1994.

In 1995, the field of healthcare management had become so diverse that the specialty tracks of the Board of Governors Examination did not cover all the areas required. The generic core of the exam was revised to reflect the latest requirements that candidates needed to know to perform their jobs, and the specialty tracks were eliminated.

The Current Picture

In 1999, the credentialing and reappointment process changed again. The term "Associate" was eliminated and "Member" took its place. The reason for the name change was to foster a sense of inclusion. Members were allowed to vote in Regent elections right away instead of waiting the previously required two years. The reappointment requirement was eliminated.

By 2002, an individual no longer had to have a position in healthcare management to seek Member status. Anyone who had an "interest and commitment to the field of healthcare management" could pursue membership. This allowed individuals such as nurses seeking a career in healthcare management to join ACHE as Members.

In 2003, recertification requirements changed. Formerly, Diplomates had to recertify every 6 years and Fellows every 10 years. With the revisions, both Fellows and Diplomates had to recertify every three years. This forced affiliates to keep up with their continuing education (CE) credits. To be recertified, individuals were required to have 24 total CE credits (half were to be Category I [ACHE education] credits and the other half could be from another organization) or retake the Board of Governors exam and attest to participation in community/civic affairs.

Streamlining the Process

In 2005, ACHE's Board appointed a Credentialing Task Force to examine ways to

> **Sidebar 4-5. The Leader-to-Leader Campaign**
>
> To help grow membership, ACHE launched the Leader-to-Leader Campaign, which awards points to affiliates for recruiting new Members or encouraging existing Members to become Diplomates or Fellows. These points can be redeemed for rewards. In 2006, the program brought in more than 1,179 new Members, 270 new Diplomates, and 40 new Fellows.

encourage more Members to become credentialed. ACHE hired Knapp and Associates to conduct research and make a recommendation on the credentialing program. Following a two-year study, the Credentialing Task Force made recommendations for change. The task force concluded that ACHE must raise the bar for the credentialing program to elevate the standards in the field. Given the varying educational and experiential backgrounds of individuals entering healthcare management, a commitment to credentialing and CE was critical to the profession. The task force recommended that the credentialing program be combined to one credential, the FACHE, in the belief that the field would be better served by removing the ambiguity of a two-credential program while elevating the standards.

While the previously required Fellow projects were useful to many candidates, they did not measure competency and therefore were not valid indicators for attaining a credential. The new credentialing system replaces Fellow projects with other criteria, such as increased CE requirements. In addition, beginning in 2009, Fellow candidates will need a master's degree or higher.

The Board of Governors exam remains one key indicator that a candidate is eligible for board certification in healthcare management. The exam is valid, reliable, and, with only a 70 percent pass rate, distinguishes those who have the knowledge to attain the credential. Additionally, by having to continually recertify their credential, affiliates are committing to lifelong learning and professional development.

The changes in the credentialing system were effective January 1, 2007. The major criteria for earning the FACHE credential include:

- A postbaccalaureate degree (this requirement will be effective January 1, 2009)
- Three years' tenure as an ACHE Member/Diplomate
- A passing score on the Board of Governors Examination in Healthcare Management
- Five years of healthcare management experience
- 40 total CE credits in the previous five years; at least 12 Category I credits
- Three references from Fellows, one of which must be a structured interview
- Professional and community/civic participation

Creating Chapters

One of the most significant developments in modern ACHE history was the creation of local chapters. With the establishment of these chapters, ACHE has the infrastructure to deliver networking, education, and career service opportunities on a local level. In doing so, ACHE can better address both local and national healthcare management needs, enhancing the benefits it offers to healthcare executives.

The concept of using local organizations for service delivery began in 1989 with the recognition of Healthcare Executive Groups (HEGs) and Women's Healthcare Executive Networks (WHENs). These were groups that already existed and presented a venue for local service delivery. However, the affiliation agreement with ACHE for the HEGs and WHENs was very loose, and ACHE did not provide much support for the organizations. In addition, the HEGs and WHENs were not evenly distributed throughout the country. For example, most affiliates in rural areas did not have access to a HEG or a WHEN, and individuals in metropolitan areas sometimes had access to more than one.

In 1999, ACHE Chairman Mark J. Howard, FACHE, and the Board of Governors decided to initiate an informed independent audit of ACHE's structure and governance, to be certain that ACHE would be best positioned to deal effectively and efficiently with both present concerns and the many new issues that would surface. The Consensus Management Group (CMG) was retained to conduct this study. CMG worked extensively with the Governance Task Force (see Sidebar 4-6) to complete the audit.

In 2001, based on the recommendations of the audit and the Governance Task Force, ACHE decided to formally create a network of local chapters and increase the national organization's presence and relevance on a local level. ACHE developed a framework for this chapter network based on the principles listed below.

- ACHE's chapter network will consist of independent, separate corporations bound by the same voluntary agreement to a reciprocal, mutually beneficial relationship.
- ACHE's chapter network will be developed initially by converting existing affiliated groups into chapters and then by developing new chapter organizations as necessary.
- ACHE's chapter network will be deployed in a way that gives every ACHE affiliate an opportunity to join and participate in an ACHE chapter.
- ACHE chapters will be independent organizations committed to supporting ACHE's mission within mutually exclusive, geographically defined markets.
- To its chapters, ACHE will deliver effective, easy-to-use guidelines, manuals, programs, and products that can be "customized"—with the help of ACHE staff—to the individual needs and requirements of chapters.

- ACHE chapters will provide professional education, networking, and career development services to their members on a local level and will promote membership and advancement within ACHE.
- ACHE will encourage local chapter membership by promoting the value chapter membership will provide to ACHE affiliates.
- ACHE will continually improve the quality of products and services offered to chapters by soliciting and acting upon the feedback and input of chapter leaders.

In 2007, the local chapter network achieved 100 percent coverage.

When designating a local chapter, ACHE uses a contract that defines the respective rights and obligations of ACHE and the local chapter as independent, separate organizations. Under the agreement, an ACHE chapter is granted a charter to operate within a defined geographic territory and to identify itself as "An Independent Chapter of ACHE." The chapter is obligated to do the following:

- Promote membership in ACHE
- Communicate that membership in the chapter and membership in ACHE are not synonymous
- Promote and encourage the use of ACHE programs, products, and services
- Maintain appropriate liability insurance
- Comply with the criteria for chapter status

ACHE is obligated to do the following:

- Permit the use of ACHE's name and corporate identity by the chapter
- Rebate a portion of ACHE dues paid to ACHE by ACHE affiliates who are members of the chapter
- Dedicate ACHE staff to manage the relationship between the chapter and ACHE
- Make products and services available to chapters to help them carry out their responsibilities under the contract
- Notify the chapter of any ACHE activities that will be conducted in the territory of the chapter

- Notify the chapter of any changes to the criteria for chapter status or the dues rebate program

The agreement can be terminated by either party with appropriate notice.

One of the goals for the local chapter strategy has been to reach the early careerist—those individuals just starting in the field of healthcare management who may not be able to travel to national meetings and continuing education events. The chapter network is designed to provide convenient resources that are close to home and offer exposure to the national organization. Before the creation of chapters, ACHE had not effectively reached this early careerist market segment.

Partners for Success

In 2003, ACHE launched the "Partners for Success" project with the goal of developing a network of local independent chapters that would provide the opportunity for 100 percent of U.S.-based ACHE affiliates to join and participate in a local chapter. The inaugural 60 chapters were chartered in February 2004, and 78 percent of all U.S.-based affiliates worked within the territories assigned to these chapters. Total chapter membership was about 14,000, with slightly more than 9,000 members being ACHE affiliates. In other words, approximately 27 percent of ACHE affiliates had joined their local chapter. By March 2007, 83 chapters had been chartered and nearly 100 percent of all U.S.-based ACHE affiliates worked within the territories of chapters. Chapter membership had grown to 17,128, and 13,628 members were ACHE affiliates, meaning that approximately 41 percent of ACHE affiliates had joined their local chapter. This rapid growth in the number of chapters generated the necessary conditions to create significant value for ACHE affiliates by providing the means for close-to-home and convenient educational, networking, and career development services.

Since the creation of the chapter network, ACHE has continued to support it. ACHE developed an annual chapter leadership conference; created audio conferences on topics such as chapter management, how to put on a management program, and how to engage students; and devised a manual for chapter management. Posted on ache.org is a chapter service center that houses many resources that help provide education and networking opportunities and facilitate communication.

This support, along with the dedicated work of more than 700 chapter volunteers, resulted in the provision of significant value to ACHE affiliates. By the end of 2006, more than 20,000 healthcare executives were attending the more than 450 chapter events offered annually. More than 3,800 of these attendees earned Category I (ACHE education) credits in 2006. Most chapters provide quarterly newsletters, online membership directories, and have chapter web sites to communicate with their members.

Combined Membership Structure

In 2006, ACHE embarked on the creation of a more unified ACHE-chapter membership structure to better serve ACHE affiliates. Previously, ACHE affiliates were required to make an affirmative decision to join their local chapter, which usually required the payment of local chapter dues in addition to ACHE dues. As a result, less than half of ACHE affiliates were choosing to join their local chapter. In addition, chapters were permitted to maintain a "local only" membership, and often this "local only" membership represented a significant proportion of the total membership of certain chapters. In June 2007, the Board of Governors decided to implement a combined membership structure by January 1, 2009. The combined membership structure meant that all ACHE affiliates were automatically members of the local chapter serving their geographic area without paying any additional local dues, and all chapter members were required to be ACHE affiliates. While this was a controversial decision, it was generally well accepted by most chapters. At that time, chapters received up to 10 percent of the dues paid to ACHE by the ACHE affiliates who were members of the chapter to help replace the revenue previously collected by chapters as local chapter dues. This change resulted in very rapid growth in the membership of chapters, providing chapters with the opportunity to provide educational, networking, and career services to a greatly expanded base of members. In this way, ACHE affiliates received more local opportunities and gained greater value without being required to make multiple decisions to join and pay more than one annual dues amount.

The creation of local chapters was a revolutionary change for ACHE both culturally and structurally. The organization went from a national, prestige-driven, exclusive organization to a more accessible and inclusive organization that was also more corporate. Information and resources were provided on the local level, and members and potential members were given the tools they needed to achieve success. This change, coupled with the changes in membership and credentialing, made the organization more relevant to its members.

Council of Regents

Over the period of time beginning with the 2000–2001 Governance Task Force's recommendation and continuing through 2007, the governance of ACHE changed significantly to meet the demands of managing a modern professional membership society in a rapidly changing healthcare and social environment. The Council of Regents acted in 2002 to amend the ACHE *Bylaws* to transfer to the Board of Governors the authority for amending the ACHE *Bylaws* and the ACHE *Regulations* that governed the qualifications for membership in ACHE and the requirements for professional credentialing. These changes also shifted the composition of the Board of Governors from geographic representatives to a body of representatives elected at large to ensure that the Board was comprised of the most effective available leaders in the field, in the judgment of the Nominating Committee. From that point, the members of the Board of Governors have served as the chief pol-icymakers for the entire association and were able to act quickly in anticipa-tion of rapid societal and healthcare field changes.

The Council of Regents retained the authority to elect the Chairman Officers, Governors, Regents-at-Large, and Nominating Committee members so that the Regents, elected directly by affiliates, were involved in the selection of the ACHE volunteer leadership. In addition, the Council of Regents increas-ingly served an important role in advising the Board of Governors on key pol-icy decisions based on their perceptions of affiliate needs and desires.

As the role of the Council of Regents, as a body, changed from pol-icymaking to policyadvising, the individual role of Regents changed as well. Prior to the formation of chapters, Regents were largely responsible for the delivery of services to affiliates locally through education programs, encourage-ment to advance professional credentials, quarterly newsletters, and career advice. After chapters were formed, the Regent's role as ACHE's local liaison to other organizations such as state and local hospital associations was expanded to include chapters and other professional society chapters. Individual Regents served as change agents throughout the process of developing chapters and increased their capabilities to serve affiliates. As recognized senior leaders within their local communities, individual Regents were able to help chapters develop contacts with other organizations and other senior healthcare executives and represent the interests of ACHE affiliates with respect to chapter programs and services. Regents played a key role in keeping both ACHE and the local chap-ters focused on the mission, vision, and values of ACHE.

As the individual roles of Regents changed, the Council of Regents was reduced in size to increase its ability to serve effectively as adviser to the Board of Governors. A Regent consolidation plan grew out of the original 2000–2001 Governance Task Force reports that reduced the Council of Regents from 100 members to 76 by increasing the number of affiliates represented by each Regent. Controversial at the time, this reduction was largely accomplished by attrition as Regents completed their terms of office between 2005 and 2008.

The streamlining of the membership and credentialing process and the creation and continuing support of chapters have made ACHE more inclu-sive and have enhanced the diversity of the organization. Chapters 5 through 8 continue this discussion and look at how ACHE has addressed issues of education, publications, and other important services.

Endnotes

1.   Agnew, G. H., "Training in Hospital Administration." *Hospitals*, Vol. 13, No. 7, July 1939.

2.   Kipnis, I. A. *A Venture Forward: A History of the American College of Hospital Administrators.* Chicago: ACHA, 1955, p. 13.

3.   ACHA *Minute Book*, Vol. 1, Oct. 7, 1932; Kipnis, I. A. *A Venture Forward: A History of the American College of Hospital Administrators.* Chicago: ACHA, 1955, p. 10.

4.   Kipnis, I. A. *A Venture Forward: A History of the American College of Hospital Administrators.* Chicago: ACHA, 1955, p. 13.

5.   ACHA *Minute Book*, Vol. 1, Feb. 14, 1933; Kipnis, I. A. *A Venture Forward: A History of the American College of Hospital Administrators.* Chicago: ACHA, 1955, pp. 14–15.

6.   The other members were Fred Carter, Robert Neff, John Smith, and Robin Buerki. Executive Committee Minutes, ACHA *Minute Book*, Vol. 1, May 3, 1934; also Kipnis, I. A. *A Venture Forward: A History of the American College of Hospital Administrators.* Chicago: ACHA, 1955, pp. 15, 31–32.

7.   Kipnis, I. A. *A Venture Forward. A History of the American College of Hospital Administrators.* Chicago: ACHA, 1955, p.15.

8.   Ibid.; First Annual Report to the Board of Regents, ACHA *Minute Book*, Vol. 1, 1937.

9.   Kipnis, I. A. *A Venture Forward: A History of the American College of Hospital Administrators.* Chicago: ACHA, 1955, p. 17.

10.   Ibid., p. 20. Direct election to Fellowship for administrators of recognized standing would remain open until Jan. 1, 1940.

11.   Board of Regents Meeting, ACHA *Minute Book*, Vol. 1, Sept. 23, 1934, p. 89; Kipnis, I. A. *A Venture Forward: A History of the American College of Hospital Administrators.* Chicago: ACHA, 1955, pp. 19–20.

12.   This decision was re-reviewed with respect to changing the name of ACHE to Healthcare rather than Hospital Administrators. "Regents Rebel, Veto Name Change Proposal." *Modern Healthcare*, Oct. 1981, pp. 77–78; Wesbury, S. A., "Background Information Concerning the Proposal to Change the Name and Objects of the American College of Hospital Administrators," ACHA, April 1981.

13.   "Regents Rebel, Veto Name Change Proposal." *Modern Healthcare*, Oct. 1981, p. 77.

14.   Constitution and Bylaws, ACHA *Minute Book*, Vol. 1, 1934; Kipnis, I. A. *A Venture Forward: A History of the American College of Hospital Administrators.* Chicago: ACHA, 1955, p. 13.

15.   Kipnis, I. A. *A Venture Forward: A History of the American College of Hospital Administrators.* Chicago: ACHA, 1955, p. 29.

16.   J. D. Lutes interview, 1982.

17.   Kipnis, I. A. *A Venture Forward: A History of the American College of Hospital Administrators.* Chicago: ACHA, 1955, p. 120.

18.   Ibid., pp. 13, 20, 66; ACHA *Minute Book*, Vol. 1, Oct. 7, 1932, p. 3.

19.   Today these positions can be vastly more complicated than they were in the 1930s.

20.   Kipnis, I. A. *A Venture Forward: A History of the American College of Hospital Administrators.* Chicago: ACHA, 1955, p. 64.

21.   Margaret R. Barnes, consulting psychologist, University Hospitals, Cleveland; Kipnis, I. A. *A Venture Forward: A History of the American College of Hospital Administrators.* Chicago: ACHA, 1955, p. 88.

22.   Kipnis, I. A. *A Venture Forward: A History of the American College of Hospital Administrators.* Chicago: ACHA, 1955, pp. 88–96.

23.   Approved courses later became accredited courses in hospital or health administration. Those faculty with neither three years of hospital administrative experience nor a master's degree and one year of administrative experience would not qualify.

24.   Kipnis, I. A. *A Venture Forward: A History of the American College of Hospital Administrators.* Chicago: ACHA, 1955, pp. 118–119.

25.   *Bulletin of the ACHA*, Vol. 1, No. 1, circa 1934–1935. According to Kipnis, Lutes started the *Bulletin* in 1934. Kipnis, I. A. *A Venture Forward: A History of the American College of Hospital Administrators.* Chicago: ACHA, 1955, p. 58. The *Bulletin* was to become the *ACHA News* in 1938.

26.   W. R. Kirk interview, March 14, 1983; Kipnis, I. A. *A Venture Forward: A History of the American College of Hospital Administrators.* Chicago: ACHA, 1955, p. 120; "Dr. Lillian D. Terris Retires," *PES NEWS*, Vol. 4, No. 1, July 1979.

THE FUNCTIONS OF ACHE: EDUCATION

The professional must join and participate in those societies and associations which give him (or her) new ways to view his established practice. He must remove himself from practice from time to time for intensive periods of study, thereby not merely acquiring new knowledge but also gaining a broader perspective so that when he goes back into service again he views matters in a new light. He must in short use every means of continuing education available so that his worth retains the lucidity and freshness of its early years.

Richard J. Stull quoting Cyril O. Houle, 1969[1]

From its inception, the American College of Healthcare Executives (ACHE) has focused on improving the education of healthcare executives. Throughout the years, ACHE has focused on two main aspects of this education: training and educating individuals to enter the healthcare management profession and furthering the education of individuals already in the profession. This chapter examines both of these aspects, following the history of ACHE's efforts in these areas and offering a glimpse at the results of these efforts. The chapter is divided into the following sections:

• Early Training Programs
• The Growth of Undergraduate and Graduate Education Programs
• ACHE's Continuing Education Programs

Early Training Programs

Prior to 1940, few programs existed for training healthcare executives. Several colleges and universities offered short courses in hospital administration, but no school offered a degree in such a program (see Sidebar 5-1). For example, the University of Western Canada gave a nine-month course leading to a certificate, but not a degree.[2] Also, New York University gave classes on "Hospital and Institutional Management" and "Community Relations of Hospitals." However, these classes were discontinued in 1928 and 1929 for financial reasons.

In 1916, Annie Goodrich, RN, a faculty member of the department of nursing and health, in the Teachers College at Columbia University, spoke at the American Hospital Association (AHA) annual meeting of the need to train superintendents of small hospitals:

> One can conceive of no greater piece of constructive and enduringly valuable work for this Association (AHA), no greater contribution toward a rapid standardization of hospitals—than the raising of a fund sufficient to establish at least one school of hospital or institutional administration and to command the services of the most highly experienced administrator in the field for its director, with an adequate staff of lecturers and instructors.[3]

The first degree-granting program in hospital administration with a "more or less complete curriculum" was located at Marquette University in Milwaukee. The idea for this program came from Rev. Moulinier, the guiding force behind the Catholic Hospital Association (CHA)[4] and a member of the 1922 Rockefeller Commission on the Training for Hospital Executives.[5] Rev. Moulinier and a colleague set up the program at Marquette in September 1924, with courses following the Rockefeller Commission recommendations. The program was "an outgrowth of the great movement for the progressive betterment of hospitals that is taking place in the country."[6] The school was also described as "a natural outgrowth of the movement for hospital standardization."

In 1927, two students earned degrees from the Marquette program. Undergraduate, two-week graduate, and summer courses were planned, but by 1928 this program had failed.[7] The reason this program ended is not clear, but it was probably because of lack of funds.[8]

The Age of Apprenticeship

Prior to the 1930s, personal apprenticeship training was the only ongoing source of training in hospital administration. At the end of his book, *Hospital*

Sidebar 5-1. Colleges that Offered Coursework in Hospital Administration Prior to 1940

Columbia Teachers College, New York
Duke University, Durham, North Carolina
Harvard School of Public Health, Boston
Illinois Training School for Nurses, Chicago
Marquette University, Milwaukee, Wisconsin
McGill University, Montreal
Michigan State College, East Lansing
New York University
Peabody College, Nashville, Tennessee
Temple University, Philadelphia
University of Iowa, Iowa City
University of Western Canada

Sidebar 5-2. Historical Perspective

In 1919, Arthur C. Bachmeyer, MD, one of the founding Fellows of ACHE, described a proposed curriculum in hospital administration at the University of Cincinnati's College of Medicine with courses in the College of Commerce. Although this proposal was unsuccessful, Bachmeyer was prepared to endorse the idea of a graduate program in hospital administration when he moved to the University of Chicago.[9]

Administration: A Career, Michael M. Davis, PhD, presented a brief history of U.S. education in hospital administration and noted that "up to the present time [1929] the outstanding educational resource of the hospital field has been those individual hospital superintendents who have been interested not only in their own institutions, but in hospital administration as a profession, and who have made their hospitals centers for training of younger men and women by personal apprenticeship."[10]

Only a small fraction of all administrators took advantage of apprenticeships. The Massachusetts General Hospital, Johns Hopkins Hospital, Mount Sinai Hospitals in New York and Cleveland, and Grace Hospital in Detroit were among the few hospitals offering the opportunity.[11] The result of this movement was genealogies of administrators offering training to the next generation.

The University of Chicago Program

In his book, Michael Davis proposed a two-year, graduate-degree curriculum in hospital administration. The curriculum focused more on management skills than on clinical management. According to his proposal, in the first nine months the student would take the following coursework[12]:

- 6 hours of accounting
- 5 hours of statistics and methods of presentation
- 6 hours of organization and management
- 6 hours of economics and social sciences
- 3 hours of history and status of hospitals, clinics, and the health profession
- 8 hours of practical observation
- 6 hours of seminar

In the second year, the program would include the following:

- 24 hours of practical work, not coursework
- 7 hours of seminar related to the student's thesis
- 6 hours of business policy
- 3 hours of public health and labor relations

Davis had the opportunity to put his thoughts into action when he started the world's first successful master's degree program in hospital administration within the business school of the University of Chicago.[13] This course was formally approved on February 14, 1934. Looking back on his work, Davis said:

> By 1933, I had experience as an administrator, a teacher, and a consultant.... This experience had led me to several conclusions, including the very firm

Sidebar 5-3. Historical Perspective

In 1937, the University of Chicago program came very close to ending. The Rosenwald funds were coming to an end, and Michael Davis, Dean William Spencer, and Gerhard Hartman visited Robert Hutchins, president of the University of Chicago, and asked for his blessing and strategic support to seek The Commonwealth Fund financing. In Hartman's words:

When we came, he was sitting at a work table in his shirt sleeves. He said to the Dean, "Bill, what's up?" The Dean told him why we were there. Hutchins said, "Oh, yes." Then the commentary was made on why the hospital administration program should be carried forward. I won't repeat the precise profanity he used except that he called the field just G__ d__ technocracy, that it is just the antithesis of what a university should represent and that it would go forward over his dead body.

The Dean, of course, was used to working with him, but I was just innocent enough so that I spoke up and said, "As an individual enrolled, may I say that it is respectable academically." Then, I indicated some of the faculty. When I named (the economist) Jacob Viner, he asked, "Did you study with him?..." "That's my major," I said. He asked, "with Frank too?..." "Yes, Professor Knight (another noted economist) is a man I'm working with day and night. I am not obligated to take the courses, but they are the men from whom I learn." I threw in the names of Ruth Emerson and Louis Wirth. I said, "I would like to respectfully suggest that it be given another three-year test interval with sufficient interim reporting to you so that you know what is really happening." He smiled and said, "So be it." That was it.[19]

one to the effect that hospitals would be much better off if their administrators had training for the job.... [M]ost administrators were absorbed in institutional detail and lacked broad basic objectives toward which administration should be headed. The trustees who employed them did not in most instances expect their executive officers to be more than housekeepers.

To start the program, the Rosenwald Fund—a fund established by Julius Rosenwald, a founder of Sears Roebuck, for "investments in a more equitable society"[14]—provided from \$5,000 to \$7,000 for three years. The program was placed in the business school for practical reasons and relied heavily on existing courses.[15]

After its first three years, the University of Chicago program was supported by The Commonwealth Fund and later by the W.K. Kellogg Foundation.[16] Open to students with a bachelor's degree, it was a joint project of the business school and the University of Chicago Clinics. Applicants were interviewed by either Michael Davis or Arthur Bachmeyer, the director of the Clinics (as the hospital was called at that time).[17]

Many aspects of the Davis curriculum became prototypes for future degree programs, but 25 years would pass before master's degree programs were able to educate sufficient numbers to meet the need projected by the 1948 Prall Report.[18] The University of Chicago program epitomized the future of the profession. Like ACHE, the Chicago program was not representative of the whole field but what the field was to become.

The Growth in Graduate and Undergraduate Education

Throughout the years, ACHE has played a significant role in the formation of graduate education programs for hospital and health services administration (see Figure 5-1). The genesis of these efforts began with the Committee on Educational Policies. Chaired by Dr. Malcolm MacEachern, the first Committee on Educational Policies met on October 1, 1935, to set the basic goals of ACHE's educational program, "goals which have since been developed and greatly expanded, but which still remain the core of the College activity."[20]

The Committee focused on restructuring the training and educating of hospital administrators, moving away from ad hoc coursework toward a specialized curriculum. As Rev. Alphonse M. Schwitalla, SJ, PhD, dean of the St. Louis University School of Medicine and Editor of *Hospital Progress*, said,

> Sidebar 5-4. Historical Perspective
>
> The link between ACHE and the University of Chicago was a close one. The following points illustrate this connection:
>
> - Dr. Michael Davis was elected the first Honorary Fellow of ACHE in 1935. At this time, Davis was also medical director for the Rosenwald Fund for a year and director of the University of Chicago hospital administration program.[24]
> - Dr. Gerhard Hartman earned his doctorate degree at University of Chicago, was an instructor in the hospital administration program, and served as executive secretary of ACHE from 1937 to 1941. He also was the director for the University of Iowa's hospital administration program.
> - Dr. Arthur Bachmeyer was the second head of the University of Chicago program and active in its inception. He was also a Charter Fellow and President of ACHE from 1940 to 1941.

The hospital administrator of the future should be an executive who can advise his board and act as a policymaker and coordinator. Such an administrator could not be trained by taking a couple of (short) courses in hospital administration after securing a bachelor's degree in some other field of specialization.[21]

A subcommittee consisting of Rev. Schwitalla, Dr. Bachmeyer, and Dr. Benjamin Black—superintendent of Alameda County Hospital—was appointed to develop a proposal for a university curriculum that would lead to a degree in hospital administration. The result of this subcommittee's work was presented for the approval of the Committee on Educational Policies and published in 1937.[22]

The Committee determined that "hospital administration is validly to be considered as a special profession…and this profession demands some form of specialized preparation."[23] The Committee went on to recommend that "the hospital administrator should have at least a master's degree" and that such a degree "seems not only highly desirable but, in view of the present status in health development, practically indispensable."

FIGURE 5-1
Landmark
Reports on
Education for
Hospital
Administration
in Which
ACHE
Participated[25]

The Age of Apprenticeship or No Training

1911   F. A. Washburn, MD, and W. B. Howland, MD. "The Training of Hospital Administrators." *Transactions of the American Hospital Association.*

1916   Annie Goodrich, RN. "How Shall the Superintendents of Small Hospitals Be Trained?" *Transactions of the American Hospital Association.* Vol. 18.

1919   A. C. Bachmeyer, MD. "A Course in Hospital Administration." *Transactions of the American Hospital Association.* Vol. 21.

1922   Willard Rappelye. *Principles of Hospital Administration and Training of Hospital Executives.* Report of the Rockefeller Committee on the Training for Hospital Executives.

The Heroic Age: 1929–1945

1929   Michael M. Davis. *Hospital Administration: A Career.* New York: Privately published.

1937   Committee on Educational Policies of the ACHA. *University Training for Hospital Administration Career. A Report by the Committee on Educational Policies of the ACHA.* Chicago, ACHA.

The Age of the Practicioner: 1945–1965

1948   "The Prall Report." *The College Curriculum in Hospital Administration.* The Joint Commission on Education of the ACHA and AHA. Charles E. Prall, Director. Chicago, Physicians Record Company.

1954   "The Olsen Report." *University Education for Administration in Hospitals.* Commission on University Education in Hospital Administration. Herluf V. Olsen, Director. Washington, DC: American Council on Education.

The Age of the New Man: 1966–1980

1967   "Hospital Administration." *JACHA,* Special issue on Education, Fall 1967.

1969   T. E. Chester. *Graduate Education for Hospital Administration in the United States: Trends.* Chicago, ACHA.

1975,   "The Dixon Reports." Commission on Education for Health Administra-
1977   tion. Vol. 1, 1975; Vol. 2, 1975; Vol. 3, 1977. *A Future Agenda.* Ann Arbor, MI: Health Administration Press.

1978   *The Report of the Task Force on the Report of the Commission on Education for Health Administration.* Chicago: ACHA.

The Age of Lifelong Learning: 1980–present

1981   ACHE. *Enhancing Executive Competence: Educational and Practice Perspectives.* Chicago: ACHE.

1984   ACHE. *Report of the Task Force on Beginning and Early Career Development Programs in Health Services Administration.* Chicago: ACHE.

1984   ACHE (revised 1987). *Guidelines for Postgraduate Fellowships and Management Development Programs in Health Services Administration.* Chicago: ACHE.

1984   *First Directory of Postgraduate Fellowships and Management Development Programs in Health Services Administration.* Chicago: ACHE.

1992   ACHE, AUPHA. *Report of the Task Force on Beginning and Early Career Development.* Chicago: ACHE.

2004   AUPHA, CAHME. *Building the Profession Through Quality and Value for Health Administration Education and Practice: A Strategic Blueprint for the Future.* Chicago: ACHE.

2005   ACHE, AUPHA. *Pedagogy Enhancement Project for Entry and Early-Career Leadership Skills for Healthcare Management.* Chicago: ACHE.

The Committee also advocated that bachelor's degree preparation include prerequisites and that a fourth of the undergraduate curriculum be devoted specifically to hospital administration. Through a survey, the Committee discovered that 46 percent of current administrators were nurses and 28 percent were physicians. Because of this, the Committee recommended two separate educational tracks for these groups. The Committee stated:

> [T]he American College of Hospital Administrators is in no sense interested in discouraging doctors of medicine or graduate nurses entering the field of hospital administration; quite the contrary is the case. The College is merely interested in seeing to it that before a doctor of medicine or a registered nurse is designated a hospital administrator, he or she should have at least a rudimentary acquaintanceship with certain basic, professional and specialized aspects of the profession of hospital administration.

The Committee also recommended that a bachelor's degree program in hospital administration lead to master's degree education that would include the following subjects:

- English and preferably German
- Philosophy, including psychology
- History
- Science, preferably biology
- Accounting
- Finance
- Statistics
- Business management
- Industrial organization
- Personnel administration
- Sociology, including community organization, social problems, public welfare, and social service in hospital administration
- Socio-legal economic history, including economic history, principles of economics, and law
- Hospital administration, including hospital statistics, medical and nursing essentials, financial administration in hospitals, hospital staff organization, and legal problems

The fifth year would be taken up by an internship leading to a certificate. The sixth year, and possibly a seventh, would be committed to academic work leading to a master's degree in administration and organization, management, finance administration, or community relations. Half of these courses would be specifically related to the hospital field.

Sidebar 5-5. Historical Perspective

On October 19, 1937, Dr. Malcolm T. MacEachern sent a letter to ACHE affiliates inviting their comments on the Committee on Educational Policies' report. As can be expected, the response was mixed. At Dr. MacEachern's urging, ACHE published a number of these replies in *ACHA News*. Following is a sample of some of those replies.

Philip Vollmer, superintendent of Fairview Park Hospital, Cleveland, justified a liberal arts education on the grounds of creativity and self-understanding. He said, *"It is apparent that no profession today or of the future can be worthy of the name unless its representatives are men and women possessing a cultural background...but surely the creative professional man or woman must first understand through the medium of history, language, literature and philosophy, his world and himself, and from this proceed to concentration on the achievements and techniques of his chosen profession.*

Harvey Agnew, MD, secretary, Department of Hospital Service, Canadian Medical Association (and later director of the program at the University of Toronto), was concerned about the future of physician administrators. He said, *"On the question of relative superiority of medical, lay, or nursing administrators, I have always refrained from taking any active part. It has been my conviction that each one of these three types of administrators can fill a definite place in our general plan of hospital work, that each brings to the position of administrator a distinct viewpoint not shared as fully by the others, and that hospital administration is such a complex and varied undertaking that at best an administrator can expect to have but a portion of the qualifications required."* Agnew interpreted the report as suggesting that *"a mere handful of medical graduates scattered over the field as administrators would be adequate"* and *"that the Committee looks upon hospital administration primarily as a business."* The result of the lengthy training proposed for physician administrators would be to drive them out of this field, he believed. If there were mostly nonmedical administrators, *"the problem of cooperation with the AMA and ACS and other medical bodies would be intensified."* He wrote, *"it would be fatal if the medical profession and the hospitals became separated, or worked at cross purposes. This would be quite probable if the primary viewpoint of the hospital administrators became that of hospital economics and efficiency of organization rather than of the care of the patient."*

E. Muriel Anscombe, administrator of the Jewish Hospital, St. Louis, wrote, *"I am wondering if it might not be a good plan to supplement this report with one showing the turnover in administrative positions to give a true picture of the opportunities in this occupation. Social unrest as well as economic loss results from the overcrowding of any profession. Do you think that such a situation might develop in the field of hospital administration?"*

Asa Bacon, superintendent of The Presbyterian Hospital, Chicago, stated, *"I am sure it will need quite a campaign of education to make boards of managers (trustees) see the necessity of engaging trained people as administrators. The Committee on Educational Policies has done well not to demand 'slavish adherence to any program of preparation' but rather to point the way for a general understanding of what is needed."*

Amy Daniels, administrator, Wing Memorial Hospital, Palmer, Massachusetts, added, *"I trust...that you will also promote or provide facilities for hospital administrators who are occupying positions of responsibility to further their education and gain additional knowledge of hospital administration. I feel that [the College's] plan of regional institutes is an excellent one and will raise the standards of hospital administration."*

Sister M. Olivia, dean, school of nursing, The Catholic University of America, Washington, DC, thought the first five years for the nurse administrator were *"not feasible. Would it not be more desirable to construct a course for hospital administrators regardless of previous general or professional education?"* she asked.

S. B. Crawford, an assistant superintendent, Maryland General Hospital, who *"though having several years of college, is not a graduate,"* added, *"We are practical administrators, rather than college theorists. The result is reflected in the character of our service and in the financial statement at the end of the year. Without endowments and with a 46 percent free service, we show a credit balance at the end of our fiscal year. I personally am heartily in favor of a college education, but I do not feel that a qualified administrator should be refused admission, now or in the future, simply because he lacks 'a sheepskin.' "*

Two physicians, A. F. Anderson, MD, and A. K. Haywood, MD, wrote to express their fears that *"medical men as administrators will become a thing of the past."* According to Worth L. Howard, administrator at The City Hospital of Akron, Ohio, *"Probably 60 percent of the hospitals in the country are not of sufficient size to warrant the expenditure of employing an executive who has had this theoretical and practical training."*

For physicians who had completed their internships, it was proposed that there be one year of basic professional courses related to administration, a year of administrative internship leading to a certificate, and then one to two years of academic study leading to a master's degree in hospital administration. For nurses, there would be three years of nursing education, two years of general education, two years of professional courses related to hospital administration, and then a year of internship followed by one or two years of graduate study leading to a master's degree in hospital administration.

The Committee's proposal to not only restructure undergraduate training but also to initiate graduate education was developed at a time when there was only one degree program in existence, graduating a handful of students annually. As was to be expected, this proposal failed to define the educational future. However, it elicited widespread agreement that university education was essential for hospital administration, and laid the groundwork for future investigations.

In 1943, the Committee on Educational Policies was chaired by Dr. Arthur Bachmeyer.[26] The scope of this committee's activities included the following:

- Determination of policies for the development of institutes and reading courses
- Promotion of organized courses in universities for new entrants
- Development of educational programs for Nominees and Members seeking advancement in ACHE

- Creation of two- or three-day conferences for Fellows
- The promotion of scholarships for students

In the same year, the second master's degree program in hospital administration was started at Northwestern University in Evanston, Illinois, under the directorship of Dr. Malcolm MacEachern.

The Prall Report

In 1945, the W. K. Kellogg Foundation funded the Joint Commission on Education of the AHA and ACHA, chaired by Charles E. Prall,[27] an Honorary Fellow of ACHE. According to Prall,[28] "The Joint Commission on Education was the culmination of about 10 years of striving to upgrade the hospital superintendency." The Commission was one of several Kellogg initiatives to improve hospital management after years of stagnation during World War II. A main protagonist supporting health administration education was Andrew Pattullo, HFACHE, associate director of the division of hospitals at the W. K. Kellogg Foundation.

The Commission found that of 232 persons becoming administrators in larger voluntary hospitals, 18 percent came from occupations unrelated to health administration. Only 36 percent came to that position with experience as an assistant administrator or as an administrator of a smaller hospital, suggesting a limited amount of on-the-job learning.[29] The Commission felt that a good supply of college graduates in hospital administration would change this situation.[30, 31] After three-and-a-half years of work, the Commission produced its final report. The report focused primarily on graduate education, harkening back to the ideas of Michael Davis, and recommended a course and curriculum for training hospital administrators: *The College Curriculum in Hospital Administration*.

The Prall Report built its curriculum proposals upon its study of problems facing hospital administrators. It was therefore more practical and less academic, especially when compared to later studies. The major impact of this report was to stimulate interest in forming new graduate programs.

Concurrent with the work of the Commission, the Kellogg Foundation supported the creation of eight new university-based hospital administration graduate programs, all but one in schools of public health.[32] Like the original program at University of Chicago, these programs provided a year of internship and "curricula structured to give the student basic administrative skills with a strong emphasis on business management and the broad responsibility of the hospital in the field of public health."[33]

In the summer of 1947, ACHE reviewed the status of the ten existing degree programs in hospital administration.

1. *University of Chicago:* This program graduated 13 students in 1947, and three of these students were physicians.
2. *Columbia University:* This program, where C. W. Munger, MD, was serving as professor of hospital administration, graduated 22 students in 1947, six of whom were physicians. Munger was Chairman of ACHE from 1944 to 1946.
3. *Northwestern University:* This program was established in September 1943 and was directed by Dr. Malcolm MacEachern. In 1947, the program graduated students at both the bachelor's and master's degree levels.
4. *Duke University Medical School and Hospital:* This program opened in 1930 as a certificate program.
5. *Washington University:* Located in St. Louis, this program was the only one located in a medical school.
6. *University of Minnesota:* This program was directed by James A. Hamilton, former director of Grace New Haven Hospital, and included Ray Amberg, director of the University Hospital, on the faculty. Hamilton was Chairman of ACHE from 1939 to 1940. Amberg was a member of the Board of Regents.
7. *Yale University:* This program admitted its first class in 1947. Members of the Department of Public Health (Ira V. Hiscock, ScD, chairman) included Professor Albert Snoke, MD, director of Grace New Haven Hospital, and Clement O. Clay, MD, later director of the Columbia program.
8. *University of Iowa:* This program was also new and was jointly directed by Gerhard Hartman, PhD, superintendent of University Hospitals, and Dean E. T. Peterson of the Graduate College. Hartman was also executive secretary of ACHE from 1937 to 1941.
9. *St. Louis University:* This program, started in 1936 in collaboration with the CHA, had graduated six students by 1947.[34]
10. *The University of Toronto School of Hygiene:* This school offered a new program under the direction of G. Harvey Agnew, MD, and Leonard O. Bradley, MD,[35] associate professor. Agnew was an Honorary Charter Fellow of ACHE.

The Administrative Internship

In the 1930s, the administrative internship could exist independently of a degree program,[36] evolving easily out of the earlier administration apprenticeships. However, as previously mentioned, master's degree programs grew in the 1940s, and these programs often consisted of one academic year and one year of administrative internship or residency.

Hospital administration programs also developed links with particular administrators who served as mentors to students. These administrators were chosen because of their status as program graduates, their reputation as administrators, or their willingness to provide good learning experiences for students. If these administrators found students able, they would often be helpful in launching early careers.

By 1946, some graduate programs sought ACHE help in placing interns (some programs used the term "residencies") and students. Aware that to be a Nominee they must satisfactorily complete courses in hospital administration approved by ACHE, many students inquired whether certain internships would be acceptable to ACHE.

The Board of Regents agreed to set up a subcommittee of the Committee on Educational Policies to implement an internship approval program. The reaction to this action was mixed. Claude Munger, Chairman of ACHE in 1946, addressed ACHE as follows:

> It is my strong belief that the College should accept leadership in establishing an approval program for administrative apprenticeships, in somewhat the same manner as the American Medical Association maintains an approval program of hospitals desiring to offer medical internships. I urgently recommend that the College undertake such a project forthwith. Thought should be given also to the possibilities of initiating in the College an approval program for the hospital administration courses themselves. We already hear of plans of questionable soundness for the initiation of courses under various auspices.[37]

Dr. Prall believed that the responsibility for choosing an internship belonged to the university course director. Dean Conley, however, took the opposite view. ACHE's files on its affiliates could be a unique source of information about possible preceptors. All the existing course directors were Fellows or Members of ACHE, as were 900 chief administrators. Conley believed no

---

Sidebar 5-6. On a Personnel Note

The total number of degree graduates in the summer of 1947 was 48 at the master's level and one at the bachelor's level.[38] Many of the professors at these programs had close links to ACHE. For example, Arthur Bachmeyer, MD, Ray Brown, Claude Munger, and James Hamilton were all ACHE Chairman Officers; Malcolm MacEachern, MD, and Harvey Agnew, MD, were Honorary Charter Fellows; Michael Davis, PhD, was an Honorary Fellow; and Gerhard Hartman, PhD, was the second executive secretary of ACHE.

Sidebar 5-7. The 1947 Committee on Educational Policies

In 1947, the Committee on Educational Policies, chaired by Robin Buerki, MD, proposed a fundraising effort to achieve the following:

- Develop short-course institutes
- Improve master's degree and internship training
- Provide scholarships
- Improve criteria for selection of hospital administrators

Although little funding was available for this last component, ACHE continued to work on improving its admission and advancement criteria.[39]

developed internship program could exist without ACHE cooperation. Because membership in ACHE "was rapidly becoming essential to a successful career in hospital administration, few students would be so reckless as to accept an internship unsatisfactory to the College."[40]

As a result of ACHE's prodding, the Joint Commission on Education organized a conference in January 1947 at Columbia University to discuss the criteria for a good internship. Later that year the Commission published *The Administrative Internship in the Hospital*,[41] recommending that half the internship year be spent rotating through hospital departments.

After the end of the Joint Commission on Education's work in June 1948, ACHE continued to propose guidelines for administrative residency, as it came to be known. From 1949 to 1954, ACHE sponsored eight two day conferences for preceptors.[42]

> **Sidebar 5-8. Significant Statistics**
>
> In November 1961, there were 3,120 graduates from 16 graduate programs in hospital and health services administration.[44] Of these 3,120 graduates,[45]
>
> - 37 percent were administrators;
> - 24 percent were assistant administrators;
> - 8 percent were administrative assistants;
> - 5 percent were in other health field organizations;
> - 7 percent were in the armed forces; and
> - 19 percent were in other positions, such as department heads, teaching clinic managers, consultants, medical practitioners, and so forth.
>
> It was noteworthy that very few of the graduates had left the field.

ACHE's residency guidelines were republished regularly until 1965. After this date, with the growth of the two-year academic program, the residency was sometimes discontinued or reduced in length to a few months during the summer, and often designated as an internship.[43]

The Association of University Programs in Health Administration

The previously mentioned Joint Commission on Education of the AHA and the ACHA was "of marked assistance to various established (graduate) programs and aided in the establishment of new programs." One of the ways the Commission helped was by bringing together directors and faculty of different educational programs for discussion of common problems. The first of these discussion meetings was held at Purdue University in the fall of 1945.

By 1948, there were discussions, lead by the Kellogg Foundation, about forming an association, leading to the first formal meeting of the Association of University Programs in Hospital Administration (AUPHA) in May 1949 under the chairmanship of Dr. Arthur C. Bachmeyer of Northwestern University. The founding programs included the following:

- University of Chicago
- Northwestern University

- Columbia University
- University of Minnesota
- University of Toronto
- Washington University
- Yale University

In addition to the participating programs, standing invitations to participate went to ACHE, the AHA, and the Kellogg Foundation. When AUPHA developed professional staff in 1965, ACHE provided financial support that continued for several years.

By 1970 to 1971, the 33 member programs of AUPHA had 1,666 enrolled students.[46] In the early 1970s, AUPHA changed its name to the Association of University Programs in Health Administration to reflect the diverse interests of faculty and the varied positions taken by program graduates.[47] By 1978, AUPHA had become "an international consortium of 120 universities in 19 nations."[48] By 1982, the AUPHA consortium had grown to 153 educational programs in 144 colleges.

Since 1982, there has been tremendous growth in the number of undergraduate programs in health administration. In recent years, AUPHA has devoted substantial resources to conferences, seminars, and publications related specifically to undergraduate education. Undergraduate AUPHA membership rose from 31 programs with 3,697 students in 1996 to 45 programs with 4,268 students in 2003.[49] In 2006, the organization served 152 educational programs—91 graduate programs and 61 undergraduate programs—in 54 countries. As of July 1, 2006, full membership in AUPHA was restricted to master's degree programs that are accredited by the Commission on Accreditation of Healthcare Management Education (CAHME) and bachelor's degree programs that are certified by AUPHA. Programs that do no meet these criteria can become AUPHA affiliates, but they receive greatly restricted benefits.

The most important function of AUPHA is to provide members with the tools, research, venues, support, and forums that enable each program, as well as healthcare administration education as a whole, to evolve and thrive in a constantly changing field. The association also continues to create opportunities for leaders from the field of healthcare management education to gather and share information on educational methods and research, and it serves as an advocate for the health administration education community before various professional, legislative, and executive bodies.[50]

Throughout the years, AUPHA and ACHE have had a solid partnership, oftentimes working together to address a need or solve a problem.[51] For example, in 2004, ACHE and AUPHA partnered to examine the educational needs of early careerists. Both undergraduate and graduate programs affiliated with AUPHA educate a large proportion of the women and men who enter healthcare management positions in the United States and Canada. Recognizing the need to continuously improve the curriculum of these programs, ACHE partnered with AUPHA through the Pedagogy Enhancement Project on Leadership Skills for Healthcare Management. The project focused on the leadership knowledge and skills needed by graduates of healthcare management programs. Key elements of the project included the following:

- Identifying key leadership needs for entry-level and early-career managers in the healthcare system
- Developing organization and leadership curriculum materials to address identified needs
- Pilot testing the materials in selected AUPHA programs

Starting the fall semester of 2005, successfully piloted teaching materials were disseminated to AUPHA program faculty and other relevant professionals via a web site designed to facilitate the distribution of newly tested curriculum materials. In addition, deliverables and materials produced through this project were made available for use by ACHE.[52]

AUPHA partners with ACHE in other ways as well. For example, AUPHA participates in the ACHE Congress on Healthcare Leadership every year, holding its annual Leaders' conference there to enhance the relationship between academia and practicing executives. Conversely, ACHE sponsors a faculty forum on diversity for AUPHA, which comes together at AUPHA's annual meeting. AUPHA also has a long-standing publishing partnership with Health Administration Press (described in detail in Chapter 6).

The Olsen Report

In 1952, the W. K. Kellogg Foundation made a grant to AUPHA to establish a Commission on University Education in Hospital Administration. The Commission, chaired by James A. Hamilton (Chairman of ACHE from 1939 to 1940) and directed by Dartmouth Dean Herluf V. Olsen,[53] an Honorary Fellow of ACHE, published its report in 1954.[54]

A major component of the Commission's work was a survey of 6,000 hospital administrators, taken on by ACHE, to determine the administrators' present and future needs.[55] Within the survey, the Commission reviewed the existing 13 graduate programs and discussed issues related to research, faculty qualifications, admissions policies, teaching methods, and program costs.[56] The survey estimated that 602 hospital administrative positions would become available annually, and the Commission recommended that several additional graduate programs be established.[57] Further recommendations of the Olsen Report included the following:

- The age of admission to graduate programs should be between 21 and 27 years.[58] From 1934 to 1952, of 1,224 graduates, the average

age of an individual admitted to a graduate program was more than 30 years.[59]

- Candidates to the graduate programs should have two semesters of accounting as well as one semester each of statistics in administration, principles of administration, personnel administration, finance, marketing, business law, and general business conditions.
- Students should go directly from undergraduate training into the graduate program.
- Residency training should continue without exceptions for experience.
- Teaching in the graduate programs should be by seminar and, therefore, class size should be from 10 to 15 students. Research should be part of the program.
- Faculty should be composed of at least two full-time equivalents.[60]

Although not an explicit recommendation, the report also stated:

In the opinion of this Commission, the graduate curricula, teaching methods and materials, and personnel of the schools of business administration most nearly approximate those considered most desirable for the program that the Commission is proposing, with its emphasis on management and administration.[61]

The debate over this controversial suggestion nearly destroyed AUPHA, whose members split in their preference for a business school or a health profession–based educational program.[62] As a result, AUPHA did not publish the report of the Commission. It was published by the American Council on Education.

The Move Toward Multiyear Programs

During the late 1950s and early 1960s, the nature of graduate education programs again began to change. Some of the most prestigious programs began moving from a one-year curriculum to two years with a summer or no residency. For example, when the Cornell program started in 1958, it was a two-year academic program based in the Sloan School of Management.[63] In the 1960s, the University of Chicago program also changed to a two-year academic program, and other programs followed.[64] The shift to a two-year program occurred principally because faculty members believed that the required knowledge could not be conveyed in one academic year.

In the 1970s, three-year, two-degree programs appeared at Columbia and Yale, offering coordinated public health and business administration degrees.[65] A multiyear academic program effectively doubled the size of the on-campus student body, thereby building the economic foundation for a larger academic faculty for these programs. As these programs developed major funded research efforts, they were also able to support more full-time faculty.[66] The presence of full-time faculty tends to yield a more academic and scholarly research focus. Such a faculty brings a different perspective than one that has more administrative experience.

Sidebar 5-9. CAHME

In 1968, the Accrediting Commission on Graduate Education for Hospital Administration was incorporated in the state of Illinois as the accrediting agency in the field of graduate education in hospital administration. The joint sponsors of the agency included the following:

- ACHE
- AUPHA
- APHA
- AHA

The Accrediting Commission replaced an approval program, which had been conducted since the founding of AUPHA in 1948 and employed criteria for membership in the association as a measure of academic quality. As the field of hospital administration gained professional stature, healthcare organizations sought administrators with master's degrees from approved programs. The sponsors of the Accrediting Commission recognized the need for a more broadly based structure encompassing the rapidly growing community of interests in the field of education in hospital administration. The Accrediting Commission was modeled on The Joint Commission and was chaired by George Bugbee, FACHE.

Consequently, a plan for a formalized accreditation program was submitted and accepted in 1970 by what was then the National Commission on Accrediting (NCA). Hospital administration became the 33rd profession to gain recognition by the NCA Board, which represented university presidents.

The name of the Accrediting Commission was changed in 1976 to the Accrediting Commission on Education for Health Services Administration (ACEHSA). This name change occurred to reflect the broad spectrum of opportunities that exists within the profession of health administration.

In 1990, there were 57 accredited graduate programs and 64 in 1993.[67]

In 2001, a joint study group, which included representatives of ACHE, proposed in a document entitled "Final Report of the Blue Ribbon Task Force" a recommendation that ACEHSA be restructured. That restructuring included the creation of Corporate Members, of which ACHE was one.[68] With a new vision for the Commission, the name of the agency was changed to the CAHME in 2004. The Corporate Members, made up of professional societies, associations, and healthcare organizations, ratified a new set of bylaws in June 2005 creating a new board of directors. As of 2007, the board makes all decisions regarding accreditation of the 72 currently accredited programs. It also decides when new programs are admitted into the candidacy process.[69] CAHME has been granted formal recognition by the United States Department of Education as the only organization to accredit master's-level healthcare management programs in the United States.

Throughout the years, ACHE has provided and continues to provide valuable leadership to CAHME. In addition to having ACHE affiliates on the CAHME board of directors and in other leadership positions, many ACHE Fellows and Members serve as site visitors, providing valuable advice and guidance to program faculties.

As faculty was drawn increasingly from scholarly academic disciplines, proportionately fewer were practicing hospital administrators who could qualify for ACHE membership.[70] As more programs moved to two academic years, the linkage between academia and practice changed. As discussed in Chapter 4, just prior to 1960 ACHE responded to the growth in full-time faculty by making the following modification to its admission criteria:

Sidebar 5-10. Historical Perspective

In 1969, Professor Theodore (Teddy) Chester of the University of Manchester, England, wrote a report entitled *Graduate Education for Hospital Administration in the United States,* which ACHE published without officially endorsing its content. Although Chester found the U.S. programs in a rapid state of growth, he nevertheless concluded that the 400 students expected to graduate in 1968 were not an adequate number.

In his report, Chester stated,

It seems to me possible to divide the development of (the graduate) programs since their inception into three distinct periods: "The age of the pioneers," "the age of the practitioners," and "the age of the new man," the latter of which is just emerging. The "heroic age" can be said to have begun in 1929 with the Michael Davis book. This period, which came to an end around 1945, was characterized by the pioneering efforts and the outstanding personalities of Dr. Arthur C. Bachmeyer and Dr. Malcolm T. MacEachern.

During the subsequent period—from 1945 to 1965—students graduating from (the first) two programs became the disciples of their masters; they spread their words and their writings over the face of the United States. A substantial number of them became themselves program directors. Generally speaking, they saw as the main goal of the newly founded schools training for the practice of hospital administration. They did not bother too much about generalized theory or fundamental research, but relied on...their own practical experience and achievements as a major source of their teaching material.

The curriculum for the programs to which Chester referred consisted of one academic year, plus the residency and a thesis. "Program faculty lived at best in uneasy coexistence with the other members of the university," concluded Chester.[71] As time passed, Chester saw the picture change:

More and younger men are coming forward, some already as program directors, who themselves have a very respectable academic background, including doctorates, and who are not only anxious to put the whole teaching program on a sound theoretical basis but also to prove to all their colleagues in the university that their academic respectability is without blemish. It seems to me that it is largely against this background that the recent trend to increase the time allocated to academic studies, while decreasing practical training, has to be seen.[72]

Candidates who are duly appointed faculty members of an approved course in hospital administration at the time of their election to the College, and have completed satisfactorily an approved course in hospital administration, or have had the required years of experience in a responsible administrative position in a hospital..., have the same eligibility..., as persons actively engaged in hospital administration.

The Dixon Report

In 1972, the W. K. Kellogg Foundation funded the Commission on Education for Health Administration. As with previously discussed study groups, its purpose was to determine the state of health administration education and make recommendations for the future. The Commission was chaired by James P. Dixon, MD, a former hospital administrator and president of Antioch College, and included Charles Austin, PhD, director of the Xavier University Graduate Program in Hospital and Health Administration as its staff director.[73]

Working from 1972 to 1974 and publishing two volumes in 1975 and a third in 1977,[74] the Commission found that fewer than 25 percent of executive positions were filled by people with education in health administration. They recommended diversity in academic approaches to meet these needs.[75] The Commission's 30 percent sample of 2,402 health administration program graduates (2,100 with master's degrees, 170 with baccalaureate degrees, and 132 with associate degrees) showed the following[76]:

- 57 percent went into hospital administration
- 13 percent went into government agencies
- 7 percent went into health planning
- 7 percent went on to further their education
- 4 percent went into ambulatory care
- 4 percent went into long-term care and mental health administration
- 4 percent became university faculty
- 3 percent went into voluntary health agencies
- 1 percent went into third-party agencies

These statistics demonstrated the diversity of organizations and positions available.

Sidebar 5-11. Historical Perspective

Jon Jaeger, FACHE, writing in 1972, said,

Since its inception 50 years ago, education for hospital administration has undergone an amazing transformation. Originally a highly pragmatic, situationally oriented instruction format, course curricula by successive stages have now become increasingly theoretical with increasing reliance upon empirical rather than intuitive decision methods. And while the advantages attributed to older approaches are still wistfully remembered, the forces that have brought about the current orientation are rooted in the basic changes occurring in our twentieth-century society.[77]

Sidebar 5-12. Significant Statistics

In addition to reporting the fields program graduates entered after graduation, the Dixon Report also revealed the following:

- Program graduates felt that their graduate programs were strongest in administrative theory and weakest in financial management, systems analysis, and electronic data processing.[79]
- In the master's degree programs, 61 percent of the faculty held doctorate degrees, and the average number of full-time faculty was 5.7.
- Thirteen percent of master's program students were minorities.[80]

ACHE appointed a task force, chaired by R. Zach Thomas Jr. to study the Dixon Report.[78] This task force and ACHE leadership viewed the Dixon report as "developed largely by educators and for educators," ignoring the role of both the practitioner and ACHE in education. The report led to a discussion about how ACHE might broaden its admission and advancement criteria to fit the developing specialized areas in healthcare administration. The ACHE task force pointed out that the Dixon Commission defined healthcare administration very broadly, including the following:

- Hospital administration (17,000 to 18,000 practitioners)
- Nursing home administration (16,000 to 20,000 practitioners)
- Voluntary health agencies (10,000)
- Public health agency administration (5,000 to 6,000)
- Clinic management (1,000)
- Comprehensive health planning (500 to 1,000)

Although the Commission found that only one-fourth of these managers had education in health administration, the ACHE task force pointed out that this lack of specialized education was hardly the case for hospitals for which the supply of program graduates was abundant and perhaps even excessive.

The task force recommended that "universities should give serious attention to developing an appropriate alignment between programs of professional education and employment opportunities for graduates." Explicitly taking an administrative practitioner perspective, the task force urged that the graduate program faculty "translate the realities of administrative practice into educational endeavors." The task force report said, "Opportunities and incentives for faculty development should be geared less to scholarly endeavor in the academic tradition and more to pursuits enabling educators to keep abreast of advances in the professional practice of health administration." In addition, the task force stressed a major point, "The professional society creates an orientation and an environment conducive to the lifelong learning which undergirds development of administrative competence and leadership. Beyond this the professional society is cognizant of the educational needs of the practitioners, and is in an advantageous position to design structured educational programs responsive to these needs." The task force finally recommended that ACHE expand its educational functions "through the development of specialized examinations in major areas of health administration."

Building Bridges with Academia

While the 1970s saw the greatest separation of academia and ACHE, the 1980s saw the development of new ways to build bridges. For example, a new faculty category of ACHE affiliation was created and the membership category of "Student Associates" was started. In addition, arrangements to allow faculty to spend time in healthcare organizations were undertaken, and the appointment of faculty editorial boards for book publishing created new links.

Other initiatives to link graduate education with ACHE included a student competition, which at first invited student teams from accredited master's programs in health administration to participate in a computer simulation "game." Developed by faculty at Georgia State University, the game offered students the opportunity to play consecutive rounds. The top three programs' participants were then invited to come to the Congress on Administration to finish the game. Later, this competition was replaced by an essay-writing contest—one for students at the master's level and one for those at the baccalaureate level. A list of contest winners can be found in Appendix 3.

All the previously mentioned links with education culminated when James Hepner, PhD, the program director at Washington University, became ACHE chair from 1991 to 1992. In addition, Kenneth R. White, PhD, professor and director of the graduate program in health administration at Virginia Commonwealth University in Richmond, was ACHE Regent-at-Large from 2002 to 2004 and served on the Board of Governors from 2004 to 2007.

Another way that ACHE strengthened its link with health administration education was by playing a more active role in supporting health services research, including through the following actions:

- Becoming an institutional sponsor of the Association for Health Services Research.
- Sponsoring an annual best paper award for the Academy of Management's Health Administration Section.
- Providing the Health Management Research Award to encourage faculty from health administration programs to conduct research to enhance managerial effectiveness and career opportunities in health services administration. A list of Health Management Research Award winners can be found in Appendix 3.

More information on ACHE's role in health services research can be found in Chapter 7.

ACHE's Continuing Education Programs

Throughout the years, ACHE's role in education has not been limited to supporting and collaborating with graduate programs in healthcare administration. In fact, in the first 25 years of ACHE, one of its largest undertakings was short educational programs. The following sections provide a discussion of the variety of continuing education programs, both past and present, offered by ACHE.

ACHE Institutes

ACHE Institutes, first started in 1933, lasted up to two weeks, were usually held in conjunction with a university, and were often cosponsored by other associations. The programs were designed to be refresher courses for professionals actually involved in administration at the time.[81] As previously mentioned, early on, in the absence of degree programs, the Institutes were a major source of education in hospital administration.

The first ACHE-sponsored Institute was held from September 18 to October 6, 1933. Entitled the "Chicago Institute for Hospital Administrators," it was held under the auspices of the University of Chicago, the AHA, the American Medical Association, the American College of Surgeons, and the Chicago Hospital Association. One hundred ninety-six administrators attended.[82]

From 1933 to 1947, Institutes were held annually and continued with the same sponsoring organizations. From 1948 to the 23rd program in 1953, the Institutes were sponsored by the University of Chicago and ACHE alone. There were also five one-week Chicago Advanced Institutes from 1950 to 1954.

Beginning in 1948, other regional Institutes were held in addition to the one in

---

Sidebar 5-13. On a Personnel Note

One way ACHE and academia have merged is through the background of five of the six ACHE chief executive officers (CEOs):

1. Gerhard Hartman, PhD (1937 to 1941), was concurrently a faculty member at the University of Chicago.
2. Dean Conley (1942 to 1965) was, prior to working for ACHE, business manager of the University of Minnesota Health Service from 1935 to 1941.
3. Richard J. Stull (1965 to 1979) was the founding director of the program at the University of California, Berkeley.
4. Stuart A. Wesbury Jr., PhD (1979 to 1991), was director of the graduate program in health services management at the University of Missouri–Columbia from 1972 to 1978.
5. Thomas C. Dolan, PhD (1991 to the present), was on the faculty of the graduate program in health services management at the University of Missouri–Columbia and was director of the Saint Louis University Center for Health Services Education and Research from 1979 to 1986.

Chicago. Of the other regional Institutes, the Minnesota Institute, with 1,006 total participants in 15 Institutes, had the largest attendance (see Figure 5-2).

The topics covered in the Institutes varied. For example, the 13th Chicago Institute—held in September 1945—covered the following topics:

- Operating fundamentals of organizations
- Nursing education
- Hospital planning and construction
- Maintenance of the physical plant
- Volunteer services
- Food services
- Public relations
- Laundry and linen

FIGURE 5-2
The Institutes for Hospital Administration, 1933 to 1955[83]

Years	Number, Name, and Location of Institute	Duration of Each Institute	Total Attendance
1933–1955	23 Chicago Institutes at the University of Chicago	2 weeks	2,738
1950–1954	5 Chicago Advanced Institutes at the University of Chicago	1 week	242
1941–1954	6 Midwest Institutes at the University of Colorado at Boulder and Denver, and at Women's College	1 week	355
1939–1955	15 Minnesota Institutes at the University of Minnesota	1 week	1,006
1940–1953	6 New England Institutes at Harvard University, Brown University, La Salle University, and Yale University	10 days	443
1939–1954	6 New York Institutes at Columbia University, Cornell University, and Francis Delafield Hospital	2 weeks	528
1952	1 Southeastern Institute at the University of Tennessee	1 week	105
1939–1954	9 Southern Institutes at Duke University, the University of Tennessee, Rollins College, Medical College of Virginia, and others	1 week	625
1941–1953	4 Southwestern Institutes at Southern Methodist University, Baylor University, and the University of Houston	1 week	308
1938–1954	6 Western Institutes at Stanford University	10 days	491
1947–1951	3 Canadian Institutes at the University of Western Ontario and Queen's University	1 week	273
1940, 1944	2 Inter American Institutes in San Juan, Lima, and Mexico City, and the University of Puerto Rico	2–3 weeks	169

Sidebar 5-14. Significant Statistics

In addition to the Institutes, ACHE sponsored short courses and meetings from 1933 to 1955. Some of these courses included the following[85]:

- From 1944 to 1954, ten Fellows' seminars lasting four days each were located at universities throughout the country (255 total attendees).
- From 1945 to 1949, four Members' conferences (196 total attendees).
- From 1951 to 1955, 17 conferences on human relations throughout North America lasting two days each (883 total attendees).
- From 1949 to 1954, eight two-day meetings on graduate education for hospital administrators. These focused primarily on residency preceptor training (431 total attendees).
- In 1955, three four-day educational conferences for hospital administrators (273 attendees).

Thus, in 22 years, ACHE sponsored short courses with a total attendance of 9,313.

- Analysis of financial statements
- Purchasing
- Fundraising
- Medical records
- Public health

A large part of the two-week course was taken up with visits to Chicago hospitals. The faculty at the 13th Chicago Institute included Drs. Claude Munger, Malcolm MacEachern, Robin Buerki, and Charles Wilinsky.[84]

By 1963, the Institutes had declined in attendance, and in June 1964 the Board of Regents adopted a new educational approach: annual Assemblies in each of the eight ACHE districts plus a Fellows' Seminar. The first of these Assemblies was held at the University of California at Berkeley from June 21 to 25, 1965. In 1966, ACHE provided eight Regional Assemblies and the Fellows seminar. By 1968, in addition to the Regional Assemblies, seminars on executive skills were given across the country.

The Congress on Healthcare Leadership

The annual Congress on Administration of ACHE started in 1958. Ray Brown, a member of the Board of Regents at that time, chaired the committee to organize the first Congress. The American Hospital Association (AHA) provided a contribution of $5,000 to start it.

A Congress brought together leading thinkers on administration to share ideas. For example, the 1961 Congress included the following speakers:

- Melville Dalton and Warren Bennis on administration
- Raymond A. Bauer on motivational research
- Donald Pelz on controls
- James D. Thompson on organizational conflict

The 1983 Congress on Administration drew 3,600 attendees and listed 50 seminars. The titles reflected a competitive corporate world, addressing such issues as diversification, competition, physician recruitment, computer systems, and image management. Eighteen percent of the presentations were made by ACHE Fellows. These topics demonstrated how ACHE successfully merged general management theory with the professional life of the hospital and health services manager by the time of its 50th anniversary.

The 1993 Congress had 4,300 attendees and reflected the previously mentioned issues as well as some others. Ninety-five management seminars were offered, including general management programs and a number of seminars designed specifically for CEOs and nurse, physician, long-term care, and managed care executives. Titles reflecting ACHE's efforts to meet the needs of healthcare executives from diverse settings and disciplines included the following:

- CEO leadership in medical staff succession and transition planning
- Key planning criteria for patient care units of the future
- Developing physician support for major strategic initiatives
- Long-term care facility trends
- Ongoing management of contract relationships

In 1985, the Congress on Administration was renamed the Congress on Healthcare Management to stress the active role of management over the more passive role of administration. In 2006, the Congress changed its name from the Congress on Healthcare Management to the Congress on Healthcare Leadership to further emphasize the importance of leadership in healthcare. Healthcare leaders were invited to attend the Congress to further their professional development, learn from experts and peers, and network with colleagues. The Congress offered keynote events, group discussions, networking receptions, and career planning sessions. There were 6 general sessions and 88 seminars spread across four days. These offerings addressed a variety of topics, including the following:

- Building a quality culture
- Emergency preparedness: What CEOs have learned
- The future of Medicaid
- The IT [information technology] factor
- Managing physician relations
- Reinventing the patient experience
- Improving executive competence through 360-degree performance evaluation
- Strengthening the role of ethics in everyday decision making

To this day, the Congress remains the major educational activity of ACHE and the largest gathering of healthcare executives in the country.

Other Educational Programs

In the 1980s, ACHE offered seminars and Executive Briefings. The seminars focused on particular topics while the briefings typically consisted of six speakers, each presenting a different topic. The briefings and seminars were two or two-and-one-half days in length, and were held from 4 to 12 times a year at various sites throughout the country. Fees were charged. Non-affiliates of ACHE could attend, but at slightly higher fees.

By 1993, ACHE was meeting the diverse learning needs of healthcare executives through a wide variety of educational programs, including conferences. These were two-day programs characterized by large attendance and leading speakers on a variety of healthcare management topics. ACHE also offered Institutes, which were characterized by workshop formats, smaller attendance, and in-depth coverage of a single topic. In 1993, some of the conferences and institutes ACHE presented included the following:

- *The Healthcare Management Ethics Conference:* A program that helped raise awareness of issues related to responsible and ethical decision making
- *The Eastern and Western Conferences:* Regional programs that offered major addresses, educational seminars, skill-assessment programs, membership activities, and career-planning presentations
- *The Partnership Institute:* A three-day workshop for teams of board chairs, CEOs, and medical staff presidents
- *The Healthcare Executive Leadership Development Institute:* A five-day skill-assessment and enhancement program for senior-level executives
- *The Healthcare Executive Public Policy Institute:* A three-day workshop that provided an intensive look at the healthcare policymaking process

In addition to conferences and institutes, ACHE held 133 offerings of 23 different seminars. Among ACHE's offerings was a special Canadian seminar that addressed issues of interest to Canadian healthcare executives and a special program exclusively for Fellows of ACHE. Other ACHE seminars focused on a variety of topics, including the following:

- Healthcare reform
- Integrated delivery networks
- Community collaboration

- Managed care
- Hospital-affiliated group practices

Presented in a classroom, the seminars provided an opportunity for one-on-one interaction with faculty.

ACHE seminars today are held at programs called "Clusters," which allow participants to choose from one or two of the six or more highly rated seminars offered at one location in a single week. In 1993, 12 cluster programs were offered. For example, the January 25 to 29, 1993, Cluster in Scottsdale, Arizona, included 12 seminars that addressed the following topics:

- High-performance internal operations
- Hospital design and construction
- Executive skills
- Personal financial planning
- Communication
- Ambulatory care assessment
- Law and legislation updates
- Managing clinical resources
- Rebuilding the healthcare workforce
- Total quality management
- Participative management
- Return on investment

To help affiliates unable to travel, ACHE offers several self-directed learning programs, which are based on books published by the Health Administration Press (see Chapter 6). These Self-Study courses enable affiliates to earn continuing education credits without having to travel to conferences or seminars.

By 2007, ACHE had greatly expanded its educational offerings to reflect the changing dynamic of the healthcare leader. As previously mentioned, more individuals in leadership positions were coming from business and other nontraditional backgrounds. In addition, physicians, nurses, and other clinicians were also filling roles in healthcare leadership. ACHE needed to provide programs that addressed both the clinical and business aspects of the healthcare management role. In addition, the amount of time an individual had available for continuing education was becoming more limited. ACHE needed to provide programs that were streamlined, time-sensitive, and available at a variety of locations. Some of the new programs created to address these factors included the following:

- *CEO/COO/Physician Executive Boot Camps.* These programs are held on the Sunday before Congress and provide intensive instruction on mastering the roles of the CEO, chief operating officer (COO), or physician executive. Some topics within the Boot Camps include working with your board, ensuring quality of care, establishing positive physician and staff relationships, an overview of the essential skills needed to function as an effective COO, and how to move beyond traditional clinical training and navigate the role of a physician executive.

- *Leadership Development Institute.* Initially called the "Healthcare Executive Leadership Development Institute" discussed above, this five-day offering was retooled in 1997 as a three-day event that focuses on an individual's personal leadership skills. Through confidential individual coaching sessions with faculty, the Leadership Development Institute gives helpful and illuminating information about an individual's leadership and decision-making style and his or her impact on others.

- *Distance Learning.* Distance learning was created to reach out to individuals who cannot attend face-to-face meetings. ACHE offers audio conferences on hot topics in the healthcare field and online seminars (or "Webinars") that allow an individual to work at his or her own pace using a case study approach. Webinars also allow individuals to interact with other online seminar participants via an electronic bulletin board.

- *Senior Executive Institute.* The purpose of the Senior Executive Institute is to provide senior executives with information on how to carry out their role in the healthcare organization. It offers networking opportunities and is designed to further develop the operational, interpersonal, and overall leadership skills an individual needs for success. This in-depth educational offering takes place over three, three-day sessions across four months. Participants attend the three different sessions and have assignments to complete between each session.

- *Ethics Seminar.* This seminar uses case studies to demonstrate how improving the ethical environment of an organization can help enhance clinical and financial outcomes, while also creating patient and staff satisfaction.

- *On-Location Programs.* ACHE offers high-quality educational programs to healthcare organizations and systems, hospital associations, and ACHE Chapters through the On-Location Program. The sessions are customized to meet an organization's or community's needs and provide Category I credits. They make continuing education convenient and minimize participants' time away from the office and travel costs. Each On-Location Program is presented by experienced educators and practitioners who provide in-depth information and proven problem-solving techniques to address the issues facing executives and their organization.

- *ACHE Chapter Education Programs.* These were designed to provide high-quality educational opportunities for ACHE Chapters at low cost, while at the same time providing a focal point around which Chapter members can meet and network. Hosted locally, these programs run from one to one-and-one-half hours, while offering Category I credits. The educational programs typically are delivered as a panel presentation high-lighting "hot topics." Among the most popular topics are career position-ing, medical staff relations, the future of hospital financing, and developing and leading high-performance teams.

More than 30 educational titles are delivered through ACHE's Clus-ter Seminars. In 2007, 13 different clusters were offered throughout the country. With six to eight seminar options in each Cluster, participants have the opportunity to learn about a variety of topics in one setting. For exam-ple, the May 2007 Cluster in New York offered the following topics:

- Creating and guiding the information-driven hospital
- The path to achieving superior productivity
- Developing proactive physician alignment and employment practices
- Understanding and influencing physician behavior
- Critical financial skills for hospital success
- Achieving physician/hospital partnerships: The clinical institute model
- Ensuring patient and employee satisfaction
- Integration versus competition

Self-Study courses also continued to do well, with 28 courses available in 2007. Some of the topics covered included the following:

- Understanding healthcare financial statements
- Leadership
- Healthcare human resources
- Preparing a long-range facility investment strategy
- The role of communication in patient safety
- Healthcare strategic planning

While education is one of the most important activities in which ACHE engages, there are other aspects of the organization that are equally as important. Chapters 6 and 7 discuss some of those activities.

Endnotes

1.   Stull, R. J., quoting Cyril O. Houle. Stull, R. J., "Foreword," in Houle, C. O., "The Lengthened Line of Education," June 1969, reprinted from *Perspectives in Biology and Medicine*, Vol. II, No. 1, Autumn 1967.

2.   Davis, M. M., *Hospital Administration: A Career*. New York: Privately pub-lished, 1929, pp. 90–93.

3.   Goodrich, A. W., "How Shall the Superintendents of Small Hospitals Be

Trained?" *Transaction of the American Hospital Association*, Vol. 18, 1916, p. 361.

4.   Shanahan, R. J. *The History of the Catholic Hospital Association 1915–1965*. St. Louis, MO: The Catholic Hospital Association of the United States and Canada, 1965, p. 60.

5.   Rappleye, W. C. *Principles of Hospital Administration and the Training of Hospital Executives.* Report of the Rockefeller Committee on the Training for Hospital Executives, 1922; "Committee on Training of Hospital Executives Issues Momentous Report," *Modern Hospitals*, Vol. 19, No. 1, July 1922, pp. 1–6.

6.   Shanahan, R. J. *The History of the Catholic Hospital Association 1915–1965*. St. Louis, MO: The Catholic Hospital Association of the United States and Canada, 1965, p. 60.

7.   Davis, M. M., *Hospital Administration: A Career.* New York: Privately published, 1929, pp. 90–93.

8.   Shanahan, R. J. *The History of the Catholic Hospital Association 1915–1965. St. Louis*, MO: The Catholic Hospital Association of the United States and Canada, 1965, pp. 60–61.

9.   Bachmeyer, A. C., "A Course in Hospital Administration." *Transactions of the American Hospital Association*, Vol. 21, 1919.

10. Davis, M. M., *Hospital Administration: A Career.* New York: Privately published, 1929.

11. Ibid., p. 90.

12. Ibid. This was not the first such list. The 1922 Rappleye report listed curriculum content, and in Sept. 1920 Dr. Goldwater listed the content areas for the administrator's self-education.

13. *Michael M. Davis, A Tribute*. Chicago: Center for Health Administration Studies, University of Chicago, 1972.

14. "Julius Rosenwald." *Chicago Tribute Markers of Distinction*. [Online article; retrieved 7/16/07. www.chicagotribute.org/Markers/Rosenwald.htm

15. Davis, M. M., "Development of the First Graduate Program in Hospital Administration," in Brown, R. (editor), *Graduate Education for Hospital Administration: Proceedings of a National Symposium, Dec 12–13, 1958*. Chicago: Graduate Program in Health Administration, University of Chicago, 1959 pp. 6–21; Davis, M. M., 1938 (ACHA reprint). Davis, M. M., "Studies in Hospital Administration at the University of Chicago." *Hospitals*, Mar. 1936.

16. *ACHA News*, Jan. 1938, p. 11. "Kellogg didn't become interested until Andrew Pattullo, who was, I think, in the last class I taught with Bachmeyer [at the University of Chicago], left to join Graham Davis and Emory Morris in his [administrative] residency or fellowship at Kellogg." L. Weeks interview with G. Hartman, 1982, p. 13. Because Kellogg funded the first wave of new hospital administration programs after World War II, this is one way the Chicago program influenced education in hospital administration.

17. Hartman, G., "Graduate Education in Hospital Administration 1934–1937." *Journal of Business of the University of Chicago*, Vol. XI, No. 4, pp. 1–13, Oct. 1938.

18. *ACHA Curriculum in Hospital Administration* (Chicago: ACHA, 1948), projected a yearly need for 230 new administrators and not less than 160, pp. 77–83.

19. L. Weeks interview with G. Hartman, 1982, pp. 12–13.

20. Kipnis, I. A. *A Venture Forward: A History of the American College of Hospital Administrators*. Chicago: ACHA, 1955, p. 27.

21. Ibid., pp. 27–28.

22. Parts 1 through 4 were presented Feb. 17, 1936. Parts 5 and 6 were presented Sept. 28, 1936. Summary, Conclusions, Principles, and Recommendations were presented to the Committee on Educational Policies on Feb. 15, 1937. The whole document was published with a foreword by Rev. Schwitalla in 1937. Thus, it became known as the "Schwitalla report" and titled *University Training for Hospital Administration Careers, A Report by the Committee on Educational Policies of the ACHA*, M. T. MacEachern, M.D., chairman, (Chicago: ACHA) 1937. The members of this committee were Father Schwitalla; Robert Bishop, MD; Robert E. Neff; Nathaniel W. Faxon, MD (director of the Massachusetts General Hospital); Joseph C. Doane, MD; and Michael M. Davis, PhD.

23. "In the minds of many present-day administrators there is some anxiety lest this rapidly spreading realization of the value of adequate training for administration should undermine their own personal position. For those individuals who just drifted into administration years ago when little beyond personal acceptability was required, adequate contact with the achievements of today can be maintained by attending Institutes, not once but repeatedly." Agnew, G. H. (president of the American Hospital Association), "Training in Hospital Administration," *Hospitals*, Vol. 13, No. 7, July 1939, pp. 73–74.

24. Wren, G. R., "An Historic View of Hospital Administration Education." *Hospital & Health Services Administration*, Vol. 25, No. 3, Summer 1980, p. 34.

25. Sources: Chester, T. E. *Graduate Education for Hospital Administration in the United States: Trends*. Chicago: ACHA, 1969 (Chester's terms describe the teachers and program faculty of these times.); and Dalston J., L. D. Prybil, H. Berman, and J. S. Lloyd, "Transforming the Accreditation of Healthcare Management Education." *Inquiry*, 2005–2006, Vol. 42, No. 4, pp. 320–334.

26. The other members of the committee were Benjamin Black, MD; Robin Buerki, MD; Claude Munger, MD; James A. Hamilton; Malcolm T. MacEachern, MD; Ada Belle McCleery; and Lucius R. Wilson, MD. Consultants to the committee were Robert Elsasser, Edward Fitzpatrick, H. V. Olsen, and L. C. White.

27.   W. K. Kellogg Foundation. *The First Twenty-Five Years*. Battle Creek, MI: Privately printed, 1955. The grant was $94,700. Kipnis, I. A. *A Venture Forward: A History of the American College of Hospital Administrators*. Chicago: ACHA, 1955, p. 90.

28.   Prall was a former dean of education at the University of Pittsburgh, 1934–1938; field coordinator at the American Council on Education, 1939–1944; and later dean of the school of education, Woman's College, University of North Carolina, 1949–1958.

29.   Prall, C. *The College Curriculum in Hospital Administration*. Chicago: Physicians Record Company, 1948, pp. 75–80. This was based on a mailed questionnaire to new administrators between 1945 and 1946 from hospitals listed in the American Hospital Directory of the AHA. The sample was confined to 1,700 hospitals of between 75 and 600 beds, but it excluded federal and Catholic hospitals.

30.   Prall, C. E., "A Review of the Report of the Joint Commission on Education for Hospital Administration," in Brown, R. E. (editor), *Graduate Education for Hospital Administration: Proceedings of a National Symposium, Dec. 12–13, 1958*. Chicago: Graduate Program in Health Administration, University of Chicago, 1959, p. 30. The Joint Commission members were R. H. Bishop Jr., MD (chairman); Frank R. Bradley; Arthur Bachmeyer; R. C. Buerki; George Bugbee; J. R. Clemmons, MD; Dean Conley; Edwin Crosby, MD; James A. Hamilton; Edgar C. Hayhow; Malcolm MacEachern; Ada Belle McCleery; Claude Munger; Sister M. Patricia; J. Gilbert Turner, MD; and staff Charles E. Prall and Paul B. Gillen. Prall, C. *The College Curriculum in Hospital Administration*. Chicago: Physicians Record Company, 1948, pp. 75–80.

31.   Wren, G. R., "An Historical View of Health Administration Education." *Hospitals & Health Services Administration*, Vol. 25, No. 3, Summer 1980, p. 34.

32.   W. K. Kellogg Foundation. *The First Twenty-Five Years*. Battle Creek, MI: Privately printed, 1955. These programs were Columbia University, Johns Hopkins University (not a hospital administration program, specifically), Yale University, Washington University of St. Louis, University of Minnesota, and universities in Toronto, Chile, and Sao Paulo, Brazil.

33.   W. K. Kellogg Foundation. *The First Twenty-Five Years*. Battle Creek, MI: Privately printed, 1955, p. 108.

34.   Sister Mary Giovani of St. Joseph, Minnesota, received the first degree in 1940.

35.   Rackow, V. *50: A Fifty-Year Retrospective, Department of Health Administration, University of Toronto*. Toronto: The Department, 1997, p. 4.

36.   This was the case at Duke.

37.   Kipnis, I. A. *A Venture Forward: A History of the American College of Hospital Administrators*. Chicago: ACHA, 1955, p. 93.

38.   "HM Salutes Frank R. Bradley, MD." *Hospital Management*, Vol. 85, April 1958, p. 34. Wren, (Wren, G. R., "An Historical View of Health Administration Education." *Hospitals & Health Services Administration*, Vol. 25, No. 3,

Summer 1980, p. 36) greatly overestimates the number of graduates in 1948. In 1948 Dean Conley reported 76 program graduates, rising to 165 graduates in 1952. Conley, D. "Professional Education in Hospital Administration." *Higher Education*, Vol. 9, No. 17, May 1, 1953 (U.S. Department of Health, Education, and Welfare).

39.   M. R. Barnes, consulting psychologist, University Hospitals, Cleveland. Kipnis, I. A. *A Venture Forward: A History of the American College of Hospital Administrators*. Chicago: ACHA, 1955, p. 88.

40.   Kipnis, I. A. *A Venture Forward: A History of the American College of Hospital Administrators*. Chicago: ACHA, 1955, p. 95.

41.   Gillen, P. B., and C. E. Prall. *The Administrative Internship in the Hospital: A Manual and Guide*, Chicago: Joint Commission on Education, 1947; *The Hospital Administrative Internship: A Conference Report*, Joint Commission on Education of the AHA and ACHA, held at Columbia University, New York, 1947.

42.   Kipnis, I. A. *A Venture Forward: A History of the American College of Hospital Administrators*. Chicago: ACHA, 1955, p. 141.

43.   Filerman, G. L., "Toward a Reexamination of Education for Health Administration," in Stimson, R., and S. Taylor (editors), *Executive Development for Graduates of Master's Degree Programs in Hospital and Health Care Administration*. Berkeley, CA: Graduate Program in Hospital Administration, University of California, 1973, p. 68.

44.   Hartman, G., S. Levey, and T. McCarthy, "The Impact of Graduate Programs in Hospital Administration." *Hospital Administration*, Vol. 7, Spring 1962, Table 1.

45.   Hartman, G., S. Levey, and T. McCarthy, "The Graduate Programs and Their Alumni." *Hospitals*, Feb. 16, 1962, pp. 54–57.

46.   Brown, R. E., in *Education for Health Services Administration at the University of Michigan, Proceedings of the Workshops*, 1972, p. 27.

47.   Wesbury, S. A. "Background Information Concerning the Proposal to Change the Name and Objects of the American College of Hospital Administrators." Chicago: ACHA, April 1981, pp. 4–5.

48.   "Foreword," Filerman, G., in Quatrano, L. A., *Health Services Administration Education 1979*. Washington, DC: AUPHA, 1978, p. vii.

49.   Thompson, J., "Competency Development and Assessment in Undergraduate Healthcare Management Programs: The Role of Internships." *Journal of Health Administration Education*, Vol. 22, 2005, pp. 417–433.

50.   AUPHA Strategic Plan, Washington, DC: AUPHA, 2006.

51.   Interview with L. Reed, president and CEO of AUPHA, Nov. 9, 2006.

52.   "Final Report of the Pedagogy Enhancement Project for Entry and Early-Career Leadership Skills for Healthcare Management." Submitted to ACHE, prepared by AUPHA. Arlington, VA: AUPHA, June 30, 2005.

53.   Olsen was dean of the Amos Tuck School of Business Administration, Dartmouth College, from 1937 to 1951, and professor from 1926 to 1960. He was a member of the ACHA book award committee in 1959 to 1960.

54.   *University Education for Administration in Hospitals.* Washington, DC: American Council on Education, 1954; Kipnis, I. A. *A Venture Forward: A History of the American College of Hospital Administrators.* Chicago: ACHA, 1955, p. 106; Wren, G. R., "An Historic View of Hospital Administration Education." *Hospital & Health Services Administration*, Vol. 25, No. 3, Summer 1980, pp. 36–38.

55.   Kipnis, I. A. *A Venture Forward: A History of the American College of Hospital Administrators.* Chicago: ACHA, 1955, pp. 106–107.

56.   The Commission members were James A. Hamilton (chairman); Milo Anderson (hospital administrator, Ohio State University Health Center); Donald G. Borg (trustee); Francis J. Brown (American Council on Education); Ray E. Brown; James P. Dixon, MD (Commissioner of Public Health, Philadelphia); John E. Gorrell, MD (former assistant director of the hospital administration program at Columbia); J. Steele Gow (trustee); and Leon N. Hickernell (director, Vancouver General Hospital). *University Education for Administration in Hospitals.* Washington, DC: American Council on Education, 1954. Also, Prall, C. E., "A Review of the Report of the Joint Commission on Education for Hospital Administration," in Brown, R. E. (editor), *Graduate Education for Hospital Administration: Proceedings of a National Symposium, Dec 12–13.* Chicago: Graduate Program in Health Administration, University of Chicago, 1959, pp. 29–42.

57.   *University Education for Administration in Hospitals.* Washington, DC: American Council on Education, 1954, pp. 122–123.

58.   Ibid., p. 156.

59.   Ibid., p. 179.

60.   Ibid., pp. 156–165. Olsen accepted the residency and because of this, said, "If the program of study in hospital administration is limited to one graduate academic year, then none of that year should be devoted to making up deficiencies in these basic foundation courses [proposed for preadmission requirements]." Prall, C. E., "A Review of the Report of the Joint Commission on Education for Hospital Administration," in Brown, R. E. (editor), *Graduate Education for Hospital Administration: Proceedings of a National Symposium, Dec 12–13.* Chicago: Graduate Program in Health Administration, University of Chicago, 1959, p. 46.

61.   *University Education for Administration in Hospitals.* Washington, DC: American Council on Education, 1954, p. 89.

62.   Stephan, J. W., in Brown, R. E. (editor), *Graduate Education for Hospital Administration: Proceedings of a National Symposium, Dec 12–13.* Chicago: Graduate Program in Health Administration, University of Chicago, 1959, p. 71; Wren, G. R., "An Historic View of Hospital Administration Education." *Hospital & Health Services Administration*, Vol. 25, No. 3, Summer 1980, pp. 36–39.

63.   Wren, G. R., "An Historic View of Hospital Administration Education." *Hospital & Health Services Administration*, Vol. 25, No. 3, Summer 1980, p. 39.

64. Bugbee, G., "New Curriculum Developments: A Two-Year Program." *Hospital Administration*, Vol. 12, No. 4, Fall 1967.

65. AUPHA. *Health Services Administration Education 1979*. Washington, DC: AUPHA, 1979, p. 84.

66. In 1960 the University of Michigan program, directed by Walter McNerney, had developed a large research staff resulting in the two-volume report, McNerney, W. J., *Hospital and Medical Economics*. 2 vol. Chicago: Hospital Research and Educational Trust, 1962.

67. AUPHA. *Health Services Administration Education 1991–1993*. Arlington, VA: AUPHA, pp. 15–16.

68. E-mail interview with J. S. Lloyd, president & CEO of CAHME, Dec. 1, 2006.

69. Ibid.

70. "ACHA regulations, up to the early 1960s, prevented faculty from advancing to Fellowship or Membership. As a result, many of these individuals dropped their affiliation with ACHE and still have not rejoined, in spite of changes that permit advancement opportunities. Their position is understandable because ACHE denied their attempts to advance at the time they were prepared to do so." Wesbury, S. A. "Background Information Concerning the Proposal to Change the Name and Objects of the American College of Hospital Administrators." Chicago: ACHA, April 1981, p. 5.

71. Chester, T. E. *Graduate Education for Hospital Administration in the United States: Trends*. Chicago: ACHA, 1969, pp. 10–11.

72. Ibid., p.12.

73. Of the 16 members of the Commission, only three are listed as ACHE members in the 1981 Directory: Lloyd Detwiller, Lawrence Hill, and Joseph B. Mann. Of these three, the first two had spent a major part of their careers in hospital administration education. Dixon was a member of the Olsen Report Commission in 1947, former Commissioner of Public Health of Philadelphia, and a member of the Society of Medical Administrators.

74. The reports of the Commission on Education for Health Administration are Vol. I and Vol. II, published in 1975, and Vol. III, *A Future Agenda*, 1977, and *Summary of the Report of the Commission on Education for Health Administration*, 1974 (Chicago: Health Administration Press). Wren, G. R., "An Historic View of Hospital Administration Education." *Hospital & Health Services Administration*, Vol. 25, No. 3, Summer 1980, pp. 39–42.

75. Commission on Education for Health Administration, J. P. Dixon, chairman. *Education for Hospital Administration*. Vol. I. Chicago: Health Administration Press, 1975, p. 43.

76. Ibid., p. 58.

77. Jaeger, J., "Education for Hospital Administration: A Reconceptualization." Health Administration Perspectives Series No. A10. Chicago: Center for Health Administration Studies, University of Chicago, Dec. 1972, pp. 1–2.

78.   The other members included Everett Fox, Aladino Gavazzi, L. Russell Jordan, Stephan Morris, William N. Wallace, and David Youngdall. ACHA, "The Report of the Task Force on the Report of the Commission on Education for Health Administration." Chicago: ACHA, 1978; ACHA, "Report of the Joint Meeting of the ACHA Board of Governors/Task Force on the Report of the Commission on Education for Health Administration," Chicago: ACHA, Aug. 10, 1977.

79.   Commission on Education for Health Administration, J. P. Dixon, chairman. *Education for Hospital Administration*. Vol. I. Chicago: Health Administration Press, 1975, p. 66.

80.   Ibid., pp. 76, 78.

81.   MacEachern, M., "Institutes for Hospital Administrators." Presented before the meeting of the ACHA, Sept. 10, 1937.

82.   Kipnis, I. A. *A Venture Forward: A History of the American College of Hospital Administrators*. Chicago: ACHA, 1955, pp. 139–142. Malcolm MacEachern organized and directed that Institute, according to George Bugbee (personal communication, 1983).

83.   Source: Kipnis, I. A. *A Venture Forward: A History of the American College of Hospital Administrators*. Chicago: ACHA, 1955, pp.139–142.

84.   "Program of the 13th Chicago Institute for Hospital Administrators, September 17–28, 1945." Cosponsored by the ACHA, AHA, ACS, AMA, The University of Chicago, and the Chicago Hospital Council and held at International House of the University of Chicago. The course content largely follows that outlined by MacEachern in 1937 (MacEachern, M., "Institutes for Hospital Administrators." Presented before the meeting of the ACHA, 1937).

85.   Kipnis, I. A. *A Venture Forward: A History of the American College of Hospital Administrators*. Chicago: ACHA, 1955, pp. 139–142.

86.   Matzick, K. J. *A National Survey to Evaluate Continuing Education in the Field of Hospital Administration*. Health Care Research Series Number 5. Iowa City, IA: Graduate Program in Hospital and Health Administration, The University of Iowa, 1967, p.33.

87.   Ibid., p. 38.

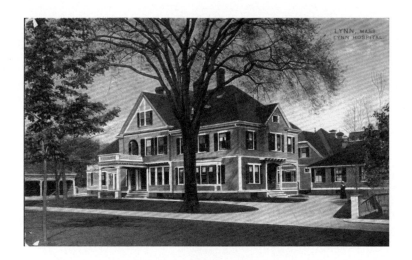

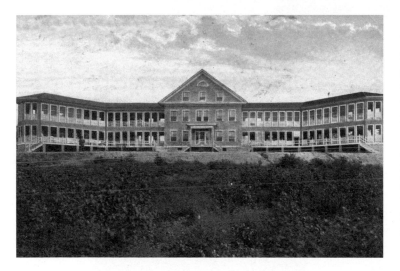

The three hospital buildings shown at left represent different styles of architecture as they evolved over the years. From top to bottom: The cottage-style hospital, represented by the Lynn Hospital in Lynn, MA; the pavilion-style hospital, represented by the Tuberculosis Hospital in Lawrence, MA; and the vertical-style hospital, represented by Hurley Hospital in Flint, MI.

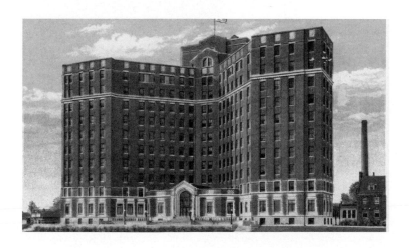

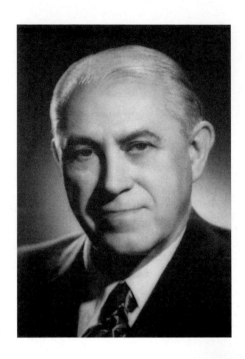

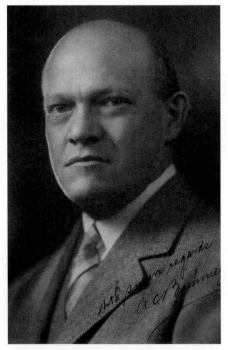

Pictured above are two founding fathers of the profession of healthcare management. *Top:* Malcolm T. MacEachern, MD, HFACHE, advocate of ACHE's founding, argued that a professional society of hospital administrators was essential to the effective management of hospitals. *Bottom:* Arthur C. Bachmeyer, MD, FACHE, was Chairman of ACHE's Committee on Future Program and Policy and in 1940 was selected to be ACHE's Board Chairman.

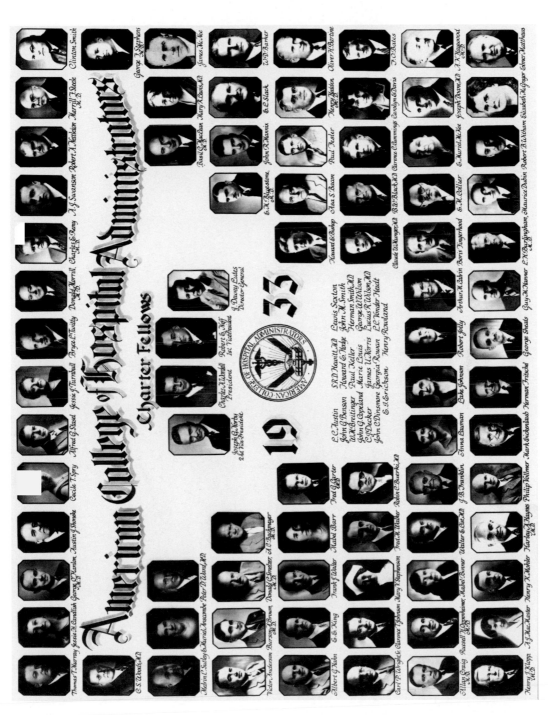

The Charter Fellows of ACHE. A full-size photograph is permanently displayed at the ACHE offices in Chicago.

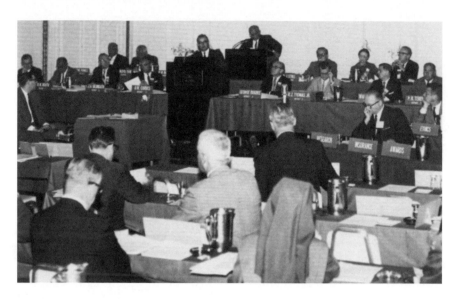

The first Council of Regents Meeting was held in 1965 at the 31st Annual Meeting in San Francisco, CA. Robert W. Bachmeyer presided.

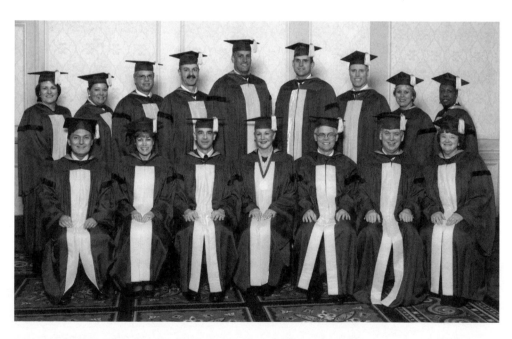

The ACHE Board of Governors shown at the 2007 Convocation Ceremony in New Orleans, LA. *Back row (left to right)*: Gayle L. Capozzalo, FACHE; Nancy A. Thompson, PhD, FACHE; Mark A. Hudson, FACHE; A. Donald Faulk Jr., FACHE; Col. Kent R. Helwig, FACHE; Rulon F. Stacey, PhD, FACHE; Christopher D. Van Gorder, FACHE; Teresa L. Edwards, FACHE; and Marie Cameron, FACHE. *Front row (left to right)*: Richard J. Henley, FACHE; Lynne Thomas Gordon, FACHE; Brig. Gen. David A. Rubenstein, FACHE, Chairman-Elect; Alyson Pitman Giles, FACHE, Chairman; William C. Schoenhard, FACHE, Immediate Past-Chairman; Thomas C. Dolan, PhD, FACHE, CAE, president and chief executive officer; and Deborah Y. Rasper, FACHE.

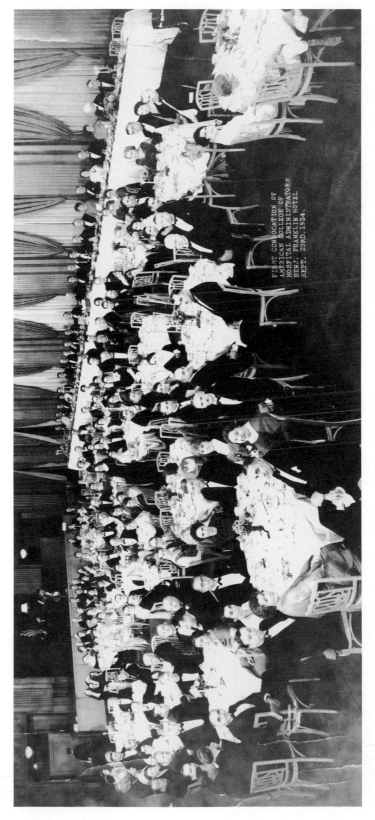

The first Convocation Ceremony of the American College of Hospital Administrators was held in 1934 at the Benjamin Franklin Hotel in Philadelphia, PA.

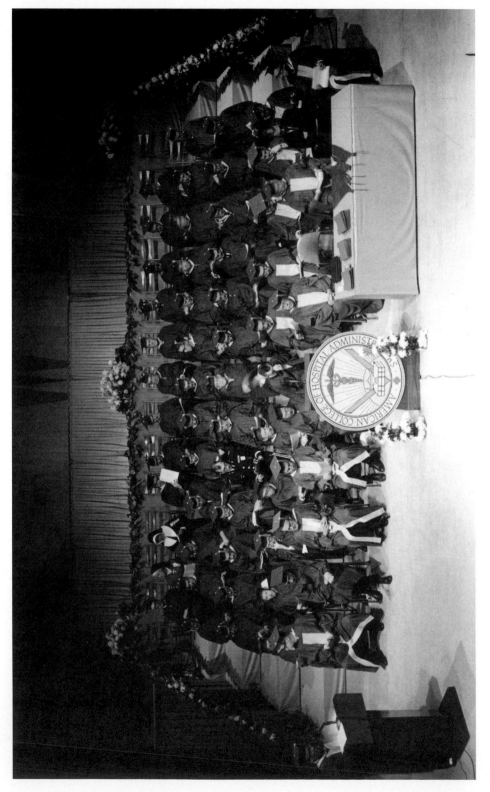

The 1965 Convocation Ceremony of the American College of Hospital Administrators was held at the California Masonic Memorial Temple in San Francisco, CA.

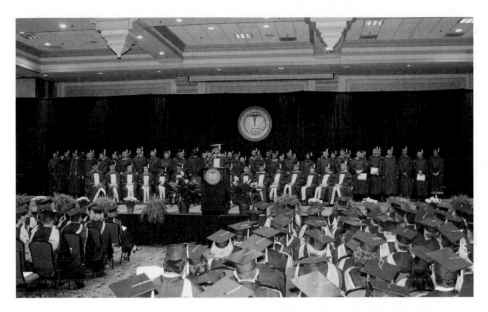

The 2007 Convocation Ceremony in New Orleans, LA. Due to credentialing changes, including the elimination of the Diplomate designation, more than 400 affiliates advanced to Fellow status.

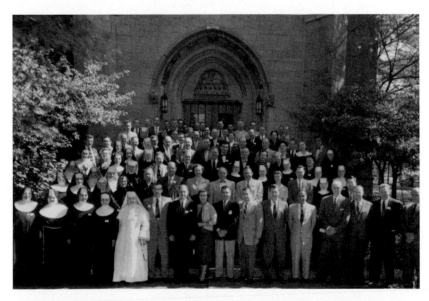

The 23rd Chicago Institute for Hospital Administrators was held in 1955 at the University of Chicago.

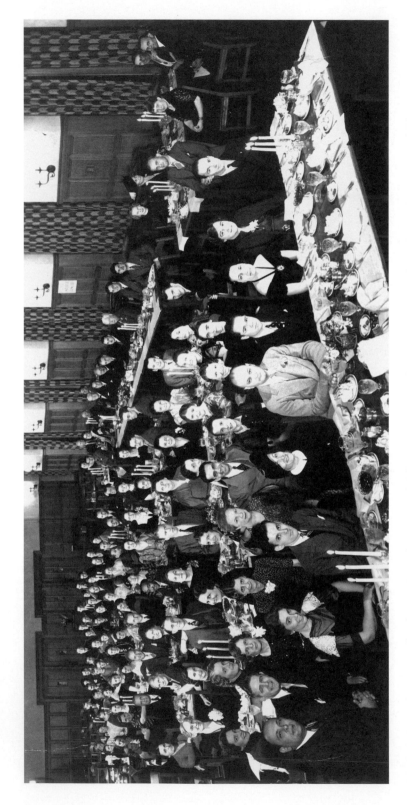

The 6th Annual Banquet for the Institute for Hospital Administrators was held in 1938 at Judson Court, University of Chicago.

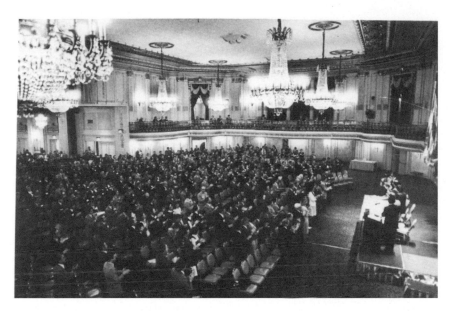

The first Congress on Administration was held in 1958 at the Red Lacquer Room in the Palmer House Hotel in Chicago.

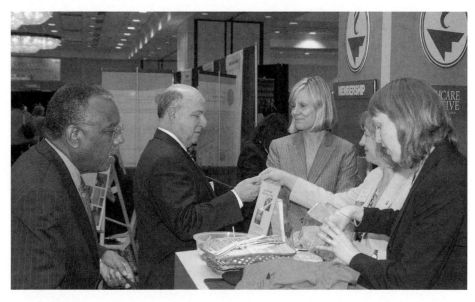

ACHE staff assist Congress attendees at the Membership booth in the exhibit hall of the 2007 Congress on Healthcare Leadership in New Orleans, LA.

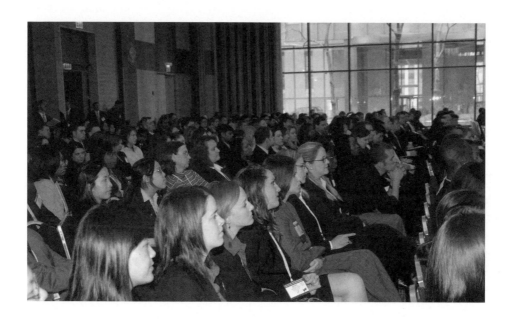

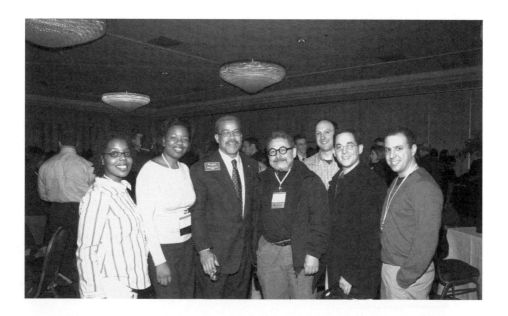

ACHE provides special events for students at Congress. *Above*: Students of healthcare management programs are shown listening to a presentation at the Student Associate Orientation during the 2006 Congress. *Below*: Attendees at the 2005 Student Associate Networking Reception are shown with Samuel L. Odle, FACHE, Immediate Past-Chairman, pictured third from left.

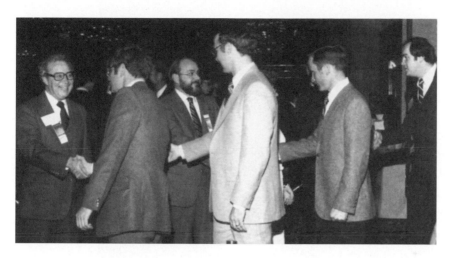

Charles T. Wood, FACHE, Chairman of the Board of Governors, and Stuart A. Wesbury Jr., PhD, FACHE, president and CEO, greet attendees at a reception during the 1982 Congress.

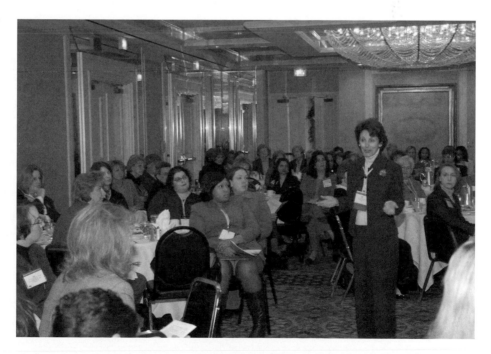

Gail Scott presents at the Women Healthcare Executives Breakfast during the 2005 Congress on Healthcare Management in Chicago.

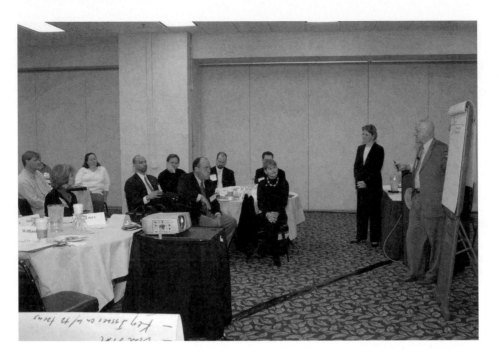

Attendees listen to a presentation by Thomas A. Atchison, EdD, and Kathryn J. McDonagh, PhD, FACHE, at the CEO Boot Camp during the 2005 Congress.

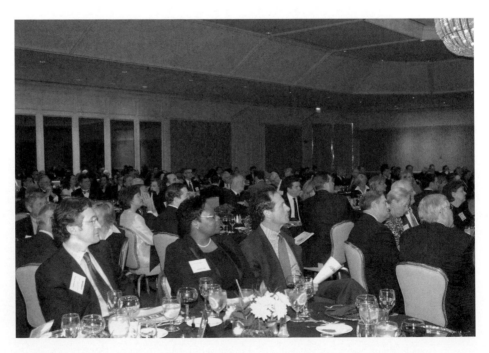

Congress participants are shown listening to a luncheon lecture at the 2006 Congress, held at the Hyatt Regency Hotel in Chicago. Luncheons often attract more than 1,000 attendees.

THE FUNCTIONS OF ACHE: PUBLICATIONS

I do not believe...that the work of the hospital superintendents is all in pota-toes and floor polish.

Dr. Hurd, 1913[1]

Since it was created, the American College of Healthcare Executives (ACHE) has been continually involved in the definition and transmittal of the body of knowledge involved in hospital and healthcare management, as well as its phi-losophy, theory, and techniques. This chapter discusses the work of ACHE regarding publications and the transmission of knowledge, notably the Admin-istrator's Library, the *Journal of Healthcare Management, Frontiers of Health Services Management, Healthcare Executive*, and Health Administration Press.

An Initial Focus

Up until the 1920s, books on hospital management were largely concerned with hospital architecture, construction, and design.[2] The typical book of this era included floor plans for hospitals. There were two reasons for this emphasis. One reason was that from 1880 to 1915, thousands of hospitals were built, and the need for books on equipment and architecture was widespread.

The second reason for the emphasis on architecture was the central problem of hospital infection called "hospitalism." As mentioned in Chapter 1, many people felt that hospital infection was a direct result of the design and location of the hospital building—if the hospital was designed and located correctly, "hospitalism" would be reduced. Thus, it was believed that architecture was the basic answer to the central problem of hospital infection. Once built, an institution was believed to require only rigorous discipline to be run successfully.

The Administrator's Library

After 1920, a shift from architecture-focused publications began to take place. More and more publications delved into a greater variety of topics (see Figure 6-1). The September 1939 issue of the *ACHA News* said,

The great lack of books on hospital administration is gradually being overcome. Ten years ago there were only a handful of worthwhile hospital texts.
Today there are a score or more good books available and nearly a dozen
more in course of preparation.

Around this same time, ACHE began to define the appropriate and
relevant literature for the hospital administrator. Of course, ACHE's Institutes and its encouragement of graduate education (see Chapter 5) also
indirectly promoted the definition of relevant managerial ideas. One of the
first manifestations of this effort was a reference library in hospital administration at the University of Chicago. In his dual capacity as cheif executive officer (CEO) of ACHE and associate director of the hospital administration course in the School of Business at the University of Chicago,
Gerhard Hartman said:

We feel privileged to bring before our members a project as farsighted and
stimulating as a reference library in hospital administration at the University
of Chicago. This library will be kept apart from the general library. [Editor's
note: The library was integrated in 1994.]

Called the "Administrator's Library," it had a twofold purpose:

1. It made available the literature of the hospital field to graduate students
    in the University of Chicago hospital administration course and to
    advanced students at ACHE Institutes. Arrangements were made
    whereby the texts and other materials were sent from the library at the
    University of Chicago to the universities at which Institutes were being
    conducted. These materials were to be used exclusively by administra-
    tors attending the Institutes.
2. As additional accessions were made and the library grew, it was
    designed to serve as a research base for hospital administration stu-
    dents.

Once the library was established, Hartman called on ACHE members
to contribute books to the library. "We feel that in doing so they will be personally adding to the strength and solidity of the educational program they
endorse through their membership in the American College of Hospital
Administrators," he said.

As part of the Administrator's Library, ACHE created a list of
appropriate and relevant literature for healthcare administrators (see Figure 6-2). The books "that should be found on every administrator's
library shelves" could be found in this list of references. All of these books
were specifically related to healthcare and not concerned with general

- Aikens, Charlotte. *Hospital Management*. Philadelphia: W. B. Saunders Co., 1911.
- Billings, John S. *Description of the Johns Hopkins Hospital*. Baltimore: Johns Hopkins Press, 1890.
- Billings, John S. *Ventilation and Heating*. New York: The Engineering Record, 1893.
- Billings, John S., and Hurd, Henry M. (editors). *Hospitals, Dispensaries and Nursing*. International Congress of Charities, Correction and Philanthropy. Section III. Baltimore: Johns Hopkins Press, 1894.
- Billings, John S., Folsom, Norton, Jones, Joseph, Morris, Caspar, and Smith, Stephen. *Five Essays Relating to the Construction, Organization and Management of Hospitals for the Use of Johns Hopkins Hospital of Baltimore*. New York: William Wood & Co., 1875.
- Burdett, Henry C. *The Cottage Hospital*. London: J & A Churchill, 1877.
- Burdett, Henry C. *Hospitals and Asylums of the World*. 4 Volumes. London: J & A Churchill, 1891–1893.
- Davis, Michael M. *Clinics, Hospitals and Health Centers*. New York: Harper & Brothers, 1927.
- Davis, Michael M., and Warner, Andrew R. *Dispensaries: Their Management and Development*. New York: The Macmillan Co., 1918.
- Galton, Douglas. *On the Construction of Hospitals*. London: Macmillan & Co., 1869.
- Hornsby, J. A., and Schmidt, Richard E. *The Modem Hospital: Its Inspiration, Its Architecture, Its Equipment, Its Operation*. Philadelphia: W. B. Saunders Co., 1914.
- MacEachern, Malcolm T. *Medical Records in the Hospital*. Chicago: Physicians Record Company, 1937.
- Mackintosh, Donald J. *Construction, Equipment and Management of General Hospitals*. London: Hodge & Co., 1916.
- Morrill, Warren P. *Hospital Manual of Operation*. New York: Lakeside Publishing Co., 1934.
- Nightingale, Florence. *Introductory Notes on Lying-In Institutions*. London: Longmans, Green, Longmans, Roberts & Green, 1871.
- Nightingale, Florence. *Notes on Hospitals*. Third edition. London: Longmans, Green, Longmans, Roberts & Green, 1863.
- Ochsner, Albert J., and Sturm, Meyer J. *The Organization, Construction and Management of Hospitals*. Chicago: Cleveland Press, 1907.
- Peabody, Francis Weld. *Doctor and Patient: Papers on the Relationship of the Physician to Men and Institutions*. New York: Macmillan, 1930.
- Rankin, W. S., Hannaford, H. E., and Van Arsdall, H. P. *The Small General Hospital*. Charlotte, NC: Trustees of the Duke Endowment, 1928 (revised March 1945).
- Stevens, Edward F. *The American Hospital of the Twentieth Century*. New York: The Architectural Record Company, 1918, 1921, 1928.
- Stone, Captain J. E. *Hospital Organization and Management*. London: Faber & Gwyer, 1927.
- Willie, W. Gill. *Hospitals, Their History, Organization, and Construction*. New York: D. Appleton & Co., 1877.
- Woolsey, Abby Howland. *Hand-book for Hospitals*. State Charities Aid Association. New York: G.P. Putnam's Sons, 1883.

FIGURE 6-1
Early Books on Health Management

FIGURE 6-2

The ACHE List of Essential Books for the Hospital Administrator in 1939[3, 4]

Davis, M. Michael. *Hospital Administration: A Career*. New York: privately published, 1929.

Chapman, Frank E. *Hospital Organization and Operation*. New York: Macmillan, 1924.

Weber, Joseph J. *First Steps in Organizing a Hospital*. New York: Macmillan, 1924.

Lapp, John A., and Ketcham, Dorothy. *Hospital Law*. Milwaukee, WI: Bruce Pub., 1926.

Bay, Emmet B. *Medical Administration of Teaching Hospitals*. Chicago: University of Chicago Press, 1931.

Rorem, Rufus C. *The Public's Investment in Hospitals*. Chicago: University of Chicago Press, 1930.

Newsholme, Sir Arthur. *Medicine and the State*. Baltimore: Williams and Wilkins, 1932.[5]

Committee on the Costs of Medical Care. "Medical Care for the American People." *Final Report of the Commission on Medical Education*. Chicago: University of Chicago Press, 1932.

MacEachern, Malcolm T. *Hospital Organization and Management*. Chicago: Physicians Record Co., 1935 (second edition 1946).

Hayt, Emmanuel, and Hayt, Lillian. *Legal Aspects of Hospital Practices*. New York: Hospital Textbook Co., 1938.

Emerson, Haven, et al. *Report of the Hospital Survey for New York*. Three volumes. New York: United Hospital Fund, 1937, 1938.

Peabody, Frances Weld. *The Care of the Patient*. Cambridge, MA: Harvard University Press, 1927, p. 48.

Ponton, Thomas R. *The Medical Staff in the Hospital*. Chicago: Physicians Record Co., 1939.

Committee on the Grading of Nursing Schools. *Nursing Schools Today and Tomorrow*. New York: privately published, 1934.

American Foundation. *American Medicine—Expert Testimony Out of Court*. New York: The Foundation, 1937.[6]

Mills, Aiden B. *Hospital Public Relations*. Chicago: Physicians Record Co., 1939.

management theory. Not one of the essential books made any reference to general management literature and almost none had footnotes or references to other literature.

Just as the profession of medicine defines its contents through its textbooks, ACHE defined hospital administration through its own list of texts. This was particularly true with respect to Malcolm MacEachern's book, *Medical Records in the Hospital*, which went through several editions and grew to enormous size. It was, for many years, the definitive textbook on hospital administration and was in active use into the 1960s. Appropriate forms for medical records and patient information were reproduced from the book, as this was the era of small hospitals when the administrator had to know details of nearly all hospital work.

Hospital Trends and Developments

As previously discussed, the role of administrators changed with the growth of hospitals and the professionalization of many areas. Until the 1940s, administrators needed an extensive knowledge of detail. Later, administrators sought competent specialized experts and created a climate for positive performance. For example, the trained dietitian, medical record librarian, laboratory technician, business officer, and nurse supervisor took on much of the work formerly performed by the administrator. The work of the administrator thus evolved into the management of professionalized workers in an increasingly large, complex, and decentralized institution.

In 1943 and 1948, instead of updating the 1939 list of publications, Arthur Bachmeyer and Gerhard Hartman edited two collections of reprinted articles about hospitals and their management:

- *The Hospital in Modern Society*[7]
- *Hospital Trends and Developments*[8]

Hospital Trends and Developments included no sample forms, which was the hallmark of the earlier era. There were extensive bibliographical references, however, and even the first regression analysis, heralding the more quantitative statistical analysis of the future.[9] The book was developed, in part, for students in "a number of our leading universities throughout the country" preparing for careers in hospital administration.

Hospitals Visualized

In 1952, Ray Brown and Richard Johnson wrote a book entitled *Hospitals Visualized*.[10] Based on the 1939 Gerhard Hartman book, *Problems and References in*

Sidebar 6-1. On a Personnel Note

Of the 149 chapters in *Hospital Trends and Developments*, at least 35 were written by people who held leadership or honorary positions within ACHE. Following are some of the individuals who contributed to the book:

- Arthur Bachmeyer, ACHE President
- Ray Brown, ACHE President
- Howard Bishop, ACHE President
- Fred Carter, ACHE President
- James Hamilton, ACHE President
- Basil MacLean, ACHE President
- Joseph Norby, ACHE President
- G. H. Agnew, Honorary Fellow
- Guy Clark, Honorary Fellow
- S. S. Goldwater, Honorary Fellow
- V. M. Hoge, Honorary Fellow
- Emanuel Hayt, Honorary Fellow
- Thomas Parran, Honorary Fellow
- Lillian Gilbreth, Honorary Fellow
- E. M. Bluestone, Charter Fellow
- George Bugbee, First Vice President
- Ray Amberg, Regent
- Otho Ball, Honorary Charter Fellow
- Malcolm MacEachern, Honorary Charter Fellow

Only a handful of articles in the publication were written by management theorists:

- Lillian Gilbreth, relating back to scientific management (see Chapter 1)
- Margaret Mead, writing about cultural anthropology
- Herbert Simon,[11] introducing a new era of thinking about organizations

Hospital Administration—described as the "first teaching document for graduate education" in hospital administration[12]—*Hospitals Visualized* was intended for the use of hospital administration students as they began their field experience. The revised version in 1957 contained roughly 2,000 questions that students might ask in 32 hospital departments. The answers to these questions, presumably obtained from knowledgeable department heads, would hopefully result in an understanding of the hospital's functioning. Some questions were simply descriptive:

- To what extent are the following fuels used in cooking: gas, steam, electricity?
- What uniform does the social service worker wear? Is it required?

Many other questions focused on hierarchical relationships:

- Who controls...?
- Who is in charge of...?
- Who is responsible for...?

Other questions related to work flow, policies, procedures, and functions such as budgeting and human resource management.

In part, *Hospitals Visualized* related back to the concern of classical management theorists with the formal organization. No human relations questions illuminated the informal organization. Instead, the text harkened back to the superintendent's era of knowledge of details. But, unlike the nurse administrator of a 40-bed hospital in the 1930s who had to teach staff, hospital department heads now had to impart knowledge to students. *Hospitals Visualized* went out of print in the mid-1960s.

The Journal of Healthcare Management

In fall 1956, ACHE launched a scholarly journal entitled *Hospital Administration*, which ACHE affiliates received as a part of their membership dues. (An ACHE journal was originally proposed in 1942 but was not initiated because of lack of funds.[13]) Early on, the journal illustrated the entry of new management ideas into the field. The first issue, for example, included articles on "Human Relations" by Oswald Hall, Samuel Stauffer, and Robert Tannenbaum.[14] Human relations concepts were evident on a frequent basis in subsequent years and addressed such topics as the following:

- Motivating hospital employees
- Human relations

- Organization as a social system
- Shared communications symbols

The social sciences were also represented in the journal, with references to the economics of patient care, the contributions of social science to hospital administration, and psychology for hospital administration. That the social sciences could contribute to good hospital management was a revelation during the 1950s. Operations research was also new, and these ideas continued with the application of game theory in 1963. Other new ideas covered in the journal included "power politics," "administration by objectives" (heralding management by objectives as a new idea), ethics and moral philosophy, and the management of research.

Many of the article topics cited above described general management theories and demonstrated their application to hospitals. The year 1962 saw articles on the differences between hospitals and other organizations, especially in terms of management principles. For example, Basil Georgopoulos and Floyd Mann built an organizational theory to explain the unique features of hospital organization.

The emphasis on human relations from 1956 to 1966 within *Hospital Administration* matched the growing size and complexity of the average hospital. It also complemented the growth of technically skilled professionals who had been given the opportunity to develop many of the functionally differentiated departments of the average hospital. The era when the superintendent had to know all the details of hospital work was over.

As Medicare and Medicaid were introduced, new concerns appeared in *Hospital Administration*. The growing complexity of the external environment of the hospital was reflected in the following topics:

Sidebar 6-2. On a Personnel Note

For 25 years *Hospital Administration* was edited first by Lynn Wimmer and then by Joyce Flory, PhD. However, in 1987, ACHE moved the journal to an external editor starting with Professor Sam Levey, PhD (1987 to 1991), and moving on to Professor Richard Kurz, PhD (1991 to 1997). James A. Johnson, PhD, served from 1998 to 2000. Kyle L. Grazier, PhD, has served as editor of the journal since 2000. The journal also has an external editorial board made up of ACHE members.

Sidebar 6-3. James A. Hamilton Hospital Administrator's Book Award

The twenty-fifth anniversary of ACHE in 1958 saw the creation of the James A. Hamilton Hospital Administrator's Book Award. The first recipient was Herbert Simon for *Administrative Behavior*.[15] The organizational decision-making concepts found in Simon's book were later represented in ACHE's journal. Later Hamilton book awards included now classic books derived from human relations and the social psychology of organizations. Authors included the following[16]:

- Chris Argyris (1959)
- Douglas McGregor (1962)
- Rensis Likert (1963)
- Daniel Katz and Robert Kahn (1968)
- Harry Levenson (1970)

A complete list of Hamilton Award winners can be found in Appendix 3.

- Area-wide planning
- Collective bargaining
- Regional medical programs
- The federal government on health
- The crisis in American healthcare

An article in 1967 on the administrator's role in computer mechanization started a series of articles on the role of the computer in the hospital, as well as the planning, scheduling, and modeling techniques requiring computers. A growing number of articles used an economic approach, and, occasionally, a political science perspective.

Nearly all of the fall issue of 1969 was devoted to health planning. New topics also included the following:

- Community participation
- Public utility status
- Regulation
- Licensure
- Regionalization

With respect to articles about hospitals themselves, the focus was on their internal organizational configuration, matrix organization, internal control, and budgeting. This is not to say that the human relations ideas vanished, but they were combined with concepts concerning participation, efficiency, and performance.

The growing number of different types of healthcare organizations was reflected in the journal's name change at the beginning of 1976 from *Hospital Administration* to *Hospital and Health Services Administration*. The 1980s brought a new series of ideas that were covered in the journal, including the following:

- Multi-institutional systems
- Marketing
- Corporate finance
- Antitrust
- Competition
- Forecasting models

Sidebar 6-4. The 1979 Bibliography

In 1979, ACHE produced "a selected bibliography for the well-read health services manager." It listed 220 books dealing with both general management and health services management. Of these 220 books, 15 were written by Fellows of ACHE. Of the 15, several were by full-time academics. The bibliography was published because "The outpouring of publications related to the profession of health services administration threatens to inundate the busy practitioner."[17]

ACHE's designation of distinguished articles and books helped define the central ideas of healthcare management as judged by managers themselves. This was yet another way for ACHE to identify the intellectual content of the field.

These words captured new developments in the field. Almost none were found in the indexes of the essential books of 1939, or in the Bachmeyer and Hartman texts in 1948. That is not to say that earlier topics disappeared completely. Instead, they were incorporated into the knowledge base of healthcare management. In fact, two areas continued to be of interest: the hospital governing board and education for health managers.

By this time, the separation between management thinking and important concepts of hospital administration ceased to exist. Hospital administration evolved into general management applied to a unique field, called either healthcare management or health services management. The need to compete with other hospitals for market share in the 1980s did not sit easily with ACHE members, as the growth of articles about ethics shows.

By the 1990s, the intellectual content of the field had changed substantially. Total quality management, a concept stemming from discussions of Japanese management methods and quality circles in the late 1980s, led to continuous quality improvement as a topic for publications, seminars, and articles in *Hospital and Health Services Administration*.[18] The 1992 national presidential campaign brought national health insurance back into the limelight and led to vigorous political debate about healthcare system reform. Increasing diversity in the workforce stimulated thinking about hospital structures, and communities and networks became important. Topics in the journal included the following:

- Transformational leadership
- Decision making
- Product-line management
- Vertical integration
- Human resource management
- Management stress

In 1998, *Hospital and Health Services Administration* was redesigned and given a new name, *The Journal of Healthcare Management*. At that time it also went from a quarterly publication to a bimonthly journal. Changes

---

Sidebar 6-5. Who Was Writing the Articles?

In 1979, Edward Eckenhoff and Stefan Harasymiw analyzed the authors of hospital literature in six journals from 1948 to 1973.[19] In 1948, more than 35 percent of the articles were written by administrators. By 1973, this number was less than 20 percent. Increasingly, professional writers were at work in magazines like *Modern Hospital* and *Hospitals*. Attorney authors increased while architect authors declined. Consultant authors increased from 1 percent to 15 percent, as did faculty member authors. Writing for healthcare management had become a field for specialists. The same trend occurred for general management. CEOs, for example, were rarely writing for *Forbes, The Wall Street Journal*, or *Harvard Business Review*.

were made to make the content more appealing and relevant to healthcare practitioners. An interview with a prominent healthcare leader was added, along with columns on current, relevant topics for quick reads of practical information.

Topics covered in the *Journal of Healthcare Management* in recent years include:

- Quality
- Patient safety
- Electronic medical records
- Cultural diversity
- Workforce issues
- Physician–executive relations
- Disaster preparedness

The *Journal of Healthcare Management* continues to be the official journal of ACHE, publishing full-length research articles that are peer-reviewed on topics of current interest to healthcare leaders. In 1998, the journal introduced a new section—the Practitioner Application, a 500-word review of the research article including the professional opinion of the Practitioner Application writer. This piece is written by a healthcare manager who is a member of ACHE and is not affiliated with the institution in which the research was conducted. These short summaries help executives evaluate the relevance of the research articles to their particular organizations.

Frontiers of Health Services Management

In September 1984, Health Administration Press began to publish *Frontiers of Health Services Management*, a quarterly journal that focuses on one topic in each issue and provides multiple perspectives on that topic. One or two feature article(s) lead the debate and are followed by three commentaries from outstanding scholars and practitioners in the field. At least five writers from different areas of healthcare are involved in each issue to provide a comprehensive understanding of the topic. For example, one issue might have an academic, two senior executives, a consultant, and a policy person writing about the same topic from their different perspectives.

The first editorial of the inaugural issue was written by John R. Griffith, FACHE. Stephen F. Loebs, PhD, was editor of *Frontiers* from 1984 to 1989, followed by Douglas A. Conrad, PhD, from late 1989 to 1994. Mary E. Stefl, PhD, served as editor from 1995 to 2001 and was followed by Leonard H. Friedman, PhD, from 2002 to 2004. In 2004, the editor role was taken on by ACHE staff member Audrey Kaufman, who has a long-standing career in healthcare publishing. Kaufman served as editor from 2004 to 2007 and in 2007 that role was transitioned back to an outside editor, Margaret F. Schulte, DBA, FACHE.

The objective of *Frontiers* is reflected in its statement of purpose: "*Frontiers of Health Services Management* is committed to providing our readers with compelling, in-depth features and commentaries that are of current importance to the practice of health services management by drawing on the expertise of the best practitioners and scholars." The journal is unique in that it provides in-depth coverage of timely topics with differing viewpoints. The well-rounded discussion of subjects helps healthcare executives better understand the big picture and the implications for their organizations.

Frontiers' excellent, high-quality content is evidenced in the number of awards it has won. From 1986 to 2006, *Frontiers* won the prestigious Dean Conley Award 13 times. The Dean Conley Award was established to recognize outstanding articles on an administrative theme published in one of the major magazines or journals serving the healthcare management field. (A full list of Conley Award winners can be found in Appendix 3.) ACHE affiliates choose whether they wish to receive the *Journal of Healthcare Management* or *Frontiers of Health Services Management* as part of their membership benefits.

Topics covered in *Frontiers* in recent years include:

- New physician roles
- Quality measurement, reporting, and implementation
- Price transparency
- Strategic planning
- Catastrophe planning
- Evidence-based management

Healthcare Executive

Published by ACHE since 1985, *Healthcare Executive* is the official magazine of ACHE. Affiliates receive the magazine as part of their ACHE membership. It is designed to inform healthcare executives about the most current trends and management innovations that affect their daily work life. The magazine replaced the earlier newsletter, *ACHA News*.

Produced six times per year, *Healthcare Executive* is now a four-color glossy publication that accepts outside advertising. Each issue contains feature stories around a specific theme, such as quality and patient safety, physician relations, technology, and careers and leadership. There also is a special feature on a timely topic, such as an interview with the incoming ACHE Chairman, reports of major ACHE research studies—such as the comparison of career attainments of men and women—or an article on a special topic, such as disaster preparedness.

Recurring columns in *Healthcare Executive* include the following:

- *Careers.* Strategies, advice, and tools for effective career management and organization development
- *CEO Focus.* Healthcare trends and issues as they specifically relate to CEOs
- *Community Health Innovations.* Programs and ideas for healthcare organizations to help improve the health status of their communities
- *Governance Insights.* Strategies for enhancing governance and board/CEO relations
- *Healthcare Management Ethics.* Approaches to addressing organizational ethics and ethics decision making faced by healthcare executives
- *Inside ACHE.* Board highlights, affiliate accolades, chapter news, and other information that tells what is new with ACHE
- *Patient Safety.* Approaches toward improving patient safety and quality, developed in partnership with the Institute for Healthcare Improvement.
- *Perspectives.* Devoted to comments of the ACHE president and CEO
- *Physician Relations.* Practical ways to work with physicians and create fruitful relationships
- *Professional Pointers.* Brief workplace strategies drawn from a variety of outside sources
- *Public Policy Update.* Analysis of the latest healthcare policy and legislative issues and how they affect healthcare organizations and their communities
- *Satisfying Your Customers.* Tips, tools, and trends to meet expectations of internal and external customers—and give healthcare organizations a competitive edge

Beginning with the September/October 2004 issue, each issue of *Healthcare Executive* has been posted on ache.org (see Chapter 7).

Health Administration Press

Health Administration Press had its origins in the early 1960s, when faculty was drawn together at the University of Michigan's hospital administration program under the directorship of Walter McNerney. This group's major research project culminated in a two-volume report, entitled *Hospital and Medical Economics: A Study of Population Service, Costs, Methods of Payment and Controls*, which was published by the American Hospital

Association's (AHA's) Hospital Research and Educational Trust in 1962.[20] Other books followed from this research, which the University of Michigan program arranged to have published.

By 1972, with the support of a $50,000 grant from the Kellogg Foundation, the publishing efforts of the University of Michigan group had become formalized as the Health Administration Press (HAP). The grant was obtained by Lewis Weeks, Gary Filerman of the Association of University Programs in Health Administration (AUPHA), and John Griffith, FACHE, professor of hospital administration at the University of Michigan. AUPHA withdrew from participation in 1984, after which time the Press was owned and operated by the University of Michigan.

By 1984, Stuart A. Wesbury Jr., PhD, president of ACHE, was considering a joint publishing venture. In addition to partnering with HAP, Wesbury had started discussions with Aaron Cohodes, head of Teach'em and Pluribus Press. Cohodes' company recorded and distributed tapes of ACHE Congress sessions. An initial thought was to link ACHE, Pluribus Press, and HAP, but these had three distinctly different corporate cultures.[21]

By 1985, discussions with Pluribus Press had come to an end but were continuing with Griffith.[22] That same year, Wesbury and Griffith developed a plan for ACHE to buy HAP, keeping the name, the staff, and the Ann Arbor editorial office, while incorporating the Press's activities into those of ACHE. Although this arrangement was satisfactory, finalizing the sale took until 1986: the university had to agree, all author contracts had to be reviewed, and all inventory had to be evaluated.

In 1996, ACHE moved HAP from the University of Michigan to ACHE headquarters at One North Franklin Street in Chicago. Over the next few years, the Press published up to 20 new titles each year, and the overall publishing operation became increasingly sophisticated. The staff now includes many seasoned healthcare and book publishing professionals. Since moving to Chicago, HAP has experienced progressive growth in part as a result of the synergy of being owned by ACHE with its many resources and its access to the healthcare executive market.

HAP publishes books for healthcare executives (its Management Series imprint) and textbooks for students in health administration programs (its textbook imprint). In 2006, HAP sold 56,927 books, the most copies sold in its history. One of the reasons for this growth is that marketing efforts have become more sophisticated to match the demands of the publishing world. Books are available for sale online through the ACHE web site as well as through Amazon.com, NetLibrary, and other major online distributors. The addition of an experienced higher education sales representative firm has also helped the Press better serve the academic community by following up examination copy requests to a much greater degree and learning more about professors' textbook needs.

As healthcare has changed and evolved over the years, so have the topics of books published by HAP, including:

- Quality and patient safety
- Patient satisfaction
- Physician–executive relationships
- Executive leadership
- Health policy
- Workforce issues
- Career management
- Financial management
- Information management
- Healthcare planning and competitive strategy
- Legal issues
- Facility design and construction

In 2004, HAP introduced a new line of books called the Executive Essentials series. These shorter books provide vital information on a current topic in 80 pages or less. The Executive Essentials books also provide a list of additional resources if the reader wants to dig deeper into the subject. The idea behind this product was to provide executives with current information that is practical and straightforward. Some of the titles in this series include the following:

- *Leadership's Deeper Dimensions*
- *Launching a Healthcare Capital Project*
- *Leading a Patient-Safe Organization*
- *Decision Making for Improved Performance*
- *Leading Others, Managing Yourself*
- *Better Communication for Better Care*
- *Consumer-Directed Healthcare and Its Implications for Providers*

Partnering with AUPHA

As mentioned in Chapter 5, HAP has a strong partnership with the AUPHA that includes a formal agreement for cooperative publishing. AUPHA members serve on the AUPHA/HAP Editorial Board, review textbook proposals, and provide other valuable input. Many high-quality textbooks have been published in the AUPHA/HAP imprint over the years.

As a major textbook publisher, HAP also provides many helpful resources for instructors. A section of the ACHE web site called "Professor Resources" is dedicated to helping professors plan their courses and includes instructor manuals and an easy-to-use order form for examination copies of textbooks. HAP is also a member of the National Association of College

Stores to keep current on the issues and needs of the college bookstores, which are major retailers of HAP textbooks.

While HAP has focused on graduate-level textbooks in the past, it has recently branched out to better serve undergraduate programs as well. An AUPHA Editorial Board for Undergraduate Studies was formed in 2005.

Self-Study Courses

As mentioned in Chapter 5, HAP offers Self-Study courses that consist of manuals with accompanying books. On average, 25 courses are available at one time, and these are promoted as being portable and convenient. Individuals can complete these Self-Study courses at home, in the office, or anywhere they choose. Six Category I (ACHE education) credits are earned for each course completed. Users purchase the course, read the course booklet and suggested chapters in the corresponding book, answer the self-graded questions, and return completed forms and the self-graded test to receive a certificate of completion. This program provides an easy way to keep up on information and earn Category I credit. New courses are added every year. Some of the most popular courses include:

- "Followership: Increasing Trust, Respect and Pride"
- "Healthcare Strategic Planning"
- "Learning to Lead"
- "The Healthcare Finance series"
- "The Healthcare Human Resources series"

Futurescan

Since 2000, HAP has published *Futurescan: A Forecast of Healthcare Trends*. This annual publication looks ahead five years

---

Sidebar 6-6. Book Companions Site

In 2006, HAP introduced the Book Companions Web site at ache.org/bookcompanions, which is designed to house the online components of textbooks. This open-access site is student oriented, and all the content on the site is closely linked to specific HAP textbooks. Students can access video clips, narrated PowerPoint presentations, and demonstrations using Excel spreadsheets. They can click through to web sites related to the subject matter of the book they are using in their course. Students can also download electronic versions of forms and exercises that are referenced in a book. Additional features and options can be added based on the ideas generated by authors or HAP. In short, the online Book Companions expand a book's presentation of information and allow HAP and its authors to deliver electronic content to students.

Sidebar 6-7. Partnering with Other Organizations

In addition to its partnership with the AUPHA, HAP has copublished books with numerous other organizations, including the following:

- AcademyHealth
- American Organization of Nurse Executives (AONE)
- American Society of Quality (ASQ)
- Center for Health Design
- Health Financial Management Association (HFMA)
- Health Information and Management Systems Society (HIMSS)
- Institute for Healthcare Improvement (IHI)
- Society for Healthcare Strategy and Market Development (of the AHA)

Sidebar 6-8. 2007 Best-Selling Books

AUPHA/HAP Textbooks

- *The Well-Managed Healthcare Organization*, Sixth Edition, by John R. Griffith, FACHE, and Kenneth R. White, PhD, FACHE
- *Health Policymaking in the United States*, Fourth Edition, by Beaufort B. Longest Jr., PhD, FACHE
- *Information Systems for Healthcare Management*, Sixth Edition, by Charles J. Austin, PhD, and Stuart B. Boxerman, DSc, FACHE
- *Health Policy Issues: An Economic Perspective*, Fourth Edition, by Paul J. Feldstein, PhD
- *Understanding the U.S. Health Services System*, Third Edition, by Phoebe Lindsey Barton, PhD
- *Healthcare Finance: An Introduction to Accounting and Financial Management*, Third Edition, by Louis C. Gapenski, PhD
- *The Financial Management of Hospitals and Healthcare Organizations*, Third Edition, by Michael Nowicki, EdD, FACHE, FHFMA
- *Human Resources in Healthcare: Managing for Success*, Second Edition, edited by Bruce J. Fried, PhD; Myron D. Fottler, PhD; and James A. Johnson, PhD
- *The Law of Healthcare Administration*, Fourth Edition, by J. Stuart Showalter, JD

Management Series Books

- *Healthcare Strategic Planning*, Second Edition, by Alan M. Zuckerman, FACHE
- *Leadership for Great Customer Service: Satisfied Patients, Satisfied Employees* by Thom A. Mayer, MD, FACEP, FAAP; and Robert J. Cates, MD
- *Leadership in Healthcare: Values at the Top* by Carson F. Dye, FACHE
- *Leading Transformational Change: The Physician-Executive Partnership* by Thomas A. Atchison, EdD, and Joseph S. Bujak, MD
- *Digital Medicine: Implications for Healthcare Leaders* by Jeff Goldsmith, PhD
- *Futurescan: Healthcare Trends and Implications* copublished with the Society for Healthcare Strategy and Market Development
- *The Six Sigma Book for Healthcare: Improving Outcomes by Reducing Errors* by Robert Barry, PhD; Amy Murcko; and Clifford E. Brubaker, PhD
- *Followership: A Practical Guide to Aligning Leaders and Followers* by Tom Atchison, EdD
- *Best Practice Financial Management: Six Key Concepts for Healthcare Leaders*, Third Edition, by Kenneth Kaufman

---

and talks about how emerging trends will impact the healthcare field. Based on a synthesis of experts' opinions and a survey of healthcare CEOs, executives, strategists, marketers, and communications professionals, this futuristic publication covers not only trends but also the implications of these trends for healthcare executives. *Futurescan* is copublished with the Society for Healthcare Strategy and Market Development of the AHA and is designed to be a helpful tool for senior management and board retreats.

Looking to the Future

From its early days housed in a building on the University of Michigan's campus to its new home in Chicago, HAP has greatly increased ACHE's role in the intellectual evolution of healthcare management. The Press is another bridge between the practitioner community and academia. As mentioned in Chapter 5, HAP's AUPHA Editorial Board provides a way for academics to play an active role in ACHE affairs. In addition, a majority of students in health administration are learning from publications offered by HAP and ACHE.

In recent years, the Press has received requests to translate books into other languages. HAP books have been translated into Chinese, Arabic, German, Greek, Italian, and Korean. In 2006, the Press hired a subsidiary rights agent to help with the requests for foreign translations.

HAP is a major player in the health administration publishing arena and is well positioned to continue to meet the future content needs of professors, students, and practicing healthcare leaders. With a new editorial board in place, HAP plans to put additional emphasis on the undergraduate market, hoping to greatly expand its offerings by the end of 2009. HAP will also increase its web site material for professors, helping them teach from a particular textbook, and for students, providing additional learning tools in various formats.

The Press has grown steadily in recent years and is well positioned for continued growth in the future. Its reputation for high-quality content and excellent customer service will ensure its continued success as a major publisher in the field of health administration.

Endnotes

1. Comment by Dr. Hurd on Hornsby, J. A., "Standardization of Hospitals." *Transactions of the American Hospital Association*, Vol. 15, 1913, p. 184. The ellipses in this quotation replace the words "with Dr. Codman" referring to Dr. Ernest A. Codman, with whom he is agreeing.
2. Ochsner, A. J., and M. J. Sturm (*The Organization, Construction and Management of Hospitals. Chicago: Cleveland Press, 1907*) devote 147 pages to management principles and 472 pages to construction and architectural plans.
3. Source: Hartman, G. "The Administrator's Professional Library." *The Modern Hospital*, Vol. 54, No. 2, Feb. 1940. These books are now very rare. Most can be found in the Rare Book Room of the Asa Bacon Library of the AHA or the National Library of Medicine in Bethesda, Maryland. These are probably the most complete libraries in the world with respect to the hospital management literature.

4.   Michael Davis was the first Honorary Fellow of ACHE after the Charter
      Honorary Fellows. Frank Chapman was the administrator of Mt. Sinai Hos-
      pital in Cleveland. John Mannix was an assistant administrator and helped
      with the book. Emmet B. Bay was a cardiologist at the University of Chicago
      Clinics and an early physician supporter of the hospital administration pro-
      gram there (Davis, M., in Brown, R. E. [editor], *Graduate Education for Hos-
      pital Administration: Proceedings of a National Symposium, Dec 12–13, 1958.*
      Chicago: Graduate Program in Health Administration, University of Chicago,
      1959). The Rorem book was part of the same series of the University of
      Chicago Press as the Bay book, which Davis edited.

      MacEachern, Emerson, and Emmanuel Hayt were Honorary College
      Fellows. Frances Peabody was a professor at Harvard Medical School.
      Thomas Ponton was a coworker and friend of MacEachern, working as his
      assistant at Vancouver General Hospital, 1918–1923, and then for him in the
      American College of Surgeon's hospital survey program (Ponton. T. R. *The
      Medical Staff in the Hospital.* Chicago: Physicians Record Company, 1939.
      2nd ed. revised by M. MacEachern, 1953).

5.   See Sir Arthur Newsholme's biography, *Fifty Years in Public Health: A Per-
      sonal Narrative with Comments* (London, 1935), cited in Eyler, J. M. *Victo-
      rian Social Medicine.* Baltimore: Johns Hopkins Press, 1979, pp. 195–196.

6.   There are apparently two volumes of this work. See Burling, T., E. M. Lentz,
      and R. N. Wilson. *The Give and Take in Hospitals.* New York: Putnam's,
      1956, p. 336.

7.   Bachmeyer, A. C., and G. Hartman. *The Hospital in Modern Society.* New
      York: The Commonwealth Fund, 1943.

8.   Bachmeyer, A. C., and G. Hartman. *Hospital Trends and Developments
      1940–1946.* New York: The Commonwealth Fund, 1948

9.   Ibid., p. 801, footnote 3.

10.   Brown, R., and R. L. Johnson. *Hospitals Visualized.* Chicago: ACHA, 1952, Sec-
      ond Edition, 1957. Another precursor to this book is Foley, M. O. *Handbook of
      Hospital Management.* Downer's Grove, IL: Privately published, 1933.

11.   Chapter One of Simon, H. A. *Administrative Behavior.* New York: Macmillan,
      1947, adapted from *Public Administration Review*, Vol. 4, Winter 1944, pp.
      16–30.

12.   Hartman, G. *Problems and References in Hospital Administration.* Chicago:
      University of Chicago Press, 1938, p. 58 (with editing by Michael M. Davis
      and Arthur Bachmeyer); L. Weeks interview of G. Hartman, 1982; G. Hart-
      man personal communication, Mar. 29, 1983.

13.   ACHA *Minute Book,* Vol. 1, Oct. 12, 1942; Kipnis, I. A. *A Venture Forward:
      A History of the American College of Hospital Administrators.* Chicago:
      ACHA, 1955, p. 51.

14.   *Hospital Administration*, journal of the American College of Hospital Admin-
      istrators, Vol. 1, No. 1, Fall 1956. It changed its name in 1976. Between

1981 and 1986, six issues a year were published with the help of ACHE's Mary W. and Foster G. McGaw Endowment Fund.

15. Simon, H. A. *Administrative Behavior*. New York: Macmillan, 1947, 1957.

16. Argyris, C. *Personality and Organization*. New York: Harper and Bros., 1957; McGregor, D. *The Human Side of Enterprise*. New York: McGraw-Hill, 1960; Likert, R. *New Patterns of Management*. New York: McGraw-Hill, 1961; Katz, D., and R. L. Kahn. *The Social Psychology of Organizations*. New York: John Wiley & Sons, 1966; Levenson, H. *The Exceptional Executive*. Cambridge, MA: Harvard University Press, 1968.

17. ACHA, *A Selected Bibliography for the Well-Read Health Services Manager*, Jan. 25, 1979, p. 50. The 15 books written by Fellows do not include those written by Honorary Fellows. There is one ACHA publication on the list.

18. Also, Kit Simpson and Curtis McLaughlin won the 1991 Health Management Research Award for "Diffusion and Adoption of Total Quality Management," and Robert Casalou won the 1991 first-place graduate division title in the Hill-Rom Management Essay Competition in Health Administration for "Total Quality Management in Health Care."

19. Eckenhoff, E., and S. Harasymirv, "Contributors to Research Literature 1948–1973." *Hospitals & Health Services Administration*, Vol. 24, No. 3, Summer 1979, pp. 11–20.

20. Walter McNerney, W. J. *Hospital and Medical Economics*. 2 vols. Chicago: Hospital Research and Educational Trust, 1962.

21. S. A. Wesbury interview, Dec. 1992; D. Grew interview, Dec. 22, 1992.

22. D. Grew interview, Dec. 22, 1992.

THE FUNCTIONS OF ACHE: OTHER IMPORTANT SERVICES

There are no static solutions to the challenges facing healthcare executives.... As the premier professional society for healthcare leaders, ACHE focuses on helping you lead your organization to excellence, grow in your career, and capitalize on educational and networking opportunities.

ACHE Annual Report, 2006

The previous chapters have discussed the work of American College of Healthcare Executives (ACHE) with regards to membership, education, and publications and have revealed how that work has progressed over the years. While these are all critical functions of ACHE, there are some equally important functions that have not yet been addressed in this book. The purpose of this chapter is to discuss these additional functions, including

- Career development
- Research
- Public policy
- Diversity
- ache.org
- Development

Career Development

While ACHE has always been interested in helping healthcare executives advance their careers, historically it did not participate in certain kinds of career development activities, such as executive search activities, because recommending one affiliate for an attractive position would probably distress others who were not chosen.

However, in the early 1980s, ACHE discovered a way to be helpful in job placement and career development without crossing ethical boundaries. At that time, Richard Dolan of the executive search firm Witt and Dolan separated from that firm to create a new company that would provide outplacement services for healthcare executives. He spoke about his new company at an ACHE Congress, and Stuart A. Wesbury Jr., PhD—then president of ACHE—followed up with him at his office. ACHE saw the acquisition of a career management firm as consistent with the plan to be more helpful to affiliates, while Dolan saw a link with ACHE as an opportunity for better access to clients. This led to ACHE's acquisition of Career Decision, Inc. (CDI), which provided the following four services:

- Executive outplacement
- Group outplacement
- Career planning and counseling
- Management assessment

After the sale, Dolan stayed with CDI for about three years, and when he left he was replaced by Michael Broscio. In 1994, ACHE transferred ownership of CDI to a management group led by Broscio. CDI eventually merged with another outplacement firm and, although no longer operating under the name CDI, Broscio continues serving transitioning professionals in the healthcare field.

Healthcare Executive Career Resource Center

During the same year that CDI was sold, ACHE created the Healthcare Executive Career Resource Center (HECRC). The mission of the HECRC is to help empower ACHE members to become effective in managing their careers. HECRC considers career management as an ongoing process that cycles through the following five major activities:

1. Self-assessment
2. Identification of an ideal next position
3. Gap analysis and preparation
4. Personal marketing
5. Periodic career audit

HECRC provides affiliates in all stages of their careers with a variety of tools and services to help in these activities. Following is a list of some of the services offered. Beginning in 1999, HECRC, together with ACHE's Division of Communications and Marketing, began moving some of these tools and services to ACHE's web site (ache.org).

- *Job Bank*. This service enables affiliates to search job opportunities online for free. Any healthcare employer can post job opportunities at no charge, giving affiliates access to a variety of job opportunities. Prior to 1999, this service was called Career Mart and consisted of a printed list of job opportunities to which the affiliate could subscribe. An average of 1,000 jobs appear on the Job Bank each month.

- *Résumé Bank.* This tool enables affiliates to develop, edit, and post résumés online for free. In addition, healthcare employers can search posted résumés online. On average, nearly 3,600 résumés are posted to this area of ache.org each month.
- *Résumé critique service.* Affiliates can e-mail, fax, or mail their current résumé to the HECRC, and HECRC staff will review the résumé and send back a personalized critique and sample résumés. This service includes further phone and fax feedback once an individual has incorporated recommendations from the initial review.
- *Internet resource links.* This benefit includes Web links to such resources as executive search firms, executive coaches, firms specializing in outplacement services, firms specializing in transitional placement services, and other employment web sites and services.
- *Executive leadership and career development books and career guides.*
- *Executive employment contracts and sample job descriptions.*
- *The Career Management Network.* This network is comprised of a group of ACHE affiliate volunteers who give affiliates seeking a career change information and advice about career transitions in healthcare management. Network volunteers can provide names of key contacts in an affiliate's chosen region or healthcare specialty, details of a local healthcare marketplace, and information on specific organizations the affiliate may be targeting.
- *Career development assessments.* Some of these assessments include self-assessments and 360-degree, personality-type, leadership, conflict management, and emotional intelligence assessments. Most are available online and at a limited number of educational Clusters.
- *Career intelligence reports.* This service offers a variety of information from different sources. HECRC searches web sites, newspapers, books, and magazines to identify information with career management value for healthcare executives. Information from sources that may wish to remain anonymous is also provided, so the sources can illuminate how covert but real practices sometimes differ from openly espoused principles.
- *Resources for early careerists and students.* In an effort to target the needs of this ever-growing market, HECRC, together with the Division of Membership, developed several resources, including networking opportunities, a postgraduate fellowship directory, scholarship information, and career overviews.

The Leadership Mentoring Network

ACHE created the Leadership Mentoring Network to expand opportunities for learning and development exclusively for ACHE affiliates. The service is designed to help healthcare executives seeking growth as leaders and professionals. The program is currently limited to ACHE affiliates who are serving in healthcare management positions.

The Leadership Mentoring Network maintains the classic one-to-one mentoring experience while relying primarily on a combination of communication media such as phone and e-mail. Face-to-face meetings are usually the exception in this networking approach. Using this approach, mentoring partnerships can develop even between individuals separated by great distances.

Sidebar 7-1. Healthcare Leadership Alliance Competency Directory

The Healthcare Leadership Alliance (HLA) is comprised of the following seven healthcare management professional societies representing more than 100,000 members across a variety of health management disciplines:

1. ACHE
2. American College of Physician Executives
3. American Organization of Nurse Executives
4. Healthcare Financial Management Association
5. Healthcare Information and Management Systems Society
6. Medical Group Management Association (MGMA)
7. MGMA's certifying body, the American College of Medical Practice Executives

In 2005, the HLA created the HLA Competency Directory, an interactive tool designed to ensure that future healthcare leaders have the training and expertise they need to continue meeting the challenges of managing the nation's healthcare organizations. The project also helps determine the commonalities and distinctions in credentialing and professional certification among the various associations.

Based on extensive job analyses and research, the Directory identifies competencies that are important across diverse professional roles within healthcare management. Three hundred competencies are categorized under five major domains:

1. Leadership
2. Communications and relationship management
3. Professionalism
4. Business knowledge and skills
5. Knowledge of the healthcare environment

The Competency Directory is organized as a relational database, which allows users to look at a complex array of information in meaningful ways.

HLA member organizations use the Directory to further enhance their certification and continuing education programs, as well as to advise their members regarding needed skills for professional development. The Directory is also used by university educators in health administration to design curricula, as well as by other professionals in the health management field, such as human resources professionals, who may use it to better define the requirements for management positions.[1]

Mentoring partnerships initially are expected to be established with a specific purpose and for a limited time. Successful mentoring partners are encouraged to expand their focus and continue their relationship as long as they wish. Prospective mentors and protégés file a personal profile with the HECRC so that it may identify appropriate matches. Since its inception, HECRC has matched 400 mentors with protégés, all of whom were ACHE affiliates.

ACHE's Healthcare Executive Competencies Assessment Tool

ACHE's Healthcare Executive Competencies Assessment Tool was developed as an instrument for healthcare executives to use in assessing their expertise in the critical areas for healthcare management. The competencies provide a guideline for the knowledge and skills that are required of health executives regardless of work setting or years of experience. The competencies are categorized into five critical domains: (1) communication and relationship management, (2) leadership, (3) professionalism, (4) knowledge of the healthcare environment, and (5) business knowledge and skills. These competencies were derived from the HLA Competency Directory, created by the HLA.

The self-assessment tool can be used to identify possible areas for growth or excellence for a healthcare executive. Organizations may also use it to develop teams, prepare education material/curricula, and identify specific job requirements. In addition, individuals may use the self-assessment tool to rate themselves based on their own perceptions, compare that to the scores given by their employer, and implement a self-development plan.

Executive Search Firms

ACHE works with healthcare executive search firms to increase the firms' knowledge about the value of putting forth candidates who are committed to professional development, as represented by ACHE membership and board certification. To foster communication between ACHE and healthcare executive search firms, each year ACHE hosts representatives from leading healthcare executive search firms at its offices for Executive Search Firm Day. On ache.org and in advertisements, ACHE also highlights executive search firms that value board certification when placing candidates.

Recruiting Future Leaders

In 2003, ACHE launched a web site designed to encourage young people to enter the healthcare management profession. Visits to the site, Health-ManagementCareers.org, grew to more than 70,000 in 2006. In addition, ACHE developed a DVD designed to expose high school students and undergraduates to the healthcare management profession. The program was provided to the National Educational Telecommunications Association for distribution to their member stations and is available to view on Health-ManagementCareers.org. In addition, the DVD was distributed to ACHE voluntary leadership for use in presentations to high school and undergraduate audiences.

The CEO Circle

Just as it has focused resources for early careerists, ACHE has also created a focused resource package for chief executive officers (CEOs). This package includes the following benefits:

- *Chief Executive Officer*, a quarterly newsletter that highlights management trends and challenges of interest to healthcare CEOs
- A subscription to *Frontiers of Health Services Management*, a quarterly journal that addresses critical management issues (see Chapter 6)
- Four publications annually from Health Administration Press that cover timely healthcare management topics and offer practical guides to busy executives
- CEO white papers summarizing ACHE research studies
- CEO-focused educational and networking opportunities
- Free admission to the CEO Circle Session, a program focusing on critical management issues at ACHE's annual Congress on Healthcare Leadership
- Reduced registration fee for the CEO Circle Forum, an exclusive educational and networking program for CEOs

Individuals must pay additional dues for this program.

Research

ACHE's Division of Research was formed in 1969 as the Division of Project Development and Special Studies. It was consciously named this because many administrators were wary of supporting functions in ACHE that were thought to be impractical or not directly useful to practicing managers. In 1983, after realizing the practicality of the work of the division, the name was changed to the Division of Research and Development. In 2007, the name was shortened to the Division of Research.

The Division of Research has functional responsibility for generating new

---

Sidebar 7-2. Engaging Trustees

ACHE engages in a number of activities designed to increase understanding among trustees of healthcare organizations regarding the significance of leaders who are ACHE affiliates and board certified in healthcare management. These activities include cultivating cooperative relationships with leading healthcare governance organizations, including the Center for Healthcare Governance and The Governance Institute. ACHE engages in an article exchange with both of these organizations; each organization writes articles for *Healthcare Executive*, and ACHE representatives write for their publications. ACHE's CEO has also become a frequent presenter at the meetings of these organizations. In addition, ACHE has placed advertisements specifically targeted at the trustee audience.

information and reporting existing information concerning healthcare executives and their activities. Throughout the years, these have become significant activities for ACHE. The division engages in a variety of work, including the following:

- *The annual affiliate needs survey.* This mailed survey gauges affiliate interest in existing and proposed products and services.
- *Health executive career studies.* The Division of Research has an ongoing commitment to study the careers of healthcare executives, contrasting the attainments of women and men, as well as whites and persons of color. The first career-related study was conducted in 1990. As of 2007, the division has completed the fourth study comparing the career attainments of men and women. A fourth study comparing the attainments of racial/ethnic minorities and whites is planned for 2008.
- *CEO fax surveys.* Six times a year the division conducts a hospital CEO fax survey on topics of immediate interest to CEOs. Such topics have included disaster preparedness, use of electronic medical records, and physician issues. The division also sends fax surveys to other affiliate groups, including early careerists and the membership as a whole to obtain information that ACHE uses in such areas as strategic planning, program improvement, and so forth.
- *Research on CEO turnover rate.* The division conducts research on the annual turnover rate of hospital CEOs using data obtained from the American Hospital Association (AHA).
- *Affiliate database.* Since 1982, ACHE has used its database of affiliate information to provide data on the demographics and educational and professional activities of affiliates. This unique database helps provide a clear picture of healthcare executives' role in shaping American healthcare. Data from the database are published on ache.org.
- *Congress poster session.* The Division of Research acts as the central clearinghouse for managerial innovations and sponsors a poster session at the annual Congress on Healthcare Leadership.
- *White papers.* The division prepares white papers on topics of interest to CEOs. Special analyses are conducted that shed light on issues and suggest strategies that might be employed by CEOs in their own organizations. Some recent white paper topics include strategies to increase the satisfaction of racial/ethnic minority executives, methods and techniques to ensure effective CEO succession planning, and strategies to increase the satisfaction of women executives in healthcare organizations.
- *Healthcare Management Research Award.* This $25,000 award is provided by ACHE on a competitive basis. As mentioned in Chapter 5, the award is available to full-time faculty members of health administration programs that are affiliated with ACHE.

Sidebar 7-3. The Delphi Studies

In 1984, ACHE began a series of three collaborative studies, called the Delphi Studies, with Arthur Andersen & Company. Conducted in 1984, 1987, and 1990, the studies were initiated to obtain some indication of leaders' perceptions of changes that would come about as a result of a major change in the way hospitals were reimbursed, and later, the impact of the growth of managed care.

No Delphi studies have been conducted since that time; however, the Division of Research, in conjunction with the Society for Healthcare Strategy and Market Development of the AHA, does conduct an environmental survey in which environmental trends are postulated and then reacted to by a sample of hospital CEOs. The results are published in the annual publication *Futurescan: Healthcare Trends and Implications*. This scan is very popular because it allows healthcare leaders and others interested in healthcare delivery to discern trends and conduct strategic planning in a more informed way.

Public Policy

For the first 40 years of its existence, ACHE chose not to take positions on public policy, such as government legislation and regulation, leaving this activity to the AHA. This changed in 1973 with the acceptance of the Report of the Board of Governor's Special Task Force, "The Role of the ACHA in the Legislative Process," by Everett Johnson (chairman), Boone Powell, Frank C. Sutton, MD, and R. Zach Thomas Jr. This report recommended that ACHE not become involved in lobbying nor open a Washington, DC, or Ottawa office; however, it did recommend that ACHE introduce position papers and ensure that they be brought to the attention of appropriate legislative bodies. For example, in 1974 several position papers on national health insurance resulted from a Board of Governors' Special Study Commission chaired by Peter Terenzio. At the same time, Professor Odin Anderson was commissioned to write a position paper on the implications of national health insurance for hospital management.

In 1980, ACHE reached an accord with the AHA, which resulted in a major departure from ACHE's past philosophy of political inactivity. The two organizations agreed to "have mutually supportive roles in the development and advocacy of policy affecting healthcare institutions and the professional management of these institutions."[2] This accord reflected a continuing close relationship between these two organizations.

After this accord, ACHE's first venture into the support of public policy was to deliver testimony before the U.S. Treasury Department on deferred compensation for managers in nonprofit organizations.[3] In 1982, ACHE also produced a press release and backgrounder on the ethical conflicts arising through healthcare rationing. "The question of whether life should be preserved at all costs will be the most difficult ethical decision facing hospitals in the 1980s," the material stated.

In 1983, a standing committee on public policy was started. In 1984, another ACHE/AHA agreement was signed, whereby AHA would provide

Washington representation for ACHE.[4] AHA would focus on institutional concerns while ACHE would focus on professional and societal concerns.

Starting in July 1985, ACHE produced a series of policy statements relevant to healthcare executives. The aforementioned policy committee monitored issues and developed, with the help of the staff, position statements that went to the Board of Governors for approval before release.

Since 1985, ACHE has continued to focus on educating members on issues and how to get involved rather than actively influencing policy. Public policy formation is not in the purview of the organization. Trade organizations such as the AHA are more suited to lobbying efforts. ACHE continues to release public policy statements, which state ACHE's position on certain healthcare issues and suggest ways in which individuals can address them in their organization and community. Once a new or revised statement has been approved by the Board, it is made available to all affiliates in the subsequent issue of *Healthcare Executive* magazine and in the Annual Report & Reference Guide.

ACHE's current public policy statements address a variety of issues, including the following:

- *Access to Healthcare*. Released in May 1986 and most recently updated in November 2005
- *Healthcare Executives' Responsibility to Their Communities*. Released in July 1989 and most recently updated in November 2006
- *Healthcare Executives' Role in Emergency Preparedness*. Created in November 2006, this is the most recently developed public policy statement
- *Organ/Tissue/Blood/Marrow Donation*. Released in November 1986 and most recently updated in November 2006
- *Strengthening Healthcare Employment Opportunities for Persons with Disabilities*. Released in May 1992 and most recently updated in November 2006

In addition to developing policy statements, ACHE is also involved in two public policy campaigns that address long-standing issues on which ACHE focuses: organ/tissue/marrow donation and covering the uninsured. The purposes of the campaigns are to educate affiliates on the topics, provide best practices in those areas, and offer resources for further information. ACHE also collaborates with other organizations to help build awareness on these issues. For example, ACHE supports the U.S. Department of Health and Human Services "Gift of Life" initiative and urges affiliates to advocate organ donation and develop organ donation programs in their own organizations. Likewise, ACHE works with the Robert Wood Johnson Foundation and supports the "Cover the Uninsured" Week and "Covering Kids and Families" program.

Diversity

In an address to the AHA in 1968, Whitney Young, a dynamic African-American leader, spoke to the General Assembly stating that he did not see many black faces in the audience. He urged the encouragement of young African-Americans into the profession of hospital administration.

One result of this speech was the creation of a Task Force on Minorities within ACHE. During this time, there were about 50 black members of ACHE. Many of them were instrumental in founding the National Association of Health Services Executives (NAHSE) in 1968[5] (see Sidebar 7-6).

Dr. Albert W. Dent was the first black Fellow of ACHE and was president of Dillard University from 1941 to 1969. ACHE now offers a scholarship in his name. Another black Fellow of ACHE, Charles E. Burbridge, was the first graduate of the doctoral degree program at Iowa, and thus, the first person to be awarded a doctorate in hospital administration. From 1971 to 1980, he was executive director of Freedman's Hospital in Washington, DC.[6]

In 1990, ACHE established an ACHE Minority Internship available to Student Associates of ACHE who had completed one year in an ACEHSA (now CAHME)-accredited graduate program. During the three-month internship, the intern rotates through all major divisions of ACHE.

Since 1990, the issue of diversity in healthcare management has become an even more important one for ACHE. ACHE has focused on increasing diversity within its own organization as well as creating and collaborating with other organizations to improve healthcare opportunities for minorities and expand healthcare leadership opportunities for ethnically, culturally, and racially diverse individuals.

Institute for Diversity in Health Management

In 1992, a study (see the description in the Research section) comparing the career attainments of black and white healthcare executives, conducted by ACHE and NAHSE, showed that black healthcare executives with similar education and experience earned lower incomes, held proportionately lower positions, and expressed less job satisfaction than their white counterparts.[8]

The study prompted three healthcare organizations, the American Hospital Association (AHA), ACHE, and NAHSE, to create the Institute for Diversity in Health Management (IFD). The Association of Hispanic Healthcare Executives joined shortly after, as did the Catholic Health Association.

The creation of IFD was based on the idea that an increasingly diverse workforce serving a diverse population needs more diversity in its management to meet the varying needs of its patients, employees, and communities. Since its inception in 1994, the Institute has engaged in a variety of activities, including the following:

- Bimonthly teleconferences with expert panels discussing important diversity topics
- A quarterly newsletter with practical tips on addressing diversity in the workplace
- Multicultural leadership breakfasts that bring minority healthcare executives together for discussions and networking
- A biennial leadership conference
- A searchable job database to link job searchers with recruiters of healthcare organizations
- Scholarships for undergraduate and graduate students
- Summer internships in which a student is paired up with a hospital for an internship program. According to Frederick D. Hobby, president and CEO of IFD, "This internship is often the first healthcare job experience for the student and the hospital's first experience with a minority executive." Individuals who take advantage of this program are often pursuing an advanced degree in health or hospital administration.

Sidebar 7-6. NAHSE

Founded in 1968 as a nonprofit association of black healthcare executives, the purpose of the NAHSE is to advance and develop black healthcare leaders and elevate the quality of healthcare services rendered to minority and underserved communities. This organization provides a vehicle for black people to effectively participate in the design, direction, and delivery of quality healthcare to all people.

The main objective of NAHSE is to ensure greater participation of minority groups in the healthcare field by developing and maintaining a strong viable national body that has productive input in the national healthcare delivery system. NAHSE's commitment to its members is displayed through the following activities:

- Professional programs/workshops
- Educational programs
- Job bank/mentoring
- Scholarships
- Student internships
- Community service projects
- Health policy impact

In addition to the previously mentioned activities, IFD collaborates with leading healthcare affinity groups to help expand healthcare leadership opportunities for ethnically, culturally, and racially diverse individuals. Some of these groups include the following[9]:

- NAHSE
- National Forum for Latino Healthcare Executives (NFLHE). NFLHE was incorporated in July 2005 to increase the representation of Latinos at the executive level of U.S. hospitals and health systems and to provide a resource base of input from Latino executives in the areas of legislation, regulation, and policy affecting the health and healthcare of U.S. Latino communities.
- Alliance of Pan Asian Healthcare Leaders (APAHL). The APAHL is an organization whose goal is to increase the presence of Pan-Asian executives in the healthcare field and to enhance the quality of patient care provided for Pan-Asian populations.

The IFD also sponsors the American Leadership Council on Diversity in Healthcare, which brings the most advanced diversity practitioners in healthcare together to develop standards of practice and share information about new initiatives. The Council functions as an advisory group that provides insight and perspective to IFD and to the field of healthcare diversity management.

In 2006, the Council began developing a Diversity Practitioner Proficiency Certificate Program to set standards of practice in healthcare diversity management and establish diversity management as a professional discipline in healthcare. The program is designed to provide the diversity practitioner with a practical learning experience in all aspects of designing, implementing, and measuring the effectiveness of a diversity initiative. Upon completion of the program, the participant receives a certificate of proficiency from the Institute.

Since the creation of IFD, ACHE continues to provide financial support for the organization and helps with logistics for the IFD's national conference. ACHE has actively recruited members to the organization, and membership in the IFD has grown to 600 hospitals.[10] Both elected leaders and staff of ACHE have served on the IFD board and have been advisers to IFD.

ache.org

The precursor to ACHE's web site was the fax-on-demand service called ACHE FAX, which allowed affiliates and other interested individuals to dial

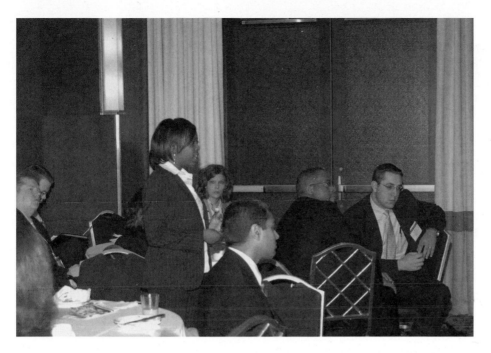

Early careerists attend a breakfast meeting during the 2006 Congress on Healthcare Leadership in Chicago.

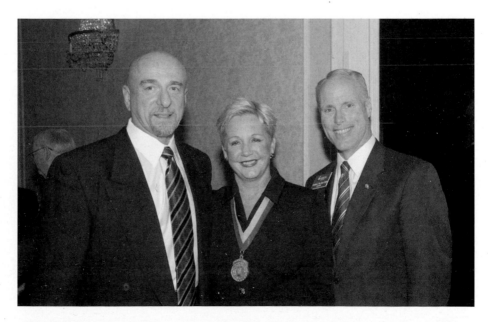

William Giles, Alyson Pitman Giles, FACHE, Chairman, and Christopher D. Van Gorder attend a 2007 Congress reception.

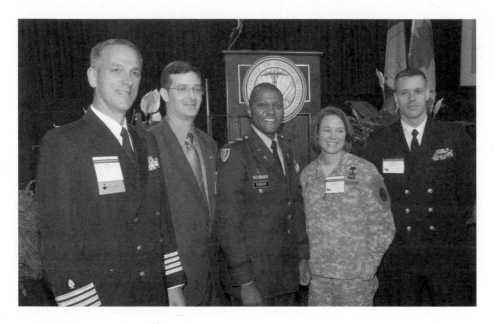

Lt. Col. Jessie L. Tucker III, PhD, FACHE (center), won the American College of Healthcare Executives's 2007 Robert S. Hudgens Memorial Award for "Young Healthcare Executive of the Year."

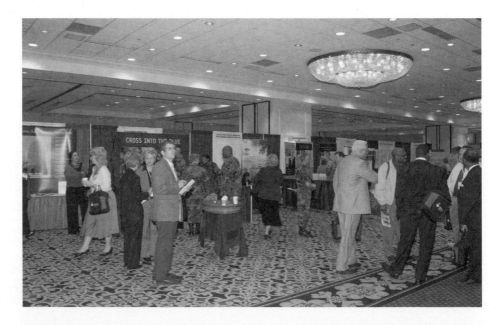

Congress attendees explore the exhibit hall at the 2007 Congress on Healthcare Leadership in New Orleans, LA.

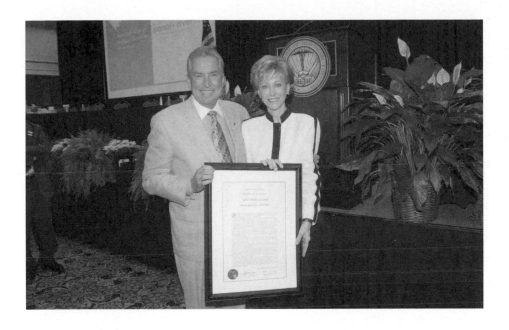

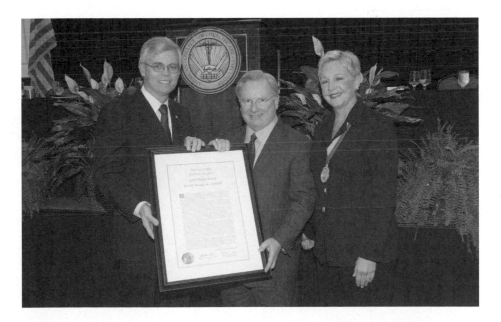

Each year at Congress, ACHE presents a number of awards for excellence in the field of healthcare management. These photos show the recipients of the 2007 Gold Medal Awards for outstanding leadership in the field. *Above*: Diane Peterson, FACHE, Past Chairman, shown with her husband, Larry L. Mathis, LFACHE, Past Chairman and prior Gold Medal Award recipient. *Below*: Jack O. Bovender Jr., FACHE, chairman and CEO of HCA, shown at center with William C. Schoenhard, FACHE, Immediate Past-Chairman, and Alyson Pitman Giles, FACHE, Chairman.

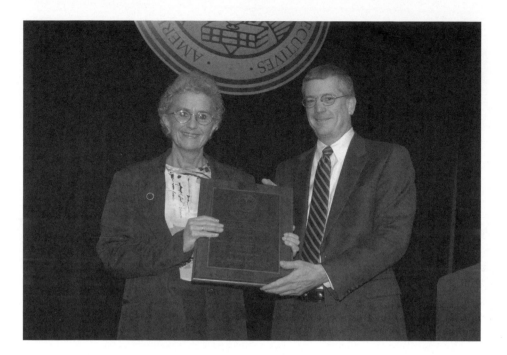

The 2006 James A. Hamilton Book of the Year Award is presented to Patrice L. Spath for her book *Leading Your Healthcare Organization to Excellence: A Guide to Using the Baldrige Criteria*. The award is presented by Gregory P. Hart, FACHE.

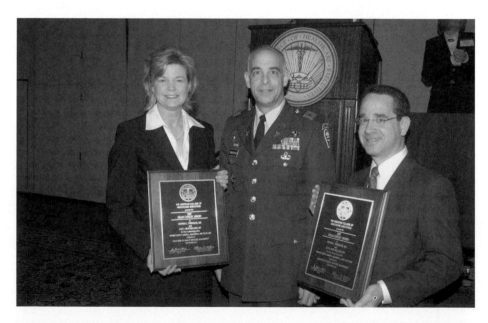

The 2007 Dean Conley Award is presented to Kay J. Beauregard, RN, and Steven C. Winokur, MD, for their article "Patient Safety: Mindful, Meaningful, and Fulfilling," which appeared in *Frontiers of Health Services Management*, 2005. The award is being presented by Brig. Gen. David A. Rubenstein, FACHE, Chairman-Elect.

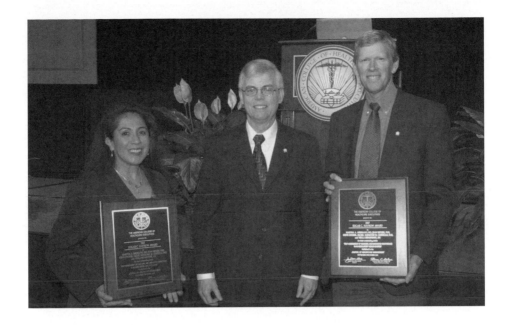

The 2007 Edgar C. Hayhow Award for best article from the *Journal of Healthcare Management* is received by Martha A. Medrano, MD, MPH, and Steven L. Enders, FACHE, for their article, "Self Assessment of Cultural and Linguistic Competence in an Ambulatory Health System." Presenting the award is William C. Schoenhard, FACHE, Immediate Past Chairman of ACHE.

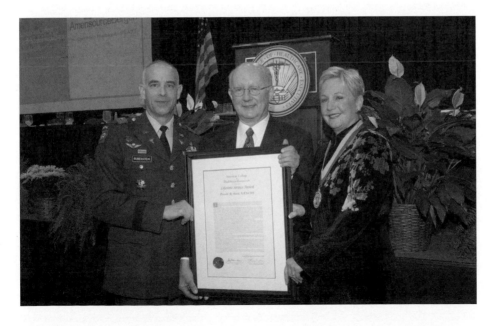

The 2007 Lifetime Service Award is presented to Donald S. Good, LFACHE, by Brig. Gen. David A. Rubenstein, FACHE, Chairman-Elect, and Alyson Pitman Giles, FACHE, Chairman.

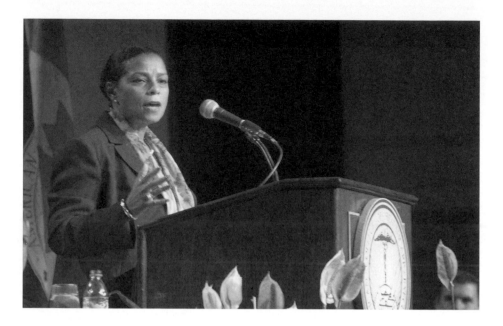

Risa Lavizzo-Mourey, MD, president and CEO of the Robert Wood Johnson Foundation, presents the 2007 Arthur C. Bachmeyer Memorial Address, "Access and the Business of Medicine: The Path Ahead."

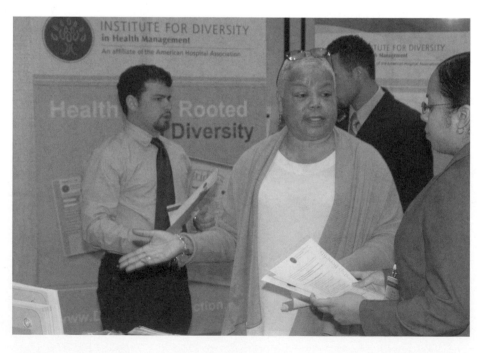

Attendees at the Institute for Diversity booth in the exhibit hall of the 2007 Congress for Healthcare Leadership in New Orleans, LA.

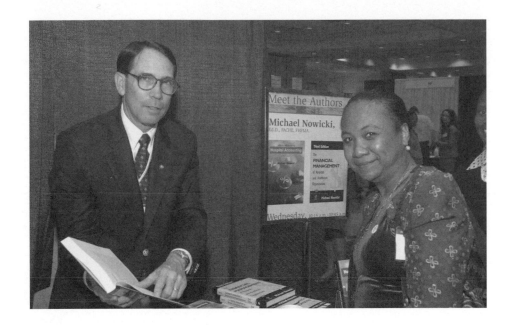

Michael Nowicki, EdD, FACHE, FHFMA, author of *The Financial Management of Hospitals and Healthcare Organizations*, signs copies of his book at the Health Administration Press bookstore in the Congress exhibit hall.

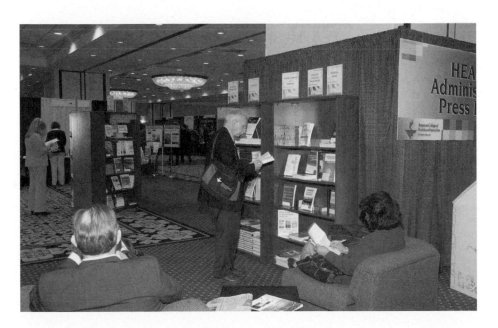

Congress attendees browse the Health Administration Press bookstore during the 2007 Congress on Healthcare Leadership in New Orleans, LA.

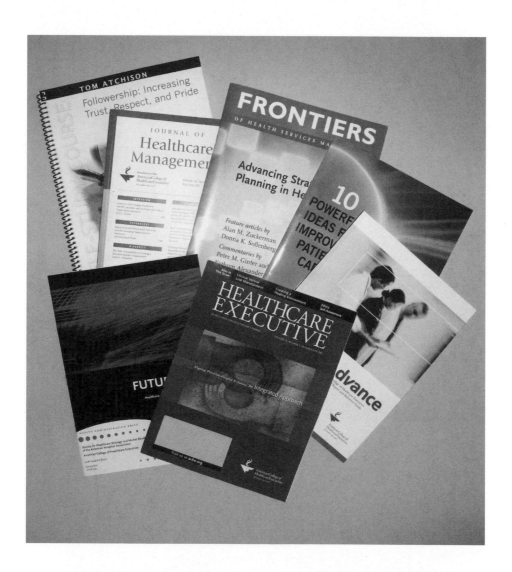

ACHE publications include *(clockwise from top left)*: Self-Study courses, the *Journal of Healthcare Management*, *Frontiers of Health Services Management*, the Executive Essentials Series, the Annual Report, *Healthcare Executive* magazine, and *Futurescan* (ACHE's guide to healthcare trends, produced in conjunction with the Society for Healthcare Strategy and Market Development of the AHA).

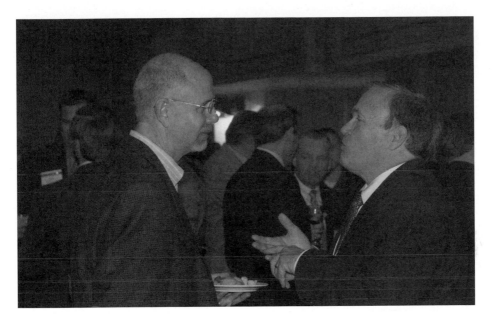

Networking is an important part of Congress, as shown at the 2007 Congress.

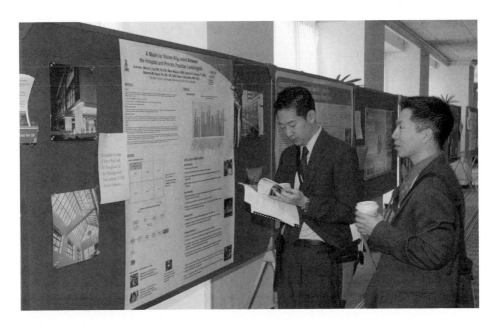

Congress attendees browse the Management Innovations Poster Session at the 2007 Congress on Healthcare Leadership in New Orleans, LA.

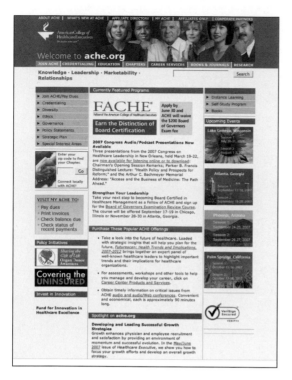

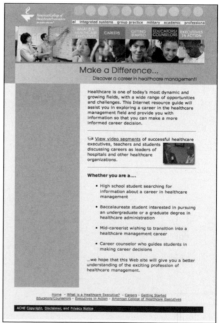

ACHE embraces the opportunity to provide Internet resources to its affiliates and those interested in healthcare management. *Left*: The ACHE homepage at ache.org is a popular and extensive resource for affiliates. *Right*: The homepage of Health Management Careers at healthmanagementcareers.org is designed for high school and college students interested in the field of healthcare management.

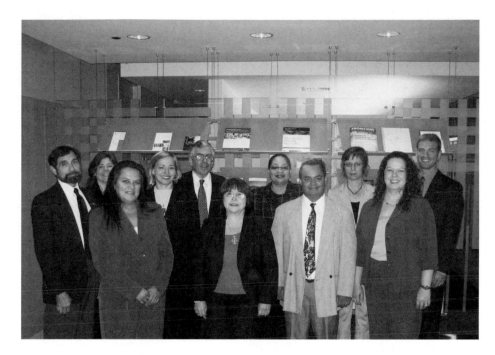

Alton E. Pickert Award winners are staff who were chosen as employees of the year (two per year). *Back row (left to right)*: Reed L. Morton, PhD, FACHE; Christine M. Sawyer, CAE; Cynthia A. Hahn, FACHE; Peter A. Kimball; Kimberly J. Mosley, CAE; Heidi M. Korthase; and Alec S. Rosofsky, CMP. *Front row (left to right)*: Patricia M. Sarno, Oriana Y. Wise, Alex Soto, and Eileen S. Petropulos.

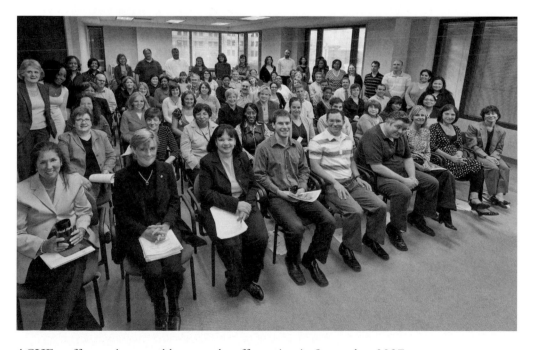

ACHE staff attend a monthly general staff meeting in September 2007.

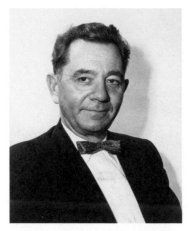

J. Dewey Lutes, 1933–1937

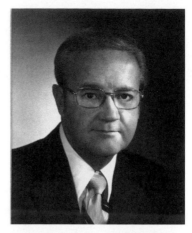

Richard J. Stull, 1965–1979

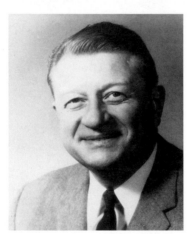

Gerhard Hartman, PhD, 1937–1941

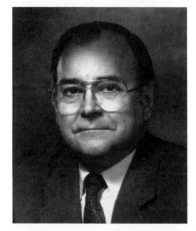

Stuart A. Wesbury Jr., PhD, 1979–1991

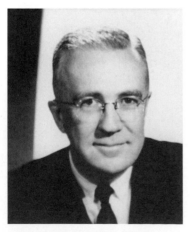

Dean Conley, 1942–1965

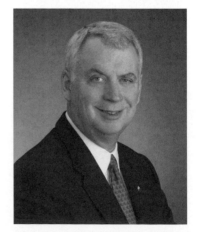

Thomas C. Dolan, PhD, 1991–present

The Chief Executive Officers of the American College of Healthcare Executives, from 1933 to the present.

in and request more than 100 documents, brochures, applications, and forms. This service was discontinued on January 1, 2003. In January 1996, ACHE launched its web site called ACHE Homepage (Also during 1996, ACHE launched ACHE Online via CompuServe, which was later incorporated into the main web site). In 1999, the name of the web site was changed to ache.org to more accurately reflect its scope.

With more than 8,000 pages of information, ache.org is a comprehensive source of information for healthcare executives. Sections of ache.org include the previously mentioned job and résumé banks. The online versions of *Healthcare Executive*, the *Journal of Healthcare Management*, and *Frontiers of Health Services Management* are also available to affiliates. The Ray E. Brown Management Resource Center is an online resource divided into four main sections: strategies for excellence; databases, statistical resources, and research; periodicals and newsletters; and association, foundation, and agency links. Other sections of the web site include the following:

- Membership
- Credentialing
- Education
- Chapters
- Career services
- Publications
- Research

The web site also allows ACHE to be transparent about its governance, providing profiles of its leaders, event announcements, the strategic plan, and other relevant information.

Since its original introduction, ache.org has become more than just a repository of information. Affiliates can now participate in online educational offerings or "Webinars," register for face-to-face seminars and conferences, and engage in online commerce, such as purchasing books and journals. The "My ACHE" section of the site allows individuals to access information about their membership status, past educational programs they have attended, upcoming programs for which they are registered, their continuing education credits, their past purchases, and so forth. The site ache.org has become an interactive and indispensable tool that helps healthcare executives navigate ACHE.

Development

In 1992, in an effort to diversify revenue sources, ACHE implemented a Sponsorship Program. In 2001 that Sponsorship Program was replaced by the Corporate Partnerships Program, which was designed to establish year-long relationships with companies through comprehensive and interactive benefits. The Voluntary Giving Program was launched in 2005 to provide contributed support to the Fund for Innovation in Healthcare Excellence. In 2007 both the Corporate Partnerships Program and the Voluntary Giving Program were integrated into the newly created Development Program.

Corporate Partnerships

Like many other associations, ACHE has long had strong relationships with corporations within the field. In the 1990s, ACHE began receiving corporate contributions for different events throughout the year, including Clusters, seminars, coffee breaks at the annual Congress on Healthcare Leadership, and columns in *Healthcare Executive*.

In 2001, ACHE hired IEG, a sponsorship consulting company, to revamp the corporate sponsorship program. IEG moved ACHE from an a-la-carte partnership philosophy to one that involved a year-long partnership commitment. While this decreased the number of companies from 35 in 2000 to 10 in 2001, it did increase the revenue generated. In 2006, ACHE took this concept one step further and decided to limit the number of corporate partners to 12 companies. ACHE also created two types of corporate partnership opportunities: premier corporate partners and corporate partners, with premier corporate partners paying more and receiving greater benefits.

The partnership program provides the opportunity to bring providers and suppliers together in a nonsales environment. It allows corporate partners to network with affiliates, identify affiliate needs, and create solutions to enhance healthcare. ACHE has an 80 percent retention rate on its corporate partnership program, and 23 percent of current partners have been partners for the entire length of the program. When it was first launched, the corporate partnership program was designed to achieve business development objectives. However, over the years ACHE has realized the importance of the educational aspect of the program. Sponsoring companies learn from affiliates as they attend seminars, go to Congress, and so forth. Corporate partner participation helps partners

---

Sidebar 7-7. 2008 ACHE Corporate Partners

Premier Corporate Partners
- AmerisourceBergen Corporation
- ARAMARK Healthcare
- Cardinal Health
- GE Healthcare
- HCA
- Johnson Controls, Inc.
- Roche Corporation
- sanofi-aventis
- Siemens Medical Solutions USA
- Trane

Corporate Partners
- McKesson Corporation
- Philips Medical Systems

understand the issues affiliates are facing, and this understanding helps create better solutions to identified needs.

Fund for Innovation in Healthcare Excellence

In November 2005, ACHE created the Fund for Innovation in Healthcare Excellence. This is a volunteer giving opportunity for affiliates to contribute money, outside of their dues, to support the field of healthcare and give back to further its development. Individuals can give money to support efforts in one of the following three areas:

- *Importing Innovation.* Innovation in healthcare can be stimulated by importing ideas from other industries and examining their applicability to healthcare organizations. The Fund supports obtaining knowledge from other industries by sponsoring structured roundtable discussions among healthcare leaders and those outside the field. Resulting white papers and educational sessions provide ACHE affiliates with concrete approaches to applying specific innovations and best practices from external industries.
- *Implementing Innovation.* To accelerate change in healthcare delivery, it is important to understand and test approaches that will improve quality, broaden access to care, and decrease costs. The Fund encourages collaboration between health services researchers and individual healthcare organizations. Just as clinicians translate research from the laboratory to the bedside, the Fund supports grants to move management research from academic settings to the practical setting of a healthcare organization.
- *Integrating Innovation with Future Leaders.* Ensuring that healthcare organizations continue to be led by highly skilled and creative executives involves exposing new and emerging managers to the latest innovations in the field. The Fund supports transformational education experiences for emerging, diverse leaders, providing them with comprehensive cohort-based and peer-to-peer programming to improve functional and leadership skills, as well as a group of colleagues upon whom they can call as they progress in their careers.

All the programs discussed in this chapter illustrate how ACHE is moving toward a more accessible, service-driven, and diverse organization. In recent years ACHE has repositioned itself to be a critical resource for healthcare executives at all stages of their career and a driving force in the improvement of healthcare across the United States.

Endnotes

1.   "HLA Competency Directory Users' Guide." Healthcare Leadership Alliance. [Online article; retrieved 1/15/07.] www.healthcareleadershipalliance.org/ HLA_Competency_Directory_Guide.pdf

2.   ACHA, "Accord on the Roles and Responsibilities of the American Hospital Association and the American College of Hospital Administrators in the Development and Implementation of Public Policy," approved July 1980.

3.   ACHA, "Statement of the ACHA on Deferred Compensation," to the Subcommittee on Select Revenue Matters of the Committee on Ways and Means, United States House of Representatives," Apr. 24, 1980. S. A. Wesbury interview, 1983.

4.   White, E. "The History of the American College of Hospital Administrators and Public Policy," Chicago: ACHA, Mar. 1985, p. 9.

5.   W. R. Kirk interview, March 14, 1983.

6.   Ibid.; L. Weeks interview with G. Hartman, 1982, p. 24. Gerhard Hartman received his doctorate in business administration from the University of Chicago in 1942, with a concentration in hospital administration. His doctoral dissertation "Hospital Malpractice Insurance" was published in *The Journal of Business* of the University of Chicago, Vol. 16, No. 4, Part 2, Oct. 1943 and was specially reprinted by the ACHA. With respect to the Iowa doctoral program in hospital administration, see Hartman, G., and J. C. Weaver, "Role Diversification: Hospital and Health Administration Graduates of the Iowa Doctoral Program." *Hospital Administration*, Vol. 10, No. 3, Summer 1965; and Hartman, G., and S. Levey, "Doctoral Study in an Emerging Profession: Hospital Administration. " *Journal of Medical Administration*, Vol. 37, No. 4, Apr. 1962.

7.   W. R. Kirk interview, March 14, 1983.

8.   ACHE and National Association of Health Services Executives. *A Racial Comparison of Career Attainment in Healthcare Management: Findings of a National Survey of Black and White Healthcare Executives.* Chicago: ACHE, 1993.

9.   "Leadership Initiatives." Institute for Diversity. [Online article; retrieved 1/25/07.] www.diversityconnection.org/diversityconnection_app/leadership-initiatives/Leadership-Initiatives.jsp?fll=S4

10.   F. D. Hobby, president and CEO for the Institute for Diversity in Health Management, interview, Nov. 13, 2006.

THE LEADERSHIP OF ACHE

For the man or woman who intends to make a career in hospital or health services administration, affiliation with the American College of Hospital Administrators is paramount.... Membership in the American College of Hospital Administrators is one obvious measure of a person's level of achievement in the health administration field and a reflection of one's interest in and commitment to self-development.

ACHA, "A Brief Description," 1979

One means of viewing the evolution of the American College of Healthcare Executives (ACHE) and its organization is to consider the periods of its six chief executive officers (CEOs). J. Dewey Lutes (1933 to 1937) and his friends created the organization. Gerhard Hartman, PhD (1937 to 1941), brought more of the field's leaders into affiliation with ACHE and developed close links with university education for hospital administration. These two periods resulted in substantial growth in seminar education for hospital administration.

Dean Conley (1942 to 1965), the first full-time CEO of ACHE, provided stability and a formal structure for ACHE. His tenure saw a growth in the number of male administrators, in part promoted by World War II and the proliferation of graduate programs. Richard J. Stull (1965 to 1979) brought financial solvency to ACHE and saw it through its corporate restructuring of 1965 and the growth of the hospital field in size, complexity, and costs.

Stuart A. Wesbury Jr., PhD (1979 to 1991), saw both growth and new directions in education, publications, and public policy. Thomas C. Dolan, PhD (1991 to the present), has brought more diversity into ACHE and has made it more accessible to all individuals interested in healthcare management. Under his tenure, ACHE has been restructured to include chapters, and the use of the Internet has broadened the reach of the organization.

The Years of J. Dewey Lutes, 1933 to 1937[1]

Presidents (Chairman Officers)

1933–1934 Charles Wordell	1935–1936 Fred G.Carter, MD
1934–1935 Robert Emery Neff	1936–1937 Basil C. MacLean, MD

Background

J. Dewey Lutes and his friends Maurice Dubin, Ernest Erickson, L. C. Vonder Heidt, and Charles A. Wordell defined ACHE and saw to its creation. As described in Chapter 3, the core components of ACHE were developed at the outset and remain in place to this day. The importance of membership, periodic meetings, and the focus on continuing education remain at the heart of ACHE.

State of ACHE

In the beginning, the organization of ACHE was conceived with a Board of Regents (15 members) and an Executive Committee, consisting of the President (later called Chairman), First Vice President, Second Vice President, and Director General (combining the functions of secretary and treasurer—this was the role Lutes filled.) plus three other members.[2] In addition, there was a Committee on Constitution and Bylaws and a Nominating Committee,[3] plus a secret Credentials Committee that would later have regional subcommittees.

Because expenses had to be limited, the Executive Committee handled problems of major consequence.

On February 15, 1937, the Board of Regents approved the establishment of the first headquarters for ACHE at 18 East Division Street in Chicago. At that time, responsibilities of the director general were so great that a full-time executive secretary was needed, a need that was not satisfied until 1942.

J. Dewey Lutes spent a great deal of time traveling around the country, often at his own expense, to spread word about ACHE. At its February meeting, the Board agreed to pay him $100 a month.[4]

The Years of Gerhard Hartman, PhD, 1937–1941

Presidents (Chairman Officers)
1937–1938 Howard Elmer Bishop
1938–1939 Robin Carl Buerki, MD

1939–1940 James Alexander Hamilton
1940–1941 Arthur Charles
    Bachmeyer, MD

Background

At the time Gerhard Hartman was appointed part-time executive secretary of ACHE, he was working on his doctorate degree in business administration at the University of Chicago, where he was a teaching assistant and instructor with the graduate program in hospital administration.[6] From 1939 to 1942, he was associate director of this program under Arthur C. Bachmeyer, MD. Hartman received his doctorate degree in 1942.

He was given the job of executive secretary at ACHE[7] after Basil McLean, MD, Chairman of ACHE, came to Chicago and asked to interview Hartman for the position. Hartman said:

I very innocently appeared for the appointment and sat down on a settee. Basil was tall, elegant, and absolutely brilliant. He sat at one end of the settee, and I at the other. What I failed to notice, was that the door to the room was two inches ajar and the entire interview was conducted without the visible but with the actual presence of Dr. Fred Carter, Dr. Claude Munger, Miss Bernice Lawson, Bob Buerki, and I have forgotten, someone else.

After the interview Basil said, "What do you want for a salary?" I can't remember what I said. It was some modest sum, far less than what they were prepared to offer. I heard a roar of laughter. Then the door burst open and out came some of the others. That is the way my role in the College began.[8]

Hartman was appointed on September 13, 1937 at a salary of $300 per month.

State of ACHE

According to Gerhard Hartman, the founding fathers of ACHE were predominantly nonphysician executives concerned with the powerful position held by some of the leading physician administrators of the day. It was not an anti-physician group, but they were concerned with achieving equality of pay.[9]

Sidebar 8-2. Dr. S. S. Goldwater

According to Gerhard Hartman,

[T]he real brilliant mind in the field was Dr. S. S. Goldwater. At that time, Dr. Goldwater was the Commissioner of Health for Mayor LaGuardia of New York. I might say that concurrently Goldwater was consultant to twenty-eight large hospitals and medical centers. He had that kind of mind. Howard Bishop, administrator of Robert Packer Hospital in Sayre, Pennsylvania, knew him. So Howard called Dr. Goldwater's secretary and said he would like to bring a fellow named Hartman in for an interview not to take more than twenty minutes. We stayed for an hour and a half. The exchange among us was truly entrancing. He not only accepted the opportunity to join ACHA, but within two months thereafter, he accepted an invitation to be the principal speaker at the 1938 Dallas convocation of the College. He gave one of his best addresses. The theme I will never forget: "Hospitals Don't Practice Medicine, Doctors Practice Medicine in Hospitals." It was just right.... He gave the College an aura that stood it in massively good stead. It was then that the journals like *Modern Hospital* and the rest accepted the publication of articles that we would digest from speeches that were given.[10]

Hartman commented, "My reason for getting the physicians into ACHE was that there was nothing to be gained by any symbolic or actual schism."

One of the major purposes of ACHE during Hartman's tenure was to build the professionalism of its members through its educational programs.[11] Hartman stated:

> Absolutely, that's why my PhD studies and my University of Chicago appointment made me seem worthy. The College, born of controversy and conflict, also had a problem because I insisted that professionalism had to equate with educational identity.

Through Ray Amberg, administrator of the University of Minnesota Hospital and Regent of ACHE, Hartman helped to organize the successful annual ACHE-sponsored University of Minnesota Institute (see Chapter 5). The president of this university wrote on behalf of ACHE to other university presidents, paving the way for other Institutes at Columbia, Duke, Berkeley, Tulane, Baylor, and Harvard.[12]

After completing his tenure at ACHE, Hartman became the administrator of Newton-Wellesley Hospital outside Boston.

The Years of Dean Conley, 1942–1965

Presidents (Chairman Officers)

1941–1942 Lucius Roy Wilson, MD
1942–1943 Joseph Norby
1943–1944 Robert H. Bishop Jr., MD
1944–1946 Claude W. Munger, MD
1946–1947 Frank Richard Bradley, MD
1947–1948 Edgar C. Hayhow, PhD
1948–1949 Jessie Junkin Turnbull
1949–1950 Wilmar Mason Allen, MD
1950–1951 Frank Walter
1951–1952 Ernest I. Erickson
1952–1953 Fraser Dudley Mooney, MD, CM
1953–1954 Merrill Festus Steele, MD
1954–1955 Albert Carl Kerlikowske, MD
1955–1956 J. Dewey Lutes
1956–1957 Arthur John Swanson
1957–1958 Frank Shelby Groner
1958–1959 Anthony William Eckert
1959–1960 Ray E. Brown
1960–1961 Melvin L. Sutley
1961–1962 Burl Toliver Terrell
1962–1963 Frank Calvin Sutton, MD
1963–1964 Robert Wesley Bachmeyer
1964–1965 Ronald Donald Yaw

Background

Paul Fesler, administrator of the University of Minnesota Hospital, brought both Dean Conley and Ray Amberg into hospital administration.[13] When

Fesler moved to Chicago, Ray Amberg replaced him, and Dean Conley became administrator of the University of Minnesota student health service.

Conley had tuberculosis, although the diagnosis was not completely clear. By the time he was offered the ACHE position by Lucius Wilson with the encouragement of Ray Amberg, Conley had a pneumothorax. Periodically, air was inserted into half the lung cavity to collapse that lung and thereby presumably stop the tuberculosis.

The committee of ACHE that interviewed Conley included Lucius Wilson, Joseph Norby, and Arthur Bachmeyer, MD, formerly a chest physician who saw that Conley's disease was under control and would not hinder his work at ACHE.

State of ACHE

As of 1943, the committee structure of ACHE had expanded to reflect the larger range of ACHE activities. In addition to the Executive Committee, there were committees on Bylaws, Educational Policies, the *Code of Ethics*, Defense, Poll of Current Issues, Nominating, Credentials, and Editorial Policies. By 1957 to 1958, in addition to the boards and committees listed in the bylaws, there were the following committees[14]:

- Election Judges
- Central Committee on Institutes
- *Code of Ethics* Committee (jointly with the American Hospital Association [AHA])
- Budget Committee
- Study Committee on Admissions and Advancements
- Insurance
- Administrative Relationship with Medical Staff (jointly with the AHA)
- AHA–ACHE Joint Committee

Sidebar 8-3. Significant Statistics

At the start of ACHE, the annual dues were $25; the initiation fees were $25 for Members and $50 for Fellows. As of September 1, 1933, ACHE had a cash balance of $1,510.29.[15] By 1939, revenue from dues initiation, advancement, and other fees was about $16,000. Expenditures were as follows:

- $6,500 for salaries
- $850 for committee expenses
- $1,500 for Institutes
- $1,100 for Convocation
- $1,500 for conventions
- $700 for printing
- $800 for office expenses
- $720 for contribution to the AHA
- $600 for refunds on dues
- $431 for miscellaneous

Receipts exceeded disbursements by $1,500. This left a surplus of $1,500 for the year and a cash balance of $5,000.[16]

Sidebar 8-4. On a Personnel Note

Conley remembered J. Dewey Lutes as a dynamo who pushed himself hard. He remembered Hartman as precocious and personable, preaching and promoting educational activities. "Arthur Bachmeyer thought a great deal of him." Bachmeyer, according to Conley, was a serious, gracious, but somewhat inscrutable person.[17]

Gerhard Hartman said of Conley, "Fortunately, when Dean Conley succeeded me, he was of a far less aggressive sort than I. He was more of a coordinator."[18]

According to W. Richard Kirk, "Conley was the first true executive."[19]

Sidebar 8-5. Significant Statistics

In June 1943, the first contribution of record was received by ACHE to help support educational programs. Given by Dr. Otho F. Ball, Honorary Fellow and publisher of Modern Hospital, the contribution was for $1,000 and began a continuing flow of funds in the form of gifts or foundation grants.[21] ACHE had not sought government funding.[22] By 1945, ACHE's income was $39,034 and expenses were $30,013.[23]

As of 1955, there were 15 regions of ACHE: 13 for the United States and two for Canada. As of 1957, there were 18 regions. The active Members and Fellows of each region elected a Regent for their area for a term of three years, and these 18 people made up the Board of Regents.[20] The President of ACHE served as Chairman of the Board of Regents. The Regents, with ACHE officers serving ex-officio, held the powers of a Board of Directors and performed the following functions:

- Approved policy, budget, and financial statements
- Approved admission and advancement policy
- Selected an executive director
- Elected Members and Fellows recommended by the Credentials Committee
- Disciplined members for nonconformance with the Bylaws, but not without due process
- Appointed the Credentials Committee and the Regional Councils, which represented ACHE in their various areas

Following were the officers of ACHE during this period:

- President
- President-Elect
- Immediate Past President
- First and Second Vice Presidents
- Secretary-Treasurer

Officers were elected by all present Members and Fellows at the annual meeting.

The Executive Committee consisted of the President, President-Elect, and Immediate Past President plus four Regents elected by the Board of Regents who would act between meetings of the Board of Regents.

Standing Boards or Committees that were appointed by the Regents included the following:

- The Board of Credentials, which consisted of Fellowship, Membership, and Nomineeship divisions (consistent with the policy of 1933, the names of the members were not published).

- The Board of Examiners, which was appointed by the Regents and had regional committees. The Board of Examiners supervised written examinations and conducted oral interviews for candidates for Membership.
- The Board of Publications, which oversaw the quarterly journal, the monthly news bulletin, and *The Administrator's Digest*, which was only published in the early 1960s.
- The Board of Professional References, which oversaw the content of the *Directory* and *Roster*.
- The Board of Awards, which formulated policy related to awards and testimonials.
- The Board of Educational Policy, which oversaw all phases of hospital administration education.
- The Board of Administrative Development, which promoted activities related to increasing the quality of hospital administration.

There was also a Committee on Bylaws and a Nominating Committee. Six members served three-year terms on the Nominating Committee. Each President appointed two new members. The Past President preceding the Immediate Past President was ex-officio chairman. This committee nominated candidates for President-Elect and First and Second Vice Presidents.

Conley's era saw the heavy involvement of ACHE in Institutes, the post–World War II influx of military administrators, the creation of the Annual Congress on Administration, overseas Fellows' seminars, and the initiation of ACHE's journal, edited by Lynn Wimmer. With the assistance of W. Richard Kirk, written Membership examinations were also initiated.

Conley, with the help of Frank Bradley and Ada Belle McCleery, administrator of Evanston Hospital, obtained the first of several W. K. Kellogg Foundation grants. The first grant was to support the study of education for hospital administration. The study would be directed by Charles Prall[24] (see Chapter 5).

Sidebar 8-6. Significant Statistics

By 1953, the total annual income of ACHE had grown to $139,000 with expenditures of $137,466. Of the expenditures,

- 48.8% went to salaries
- 13.5% went to travel
- 7.9% went to special services
- 7.4% went to committees
- 3.4% went to meetings
- 2.6% went to scholarship loans
- The rest went to office costs and other[25]

In 1955, annual dues for Fellows, Members, and Nominees were $50; and fees for admission or advancement were $50.

Sidebar 8-7. On a Personnel Note

According to W. Richard Kirk, a new generation of administrators gained prominence in ACHE by the mid-1960s. This group included Ron Yaw, Boone Powell, Robert Bachmeyer, and Richard and Everett Johnson. Boone Powell, in particular, led the restructuring of ACHE from 1963 to 1966.[26]

The Years of Richard J. Stull, 1965–1978

Presidents (Chairman Officers)

1965–1966 Boone Powell Sr.
1966–1967 Peter Bernard Terenzio
1967–1968 Donald Wesley Cordes
1968–1969 Roy Zachariah Thomas Jr.
1969–1970 Arnold Leonard Swanson, MD
1970–1971 Orville Northrop Booth

1971–1972 Everett Arthur Johnson, PhD
1972–1973 William Norrby Wallace
1973–1974 Gene Kidd
1974–1975 William Stewart Brines
1975–1976 James D. Harvey
1976–1977 Henry Xavier Jackson
1977–1978 Norman Dewitt Burkett Sr.
1978–1979 Ray Woodham

Background

Richard Stull graduated from the Duke University program in hospital administration in 1942. He served as an administrator in Phoenix, Pennsylvania, and Norfolk, Virginia, and as the western representative for James A. Hamilton Associates. Stull worked for the University of California from 1948 to 1960 as director of University Hospitals and founder, director, and professor of the Berkeley program in hospital administration. From 1961 to 1965, he was vice president of the Brunswick Corporation and head of their Aloe Medical Division.[27]

With regards to coming to ACHE, Stull said:

> Boone Powell was the first to contact me about the ACHA position. I talked with Ray Brown and told him I was thinking about getting out of Brunswick. The next thing I knew he had gotten hold of Boone Powell and Ron Yaw and said, "Hey, you might be able to get Stull. He's in limbo, he can stay at Brunswick but I think he wants to get back into the health field."[28]

State of ACHE

Richard Stull's arrival in July 1965 coincided with ACHE's major reorganization. The former Board of Regents was divided into a Board of Governors and a new Council of Regents in order to improve communication at the grassroots level. The relationship between these two groups was specified through the work of a 1965 joint study committee. Its recommendations were accepted by the Council in 1966.

The Council of Regents was composed of an elected representative from each state, Canadian province, and territory, plus one from the District of Columbia. A Regent-at-Large was elected from the U.S. uniformed services. Thus, the Council of Regents could have up to 64 members.

Every active Fellow in a state was invited to be a candidate for Regent. Members and Fellows voted for the Regent in their state or province by mail ballot. Unless one candidate received a majority of the votes, the top two candidates were voted on in a second mailed ballot.

If no Regent was elected for a state or province, the members from that state were annexed to an adjacent state. Votes of Regents were weighted by the number of members in the state or province—one vote for every 50 members, but not exceeding five votes for any Regent. The Regents' terms were three years, and they met during the annual meeting of ACHE.

The Council of Regents represented the membership and had the power to do the following:

- Approve dues and assessments
- Approve regulations related to admissions and advancements
- Make Bylaws changes
- Elect members of the Board of Governors (only one Governor could be appointed from each of the seven districts)
- Elect the Nominating Committee
- Approve or disapprove reports, actions, and resolutions
- Designate the seven districts

The Immediate Past Chairman of ACHE (formerly called the President) presided at meetings of the Council of Regents. According to an ACHE promotional piece: "Regents function as the principal on-line representative of the professional society in each state or province. In the last few years their duties and responsibilities have increased substantially as they have become the major link between the headquarters staff and their constituents."

The Board of Governors, elected by the Regents, included one representative from each of ACHE's seven districts as well as ACHE's four top officers: Chairman, Chairman-Elect, Immediate Past Chairman, and president, who was a member without a vote. (Stull was the president.) The Board of Governors had charge of the property of ACHE and had the authority to control and manage the affairs and funds of ACHE. The Board of Governors functioned as a Board of Directors, described in the General Not-For-Profit Corporation Act of Illinois, and was empowered to establish committees, grant Honorary Fellowships, bestow special awards, and accept grants and contributions.

Governors were asked to do the following:

- Communicate with and assist Regents
- Generate visibility for ACHE
- Identify potential affiliates for ACHE
- Help plan educational meetings
- Encourage the Young Administrators' Groups

- Monitor ACHE educational programs
- Contribute to the literature of hospital administration

The officers of ACHE were the Chairman, Chairman-Elect, Immediate Past Chairman, president, secretary, treasurer, and, if necessary, assistant secretaries and treasurers. Thus, J. Dewey Lutes's original position was held by up to five people, all of whom were now appointed by the Board of Governors. The Council of Regents elected the Chairman-Elect, who also served as chairman of the Budget and Finance Committee. The Executive Committee of the Board included the Chairman-Elect, Chairman, Immediate Past Chairman and president (without vote), and could take action between Board of Governors' meetings.

During his tenure, Stull revamped the educational effort of ACHE, with support from the W. K. Kellogg Foundation, by creating a seminar series that continues to this day. In addition, the annual Congress grew even larger.

The written examination for membership was updated, and the oral examination was restructured. With the support of Eli Lilly Co., funds were obtained by Conley and Stull to develop an oral interview manual and examination procedures.[29] Regarding this, Stull wrote:

> The results were a programmed manual of instructions for the interviewer and a base of questions with a rating system to be employed in the oral exam. The scoring was done by an outside independent agency. By 1976, the College had begun to embark on its program of self-assessment, self-development and life-long learning.

With the growth of specialization in healthcare management, ACHE broadened its admission criteria while upgrading the educational requirements for membership.[30] According to Stull:

Sidebar 8-8. Committees of ACHE

The Standing Committees of ACHE during Richard Stull's tenure were as follows:

- Nominating
- Bylaws
- Credentials
- Audit

The Nominating Committee had 10 members (one from each District and three past Chairman Officers) and proposed candidates to the Council of Regents for the office of Chairman-Elect, the Board of Governors, and members of the Bylaws and Nominating Committees.

As of 1978, an additional committee included the Committee on Awards and Testimonials, which was the parent to committees on the Book of the Year, the Articles of the Year, and the Gold and Silver Medal Award for Excellence in Administration. The Committee on Budget and Finance oversaw the financial policies of ACHE. The Committee on Education oversaw the educational programs of ACHE. There were also the Committees on the following:

- Elections
- Ethics
- Insurance
- Membership Programs and Services
- Publications and Public Information
- The Robert S. Hudgens Memorial Award for the Young Hospital Administrator of the Year

There were some young guys who wouldn't go into government service [at the Department of Health Education and Welfare] because they couldn't get into the College. Planners, academics, and all kinds of people were coming into the field in varying health institutions or non-institutional positions. They were accommodated by changing College regulations and requirements. The largest number in the membership were still in hospitals or in the emerging multiple hospital system structures.[31]

When Everett Johnson was Chairman (1971 to 1972), ACHE initiated a series of nine task forces to examine special topics of concern for the membership.[32] Task forces reports included the following:

- "The Regents Role in Medical Care Leadership," Donald W. Cordes, chairman
- "A Statement on the Productivity of Group Medical Practice," Sister Virginia Schwager, chairman
- "Principles of Appointment and Tenure of Executive Officers," Jerome T. Bieter, chairman
- "Specialized Management in Hospital Administration," Henry X. Jackson, chairman
- "Providing Primary Care in Community Hospitals," Charles T. Wood, chairman
- "The Chief Executives' Role and Responsibility for Administrative Development," Alton E. Pickert, chairman
- "Recommendations on Standards to the Joint Commission on Accreditation of Hospitals," William S. Brines, chairman

Stull was also responsible for computerizing the membership data known as ACHE's "Administrative Profile" and the establishment of a Division of Project Development and Special Studies with Carroll M. Mickey, PhD, as its director (see Chapter 7). With a grant from Mead Johnson and Co., ACHE helped launch Young Administrator Forums around the country.[33] Stull also initiated significant steps leading to a broad approach to professional development, including the concept of self-assessment. In Stull's words, "The College had progressed to a status of an accepted and respected professional society."

> **Sidebar 8-9. Significant Statistics**
>
> When Richard Stull arrived at ACHE, its finances were in a serious state; the association was in debt by half a year's income and steadily going deeper into debt. The organization had a debt of $110,000 and a yearly income of $250,000. Within two years, Stull had wiped out the debt. By the time he stepped down in 1979, ACHE had more than $3 million in fund balances, clearly providing a firm financial foundation.[34] During his tenure, Stull raised about $2.5 million from outside funding sources. The largest gift of $1 million was from Foster G. McGaw, founder of the American Hospital Supply Corporation.[35]

In 1974, Stull had triple bypass surgery followed by a thoracotomy in 1976. His health slowed his pace, and he stepped down from ACHE in 1979.[36]

The Years of Stuart A. Wesbury Jr., PhD, 1979 to 1991

Chairman Officers

1979–1980 Chester Lee Stocks
1980–1981 Donald Richard Newkirk
1981–1982 Charles Thomas Wood
1982–1983 Earl George Dresser
1983–1984 Alton Eades Pickert
1984–1985 Austin Ross

1985–1986 William Elmer Johnson Jr.
1986–1987 D. Kirk Oglesby Jr.
1987–1988 Francis Joseph Cronin Jr.
1988–1989 David Hans Jeppson
1989–1990 H.W. Maysent
1990–1991 James Orville Hepner, PhD

Background

Like Hartman, Conley, and Stull, Stuart A. Wesbury Jr., PhD, came to ACHE with strong university and academic connections. He received his master's degree in hospital administration from the University of Michigan in 1960 and his doctorate from the University of Florida in 1972. He worked in several hospitals, including a period of service as the director of the University of Florida's Shands Teaching Hospital and Clinics. From 1972 to 1978 he was the director and professor of the graduate program in health services management at the University of Missouri at Columbia. Thus, the close relationship between university education and ACHE continued.

State of ACHE

The Wesbury era saw the development of the public policy agenda described in Chapter 7. Wesbury's interest in policy led him to resign from ACHE in 1991 to run for an Illinois seat in the U.S. House of Representatives. The Wesbury era saw the development of the self-assessment–based continuing education described in Chapter 5. It also saw the development of closer links with academia through recognized affiliations with health management graduate programs, program faculty membership, and visiting faculty fellowships.

Several significant changes occurred relative to ACHE's governance in the 1980s, most significantly, the enlargement of the Council of Regents and the Board of Governors. In 1988, a Regent was added to represent each of the active uniformed services (Army, Air Force, Navy/Coast Guard/uniformed members of the Public Health Services).

Likewise, a Governor for the uniformed services was added. This Governor and the three uniformed services Regents made up a new district—District 8.

In addition, one Regent-at-Large was added for each of the seven geographical districts. This individual was elected via the Nominating Committee process. Regents-at-Large were ideally intended to better represent women and racial/ethnic minorities in ACHE. In addition, a Governor-at-Large was elected via the Nominating Committee process. The Regents-at-Large, however, did not report to the Governor-at-Large.

States with more affiliates were allocated additional Regents. Thus, for example, a state with 501 or more affiliates was entitled to two Regents. Those with 751 or more had three Regents. Finally, the maximum term for Regents was changed from two 3-year terms to one 4-year term.

During Wesbury's tenure, formal recognition of local healthcare executive groups and women's healthcare executive networks occurred. These were the precursors to the Chapters that exist today. In addition, many Regents called on affiliates in their jurisdiction to assist them as members of a Regent's Advisory Council. This increased affiliate participation, allowed feedback from the diverse interests represented by affiliates, and encouraged affiliate participation in planning and goal setting. The creation and development of these Councils was spearheaded by D. Kirk Oglesby Jr.

ACHE's educational offerings continued to grow under Wesbury's watch. In 1991, there were 5,836 paid attendees to about 180 seminars and programs, 1,150 attendees to conferences, and 3,681 attendees at the annual Congress. In addition, 789 self-directed learning modules were sold. This era saw the acquisition of Health Administration Press and Career Decision, Inc., as described in Chapters 6 and 7. Wesbury developed the "programmatic thrusts" that became a feature of ACHE planning.

In describing Wesbury, Thomas C. Dolan, said:

A former pharmacist, hospital executive, and healthcare management professor, Stu was uniquely qualified to become president of the American College of Healthcare Executives. His rare combination of both outstanding intellectual and interpersonal skills allowed him to succeed in every arena. Under his leadership, ACHE broadened its membership both demographically by attracting woman and people of color and professionally by recruiting military officers and academics. Stu became the nation's leading statesman representing healthcare executives.

The Years of Thomas C. Dolan, PhD, 1991 to the Present

Chairman Officers

1991–1992 Paul Stribling Ellison
1992–1993 Robert Reece Fanning Jr.
1993–1994 Ronald G. Spaeth
1994–1995 William C. Head, Col. USAF, MSC
1995–1997 Garth A. H. Pierce
1997–1998 Larry L. Mathis
1998–1999 David W. Benfer
1999–2000 Mark J. Howard

2000–2001 Michael C. Waters
2001–2002 Diane Peterson
2002–2003 Mark R. Neaman
2003–2004 Larry S. Sanders
2004–2005 Richard A. Henault
2005–2006 Samuel L. Odle
2006–2007 William C. Schoenhard
2007–2008 Alyson Pitman Giles
2008–2009 Brig. Gen. David A. Rubenstein

Background

With Thomas Dolan's presidency, the links to academia continue. Dolan came to ACHE in 1986 from Saint Louis University in St. Louis, Missouri, where he directed the Center for Health Services Education and Research. Dolan has his doctorate from the health administration program at the University of Iowa. Stuart A. Wesbury Jr., PhD, chaired the Association of University Programs in Health Administration (AUPHA) in 1977 to 1978, while Dolan chaired AUPHA from 1983 to 1984.

State of ACHE

During the 1990s, the governance of ACHE again changed. Two new affiliate categories were added. In 1993, the category "International Affiliate" was designated, and in 1994, "Retired Affiliate" was added. Based on the 1995–1996 Governance Task Force recommendations, an additional Regent-at-Large was added for the uniformed services. Two additional Governors-at-Large were added so that in 1997 the Board was composed of 11 Governors plus the three Chairman Officers. The Governors-at-Large served in a governance capacity and did not represent specific geographic regions or special-interest groups. In 1998, District 3 was divided and a new ninth district was designated. In all, the Board consisted of 12 Governors and three Chairman Officers.

To open the governance process to more affiliates, in 1999 Diplomates as well as Fellows of ACHE were allowed to serve as Regents. In 2002, Regents'

Sidebar 8-10. On A Personnel Note

By August 1983, ACHE employed 52 staff persons. Of this group, 13 were healthcare management professionals by both education (master's degrees) and practical experience. Eleven other staff members held professional degrees related to their ACHE roles. In 1981, a vice president was needed. By 1993, ACHE employed a president, an executive vice president, and a senior vice president. ACHE had seven internal departments, including Health Administration Press in Ann Arbor, Michigan.

terms were shortened to three-year terms as were the terms of the Board of Governors.

As mentioned throughout this book, the goal of ACHE in recent years has been to make the organization more accessible and valuable to affiliates. To that end, Dolan helped spearhead the creation of a local chapter network, which helps provide valuable services to ACHE members at the local level. To support this network, the organization had to revisit its governance structure.

In 2002, the Governance Task Force (see Chapter 4) proposed a change to ACHE bylaws that provided for ACHE Chapters and made the Board of Governors the primary legislative body representing the affiliates. The Council of Regents served as an advisory council. Powers that transferred from the Council of Regents to the Board of Governors included the powers to make all policy decisions, approve all bylaws and governance changes, approve changes to credentialing requirements, approve all changes to the *Code of Ethics*, and designate districts.

In 2003, ACHE voting jurisdictions on the Council of Regents were modified. In addition, the Governance Implementation Task Force recommended that a Committee on Chapters be created. In 2004 to 2005, per the Board of Governors's request, the position descriptions for Governor, Regent, and Regent-at-Large were reviewed to better delineate the respective roles, particularly in relation to Chapters. Geographic size was determined not to be a factor in deciding the level of Regent representation. The bylaws were changed, empowering the Board of Governors to determine the number and configuration of ACHE administrative districts.

In 2005, Regent representation was reproportioned. One Regent represented up to 999 affiliates, two represented 1,000 to 1,500 affiliates, three represented 1,500 to 1,999 affiliates, and one additional Regent was selected for every additional 500 affiliates.

As of 2006, the Board of Governors had 15 members—the three Chairman Officers and 12 at-large members. According to Dolan, "This allows ACHE to have the best and brightest from all over the country on the Board." Board Members serve three-year terms.

In 2007, 78 members serve on the Council of Regents. Regents serve one three-year term so as to get more people involved in the governance process.

During Dolan's tenure, ACHE also revamped the Nominating Committee. The nominating process is more open than in previous eras, with each of the six districts represented along with the Immediate Past Chairman and a penultimate Past Chairman, who chairs the committee. There are no delegations anymore, and the Nominating Committee presents a single slate for voting. To remove any financial barriers to candidacy, ACHE covers the cost of candidates to appear before the Nominating Committee.

The Dolan years have seen an increase in the diversity of ACHE. For example, in 1992, only 26 percent of affiliates were women; by 2007, more than 40 percent were women. Likewise, the percentage of affiliates from minority populations increased from 4.9 percent in 1992 to 12.7 percent in 2007. In 1992, 26 percent of affiliates came from healthcare organizations other than hospitals. By 2007, this number had grown to 34 percent, illustrating the increased influence of nonhospital organizations, such as consulting firms, long-term care organizations, and group practice.

To encourage and respond to this diversity, ACHE engaged in multiple different efforts, including conducting diversity and gender studies, helping form the Institute for Diversity, and producing publications that address the changing nature of the healthcare executive and the diversity issues faced by healthcare organizations (see Chapters 6 and 7 for more information on these projects).

ACHE also modified its credentialing requirements during this era. Early on in Dolan's tenure, ACHE eliminated the requirement to move from Member to Diplomate after 10 years. Individuals were no longer required to sit for the Diplomate exam, or if they took the exam and failed, they did not lose their Membership status. Instead, affiliates could remain Members indefinitely.

In 2007, following an extensive two-year analysis, ACHE concluded that enhancements to the credentialing system would strengthen ACHE's mission to advance healthcare management excellence. As a result, the Diplomate and Fellow statuses were merged into one rigorous credentialing system leading to board certification in healthcare management. Requirements for the revised Fellow of the American College of Healthcare Executives (FACHE) credential included a postbaccalaureate degree, three years' tenure as an ACHE affiliate, five years in a healthcare management position, references from Fellows, a passing score on the Board of Governors Examination in Healthcare Management, continuing education credits, and involvement in community and professional activities.

In addition, ACHE changed its recertification rules to help affiliates keep abreast of current knowledge on healthcare management. Fellows must recertify every three years through continuing education or by retaking the Board of Governors Examination.

Other important activities that have occurred during Dolan's tenure include the following:

- *Providing ethics information, tools, and references.* These tools include policy statements, ethics seminars, a column in *Healthcare Executive*, a self audit, and a tool-kit.
- *Providing enhanced career support.* The creation of the Healthcare Executive Career Resource Center has helped drive ACHE's efforts in career

support. Tools such as the job bank, résumé bank, and the Leadership Mentoring Network all provide direction, support, and resources for affiliates no matter what their career stage.

- *Collaborating with others to improve the delivery of healthcare in the United States.* Traditionally, ACHE has worked with other organizations, such as the AHA, the International Hospital Association, the AUPHA, the Commission on Accreditation of Healthcare Management Education, and the Canadian College of Health Services, on initiatives to improve the delivery of healthcare. ACHE has increased its collaborative efforts and is partnering with organizations such as the Institute for Diversity in Health Management, the Healthcare Leadership Alliance, the Governance Institute, the Centers for Healthcare Governance, the National Patient Safety Foundation, and the Institute for Healthcare Improvement.
- *Embracing technology.* Since the beginning of Dolan's tenure, ACHE has made significant advances in its use of technology. ACHE's web site, ache.org, has more than 8,000 pages and receives more than a million visits per year.

Fiscal Year	Revenues ($)	Expenses ($)	Assets/Liabilities ($)
1934	2,215	1,510	
1937	9,116	7,334	
1941	19,033	18,868	
1945	39,034	30,013	
1950	135,925	76,548	
1953	139,069	96,347	
1957	134,109	103,804	78,868
1961	384,743	396,277	126,301
1966	480,650	427,023	N/A
1971	1,193,439	1,178,389	1,096,788
1976	2,062,809	2,017,848	2,489,433
1981	3,641,150	3,493,127	4,984,001
1986	7,769,757	7,381,154	7,755,699
1991	12,313,424	12,234,576	9,936,944
1996	14,143,753	13,665,460	20,494,814
2001	16,101,085	16,087,432	27,361,193
2006	21,326,813	19,271,756	44,716,085

FIGURE 8-1
ACHE Finances 1934 to 2006, Selected Years

The growth of ACHE throughout the years can be measured by the number of Affiliates and by its financial reports. Figure 8-1 summarizes ACHE finances for selective years from 1934 to 2006.

As the field of healthcare continues to change, so will the individuals who manage healthcare organizations. ACHE stands ready to identify and address those changes and continue to be a critical resource for healthcare executives.

Endnotes

1.   After the first edition of this book, John Mannix started work on brief biographies of all ACHE Presidents (to 1972) and Chairman Officers (1972 on). The material he collected can be found in the Mannix archives, AHA historical collection. The biographies and footnoted references build on his work.

2.   ACHA *Minute Book*, Vol. 1, Feb. 13, 1933. President Charles A. Wordell, First V.P. Robert E. Neff, Second V.P. Joseph Norby, Director General J. Dewey Lutes. The other members were Rev. Fritschel, John Smith, and Maurice Dubin.

3.   ACHA *Minute Book*, Vol. 1, Feb. 14, 1933. Constitution and Bylaws: Maurice Dubin, chairman; Robert E. Neff; John Smith; and Dr. F. G. Carter. Nominating Committee: Dr. Walter List, chairman; Howard Bishop; Dr. Herman Smith; and A. J. Swanson.

4.   ACHA *Minute Book*, Vols. 1, 2, Feb. 15, 1937; Sept. 12, 1937; Sept. 13, 1937; J. D. Lutes interview, 1982.

5.   Kipnis, I. A. *A Venture Forward: A History of the American College of Hospital Administrators.* Chicago: ACHA, 1955, p. 23.

6.   Ibid., pp. 35–36. Hartman was born in 1911; received his doctoral degree in 1942; was a teaching assistant in the University of Chicago hospital administration program from 1936 to 1937 and associate director from 1937 to 1942; ACHA executive secretary to 1941 (reported dates vary). His last signed ACHA minutes are for June 6, 1941. He was absent due to illness Sept. 14 and Sept. 15. The Board of Regents discussed a replacement for him. From 1942 to 1946 he was director of the Newton Wellesley Hospital, Newton Lower Falls, MA, and became director of the University of Iowa Hospitals (1947–1971) and professor and director of the graduate program in hospital administration, State University of Iowa, from 1947 through 1980.

7.   Hartman, G. *In First Person: An Oral History.* Lewis E. Weeks (editor). Chicago: American Hospital Association and Hospital Research and Educational Trust, 1983.

8.   Ibid., p. 11.

9.   Ibid., pp. 14–15.

10.   Ibid.

11. Ibid., p. 15

12. Ibid., p. 17.

13. D. Conley interview, Apr. 21, 1983. Hartman described Ray Amberg as follows: "Bob Buerki said that when you meet Ray Amberg don't be fooled. He said that Ray is half Irish and half Swede, that his speech may be as slow as a Swede's but his mind is as fast as an Irishman's." Hartman, G. *In First Person: An Oral History.* Lewis E. Weeks (editor). Chicago: American Hospital Association and Hospital Research and Educational Trust, 1983.

14. ACHA *Minute Book*, Vol. 5, 1957.

15. Kipnis, I. A. *A Venture Forward: A History of the American College of Hospital Administrators.* Chicago: ACHA, 1955, p. 14; ACHA *Minute Book*, Vol. 1, 1933; Lutes, J. D., "To the Members of the Board of Regents," First Annual Report of the Director-General of the ACHA, in ACHA *Minute Book*, Vol. 1, 1934, p. 3.

16. Kipnis, I. A. *A Venture Forward: A History of the American College of Hospital Administrators.* Chicago: ACHA, 1955, p. 63.

17. D. Conley interview, 1983.

18. Hartman, G. *In First Person: An Oral History.* Lewis E. Weeks (editor). Chicago: American Hospital Association and Hospital Research and Educational Trust, 1983, p. 19.

19. W. R. Kirk interview, March 14, 1983.

20. Kipnis, I. A. *A Venture Forward: A History of the American College of Hospital Administrators.* Chicago: ACHA, 1955, p. 128.

21. Ibid., p. 63.

22. S. Wesbury interview, 1983. Wesbury said at the time that there was no ACHE policy to avoid government grants or contracts.

23. Kipnis, I. A. *A Venture Forward: A History of the American College of Hospital Administrators.* Chicago: ACHA, 1955, p. 131.

24. D. Conley interview, 1983.

25. Kipnis, I. A. *A Venture Forward: A History of the American College of Hospital Administrator*s. Chicago: ACHA, 1955, pp. 130–131.

26. W. R. Kirk interview, March 14, 1983. Dean Conley took early retirement at age 60 in 1965.

27. Ibid. Richard Stull brought in John O'Conner as the financial officer for ACHE. Stull recalls ACHE's assets at the end of his tenure as over $4 million, with $3.6 million invested. Hartman, G. *In First Person: An Oral History.* Lewis E. Weeks (editor). Chicago: American Hospital Association and Hospital Research and Educational Trust, 1983, p. 46.

28. L. Weeks interview with R. J. Stull, 1982, p. 37.

29. Ibid., p. 40.

30. Ibid., p. 40.

31. Ibid., p. 41.

32.   Ibid., p. 41. W. R. Kirk interview, 1983. Kirk said there were nine Task Forces then, but there may have been ten.

33.   L. Weeks interview with R. J. Stull, 1982, p. 44.

34.   W. R. Kirk interview, March 14, 1983.

35.   L. Weeks interview with R. J. Stull, 1982, p. 45.

36.   Ibid., pp. 45–46.

EPILOGUE

This publication describes ACHE's journey from its early days through its most recent accomplishments, using the changing dynamics of healthcare and the role of the healthcare executive as a backdrop. This journey would not be complete without some discussion of the future healthcare picture and the role of ACHE in that picture. The following pages take a brief look at some of the emerging trends in healthcare and address the future role of healthcare executives and ACHE.

Emerging Trends in Healthcare

As the science of medicine evolves, more and more patients will be treated for medical conditions outside of a hospital. For example, many types of elective surgery and other procedures, including ones that previously could only happen within a hospital environment, will take place in ambulatory settings or on an outpatient basis. As noninvasive surgery, such as orthoscopic or laproscopic surgery, become more common for even complex procedures, recovery time from surgery will also decrease. In addition, treatment for chronic conditions—such as asthma and diabetes—will focus more on prevention and maintenance, shifting treatment from acute, episodic care in the hospital to chronic care in ambulatory facilities and other healthcare venues. Because of all these factors, in the future, the number of people entering a hospital for medical treatment will probably be less than it is today; however, the acuity of these patients will be much higher. In other words, patients entering a hospital of the future will be sicker than they ever have been before.

In addition to the changing acuity of the average hospital patient, the patient population of the future will also be more diverse with respect to age, culture, and ethnic background. This will reflect society as a whole, as the country becomes more diverse. Hospital employees and healthcare executives will also reflect this diversity.

Another trend taking shape for the future is a further involvement of patients and families in their own care. Recently, there has been a clear movement in this direction, and this trend will continue as care becomes more patient centered and better addresses the cultural, emotional, and physical needs of the patient and family. Physicians, nurses, and other clinicians will be more involved in talking with patients and families and educating them on all aspects of their care. More in-depth discussion of treatment options will take place as patients' perspectives become increasingly important. Healthcare facilities will be designed to further address patient and family needs. For example, more new facilities may be designed to reflect the involvement of the family in care, allowing the family to remain with the patient throughout his or her stay in the healthcare facility.

As the future unfolds, healthcare organizations will become more "wired." For example, many healthcare organizations will have electronic medical records, automated order entry systems, and computerized decision support systems in place. Technology will be used not only to improve the administration of patient care but the delivery of care, treatment, and services as well. In the next decade, growing use of genomics—mapping DNA and using genes to customize treatment—will become more prevalent and accepted.

The Challenges Facing Healthcare Organizations

One of the most significant challenges organizations will face in the coming years is the continued improvement of patient safety and healthcare quality. While work is already underway to meet this challenge, work will continue and expand in this area. Participation of all types of healthcare practitioners, as well as patients and their families, will be necessary to ensure an appropriate level of healthcare safety and quality in the United States.

Another challenge healthcare organizations will continue to face is the growing number of uninsured Americans. Currently, there are nearly 50 million people in the United States that do not have health insurance.[1] This, coupled with the high cost of healthcare, has led to a significant portion of the country's gross domestic product (GDP) being allocated to healthcare costs. As of 2007, it's looking more and more likely that there will be some form of national healthcare program in the United States to address this issue. Currently, the United States is the only developed country in the world without this type of program. As a nation, America will need to decide how to rein in healthcare costs. These costs cannot continue to grow at the current rate or they will envelop the GDP.

The Role of the Healthcare Executive

As previously mentioned, healthcare executives will be more diverse in the future, reflecting the various cultures and races served in their organizations.

In addition, over the next 20 years, as baby boomers retire, there will be a massive changing of the guard in healthcare leadership. Just as there was a dramatic change when boomers took over from pre-boomers, there will be a large perspective shift in healthcare leadership when Generation X takes over from the boomers.

The background of healthcare executives will continue to diversify as more clinicians seek healthcare management roles. Many healthcare executives have found that a clinical background brings a good perspective to healthcare management. In coming years, a further melding of business and healthcare skills will be needed, as executives will need to understand both the safety and quality issues associated with healthcare management as well as the financial and human resource issues.

In addition to a more diverse executive population, the leadership style of healthcare executives will change, shifting from the strong personalities of the past to a more "servant leader style." This style will focus less on command and control and more on teamwork and collaboration.

In years to come, healthcare executives will need to become more politically active. As previously mentioned, the need to address the uninsured and rising costs of healthcare will take center stage in public policy debates. Healthcare executives will need to represent their constituency to government leaders and the community to clearly articulate the resources needed by their organizations' patient populations.

ACHE in the Future

Just as ACHE has been there to serve healthcare executives for the past 75 years, the organization will continue to be there in the future. ACHE will address the greater variety of individuals entering the field with various backgrounds by ensuring everyone has a common base of knowledge necessary to be an effective healthcare leader. ACHE is committed to continuing its Board of Governors Examination and making sure that it tests individuals on the basic body of knowledge necessary for effective healthcare management.

ACHE will also continue to provide education to executives to help them face day-to-day challenges, including how to improve patient safety and quality, provide effective governance, and effectively work with clinicians. Given the continuous and rapid advances in technology, there will be more variation in the types of education being offered through ACHE. For example, the manner in which the organization provides education will include electronic and web-based venues, podcasts, and so forth.

In the coming years, ACHE will continue to provide practical and useful programs and services. For example, ACHE will expand educational offerings in community and public policy and continue to champion diversity in the field. To best serve constituents and stay on top of trends, ACHE will continue to conduct research on the field of healthcare. To better serve patients and society, the organization will continue to work with suppliers to bring healthcare suppliers and executives together. ACHE will continue to champion ethics in the field and make sure the *Code of Ethics* reflects the rapid change in healthcare delivery.

ACHE is committed to helping healthcare executives throughout their entire career by not only recruiting high school and college graduates into the field and helping them establish their careers but also continuing as a career ally for healthcare executives as their careers mature and flourish.

Going forward, healthcare and the role it plays in society will continue to evolve, and ACHE will evolve along with it. ACHE will always be, as it has always been, an affiliate body that works in harmony and strives for excellence in the field of healthcare management.

Endnote

1.   Center on Budget and Policy Priorities. *The Number of Uninsured Americans Is at an All-Time High.* August 29, 2006. [Online article; retrieved 5/20/07.] www.cbpp.org/8-29-06health.htm

APPENDIX 1. *Code of Ethics*

AMERICAN COLLEGE OF HEALTHCARE EXECUTIVES CODE OF ETHICS*

* As amended by the Board of Governors on March 16, 2007.

PREAMBLE

The purpose of the *Code of Ethics* of the American College of Healthcare Executives is to serve as a standard of conduct for affiliates. It contains standards of ethical behavior for healthcare executives in their professional relationships. These relationships include colleagues, patients or others served; members of the healthcare executive's organization and other organizations, the community, and society as a whole.

The *Code of Ethics* also incorporates standards of ethical behavior governing individual behavior, particularly when that conduct directly relates to the role and identity of the healthcare executive.

The fundamental objectives of the healthcare management profession are to maintain or enhance the overall quality of life, dignity, and well-being of every individual needing healthcare service and to create a more equitable, accessible, effective, and efficient healthcare system.

Healthcare executives have an obligation to act in ways that will merit the trust, confidence, and respect of healthcare professionals and the general public. Therefore, healthcare executives should lead lives that embody an exemplary system of values and ethics.

In fulfilling their commitments and obligations to patients or others served, healthcare executives function as moral advocates and models. Since every management decision affects the health and well-being of both individuals and communities, healthcare executives must carefully evaluate the possible outcomes of their decisions. In organizations that deliver healthcare services, they must work to safeguard and foster the rights, interests, and prerogatives of patients or others served.

The role of moral advocate requires that healthcare executives take actions necessary to promote such rights, interests, and prerogatives.

Being a model means that decisions and actions will reflect personal integrity and ethical leadership that others will seek to emulate.

I.   THE HEALTHCARE EXECUTIVE'S RESPONSIBILITIES TO THE PROFESSION OF HEALTHCARE MANAGEMENT

The healthcare executive shall:

A.   Uphold the *Code of Ethics* and mission of the American College of Healthcare Executives;

B.   Conduct professional activities with honesty, integrity, respect, fairness, and good faith in a manner that will reflect well upon the profession;

C.   Comply with all laws and regulations pertaining to healthcare management in the jurisdictions in which the healthcare executive is located or conducts professional activities;

D.   Maintain competence and proficiency in healthcare management by implementing a personal program of assessment and continuing professional education;

E.   Avoid the improper exploitation of professional relationships for personal gain;

F.   Disclose financial and other conflicts of interest;

G.   Use this *Code* to further the interests of the profession and not for selfish reasons;

H.   Respect professional confidences;

I.   Enhance the dignity and image of the healthcare management profession through positive public information programs; and

J.   Refrain from participating in any activity that demeans the credibility and dignity of the healthcare management profession.

II.   THE HEALTHCARE EXECUTIVE'S RESPONSIBILITIES TO PATIENTS OR OTHERS SERVED

The healthcare executive shall, within the scope of his or her authority:

A.   Work to ensure the existence of a process to evaluate the quality of care or service rendered;

B.   Avoid practicing or facilitating discrimination and institute safeguards to prevent discriminatory organizational practices;

C.   Work to ensure the existence of a process that will advise patients or others served of the rights, opportunities, responsibilities, and risks regarding available healthcare services;

D.   Work to ensure that there is a process in place to facilitate the resolution of conflicts that may arise when values of patients and their families differ from those of employees and physicians;

E.   Demonstrate zero tolerance for any abuse of power that compromises patients or others served;

F.   Work to provide a process that ensures the autonomy and self-determination of patients or others served; and

G.   Work to ensure the existence of procedures that will safeguard the confidentiality and privacy of patients or others served.

III. THE HEALTHCARE EXECUTIVE'S RESPONSIBILITIES TO THE ORGANIZATION

The healthcare executive shall, within the scope of his or her authority:

A.   Provide healthcare services consistent with available resources, and when there are limited resources, work to ensure the existence of a resource allocation process that considers ethical ramifications;

B.   Conduct both competitive and cooperative activities in ways that improve community healthcare services;

C.   Lead the organization in the use and improvement of standards of management and sound business practices;

D.   Respect the customs and practices of patients or others served, consistent with the organization's philosophy;

E.   Be truthful in all forms of professional and organizational communication, and avoid disseminating information that is false, misleading, or deceptive;

F.   Report negative financial and other information promptly and accurately, and initiate appropriate action;

G.   Prevent fraud and abuse and aggressive accounting practices that may result in disputable financial reports;

H.   Create an organizational environment in which both clinical and management mistakes are minimized and, when they do occur, are disclosed and addressed effectively;

I.   Implement an organizational code of ethics and monitor compliance; and

J.   Provide ethics resources to staff to address organizational and clinical issues.

IV. THE HEALTHCARE EXECUTIVE'S RESPONSIBILITIES TO EMPLOYEES

Healthcare executives have ethical and professional obligations to the employees they manage that encompass but are not limited to:

A.   Creating a work environment that promotes ethical conduct by employees;

B.   Providing a work environment which encourages a free expression of ethical concerns and provides mechanisms for discussing and addressing such concerns;

C.   Providing a work environment that discourages harassment, sexual and other; coercion of any kind, especially to perform illegal or unethical acts; and discrimination on the basis of race, ethnicity, creed, gender, sexual orientation, age, or disability;

D.   Providing a work environment that promotes the proper use of employees' knowledge and skills;

E.   Providing a safe work environment; and

F.   Establishing appropriate grievance and appeals mechanisms.

V. THE HEALTHCARE EXECUTIVE'S RESPONSIBILITIES TO COMMUNITY AND SOCIETY

The healthcare executive shall:

A.   Work to identify and meet the healthcare needs of the community;

B.   Work to support access to healthcare services for all people;

C.   Encourage and participate in public dialogue on healthcare policy issues, and advocate solutions that will improve health status and promote quality healthcare;

D.   Apply short- and long-term assessments to management decisions affecting both community and society; and

E.   Provide prospective patients and others with adequate and accurate information, enabling them to make enlightened decisions regarding services.

VI. THE HEALTHCARE EXECUTIVE'S RESPONSIBILITY TO REPORT VIOLATIONS OF THE CODE

An affiliate of ACHE who has reasonable grounds to believe that another affiliate has violated this *Code* has a duty to communicate such facts to the Ethics Committee.

ADDITIONAL RESOURCES – Available on **ache.org** or by calling ACHE at (312) 424-2800.

1.   ACHE *Ethical Policy Statements*

   "Creating an Ethical Environment for Employees"

   "Decisions Near the End of Life"

   "Ethical Decision Making for Healthcare Executives"

   "Ethical Issues Related to a Reduction in Force"

   "Ethical Issues Related to Staff Shortages"

   "Health Information Confidentiality"

   "Impaired Healthcare Executives"

   "Promise-Making, Keeping and Rescinding"

2.   ACHE Grievance Procedure

3.   ACHE Ethics Committee Action

4.   ACHE Ethics Committee Scope and Function

APPENDIX 2. POLICY STATEMENTS

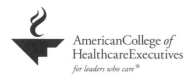

AmericanCollege *of*
HealthcareExecutives
for leaders who care®

ETHICAL
POLICY STATEMENT

Considerations for Healthcare Executive-Supplier Interactions

November 2007

Statement of the Issue

Healthcare executives share a fundamental commitment to enhance the quality of life and well-being of those needing healthcare services and to create a more equitable, effective and efficient healthcare delivery system. To accomplish these fundamental objectives, healthcare executives must rely on an intricate network of professionals that include professionals within the supplier community.

The realm of healthcare executive-supplier relationships involves not only the purchase of goods and services, but also the mutual provision of information and advice.

In interacting with current and potential suppliers, healthcare executives must act in ways that merit trust, confidence and respect, while fulfilling their duties to the public, their organizations and their profession. Further, it is important to avoid even the appearance of conflicts of interest that may seem to unduly advantage the health-care executive, the organization or the supplier. Thus, healthcare executives must demonstrate the utmost integrity as well as embrace the need for transparency in interactions with suppliers.

Policy Position

The American College of Healthcare Executives believes that healthcare executives should interact with company representatives who sell products and services to their organizations in a way that:

• Advances patient care or improves healthcare delivery;

• Is fully disclosed to the executive's organization;

• Does not damage the reputation of the organization or the profession;

• Does not violate applicable law; and

• Does not violate policies of the executive's organization.

In determining whether the nature of specific interactions meet each of the above guidelines, healthcare executives should carefully consider the issues detailed below.

1. The interaction between an executive and a supplier can be considered to enhance patient care or improve healthcare delivery when one or more of the following conditions are evident:

• It furthers the *executive's* knowledge of products or services which may improve patient care.

• It furthers the *supplier's* knowledge of healthcare needs, so that the supplier can produce better products and services.

• It facilitates the efficient and cost effective delivery of products and services to the executive's organization.

Examples of interactions that could enhance patient care or improve healthcare delivery are attendance by executives at trade show exhibits of supplier products, seminars or demonstrations produced by suppliers, and participation in supplier advisory councils, supplier surveys, or one-on-one visits with suppliers to exchange ideas.

2. Full disclosure of the supplier-executive relationship to the executive's organization should ordinarily be made to the party within the organization to whom the executive reports (e.g., a supervisor, the CEO or the Board/Chairman) or through the organization's compliance program officer. To prevent misunder-standing, it is advisable that disclosure include all remuneration arrangements, including reimbursements or perquisites (e.g., airfare or meals).

3. Even with full disclosure, damage to the reputation of the executive, to the organization or the profession may occur. The executive should avoid interactions with suppliers when this risk is present.

Considerations for Healthcare Executive-Supplier Interactions (cont.)

• Executives should avoid interaction with suppliers that could result in undue influence by suppliers in the decision-making process.

• As with any position of public trust, avoiding even the appearance of wrongdoing, conflict of interest or interference with free competition is important. Executives should take care that interactions with suppliers not result in perceptions of undue influence or other perceived impropriety.

4. Healthcare executives are subject to the federal anti-kickback statute which makes it a criminal offense to knowingly and willfully offer, pay, solicit or receive any remuneration in order to induce referrals of items or services reimbursable by federal healthcare programs.

• The anti-kickback statute interprets "remuneration" very broadly, including the transfer of anything of value, in cash or in kind, directly or indirectly, covertly or overtly.

• The healthcare executive should be aware that other statutes, which may vary from state to state, may also be applicable. If the application of a law is unclear to a proposed interaction, the executive has a duty to seek guidance from the appropriate party, who may be the person to whom the executive reports or the organization's legal counsel.

5. In addition to applicable laws, healthcare executives have a duty to be familiar and comply with their organizational policies governing interaction with suppliers. If the application of a policy is unclear to a proposed interaction, the executive has a duty to seek guidance from the appropriate party, who may be the person to whom the executive reports, the organization's legal counsel, compliance officer or ethics advisor.

The same type of relationship, such as participating in a supplier produced seminar or a supplier advisory council,

may be appropriate, or alternatively, may raise significant questions. The context and nature of the relationship can be more significant than the specific setting or type of interaction. Therefore, in addition to the above criteria, there are a number of questions healthcare executives should consider when assessing the nature of arrangements with suppliers and evaluating if a real or perceived conflict of interest is likely:

• Will the relationship affect your judgment, the judgment of your colleagues or the organization?

• Who will benefit from the relationship? Who might suffer?

• Would you be comfortable with the relationship being known to your patients, stakeholders and the general public?

• Can you defend the relationship to your colleagues and superiors?

• Does it represent a positive model for managerial, professional or organizational behavior?

• Would you expect other organizations or individuals to behave similarly?

• Is it fair to all parties?

When considering these questions, the healthcare executive should be cognizant of the need for public trust and the avoidance of even the appearance of impropriety. Furthermore, to foster knowledge and sensitivity to potential issues associated with supplier interactions, healthcare executives should promote the dissemination of this policy statement to appropriate managers within their organizations as well as to relevant suppliers.

Approved by the Board of Governors of the American College of Healthcare Executives on November 12, 2007.

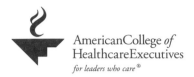

AmericanCollege *of*
HealthcareExecutives
for leaders who care ®

ETHICAL
POLICY STATEMENT

Creating an Ethical Environment for Employees

March 1992
August 1995 (revised)
November 2000 (revised)
November 2005 (revised)

Statement of the Issue

The number and magnitude of challenges facing healthcare organizations are unprecedented. Growing financial pressures, rising public and payor expectations and the increasing number of consolidations have placed hospitals, health networks, managed care plans and other healthcare organizations under greater stress—thus potentially intensifying ethical dilemmas.

Now, more than ever, the healthcare organization must be managed with consistently high professional and ethical standards. This means that the executive, acting with other responsible parties, must foster and support an environment conducive not only to providing high-quality, cost-effective healthcare, but also seek to ensure individual ethical behavior and practices.

Recognizing the importance of ethics, healthcare executives should seek various ways to integrate ethical practices and reflection into the organization's overall culture. To create such an ethical environment for all employees, healthcare executives should: 1) support the development and implementation of employee ethical standards of behavior that include ethical clinical and administrative practices, and 2) ensure effective and competent ethics resources exist and are available to all employees, such as ethics committees to clarify such standards of behavior when there is ethical uncertainty. The executive also must support and implement a systematic and organization-wide approach to ethics training as well as corporate compliance for all staff.

The ability of an organization to achieve its full potential will remain dependent upon the motivation, knowledge, skills and ethical behavior of its staff. Thus, the executive has an obligation to accomplish the organization's mission in a manner that respects the values of individuals and maximizes their contributions.

Policy Position

The American College of Healthcare Executives believes that all healthcare executives have an ethical and professional obligation to employees of the organizations they manage to create a working environment that supports, but is not limited to:

• Reviewing the principles and ideals expressed in vision, mission and value statements, personnel policies, annual reports, employee orientation materials, and other documents to test congruence;

• The development of an organizational code of ethics that includes guidelines for all employees' ethical standards of behavior and practices;

• Responsible employee ethical behavior and practices based on the organization's code of ethics and ethical standards of practice. Such expectations should be included in employee position descriptions where relevant;

• Free expression of ethical concerns;

• An available ethics resource for discussing and addressing clinical, organizational and research related ethical concerns without retribution, such as an ethics committee;

• Establish an anonymous mechanism that safeguards employees who wish to raise ethical concerns;

• Freedom from all harassment, coercion and discrimination;

• Appropriate use of an employee's knowledge, skills and abilities; and

• A safe work environment.

These responsibilities can best be implemented in an environment where all employees are encouraged to develop and adhere to the highest standards of ethics. This should be done with attention to other features of the code of ethics and appropriate professional code, particularly those that stress the moral character of the executive and the organization itself.

Approved by the Board of Governors of the American College of Healthcare Executives on November 7, 2005.

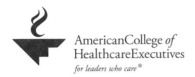

AmericanCollege *of*
HealthcareExecutives
for leaders who care®

ETHICAL
POLICY STATEMENT

Decisions Near the End of Life

August 1994
November 1999 (revised)
November 2004 (revised)

Statement of the Issue

Medical technology has shaped the circumstances of death, giving us options about when, where and how we die. Intervening at the moment of death, technology can now sustain lives, but often there is little or no hope for recovery or for a meaningful existence.

Fearful of economic dependency, prolonged pain and loss of self, patients and/or proxies are exercising more influence over decisions near the end of life. The traditional value to preserve life by all possible means is now being weighed against quality-of-life considerations.

Policy Position

The American College of Healthcare Executives (ACHE) urges healthcare executives to address the ethical dilemmas and problems surrounding death and promote public dialog that will lead to awareness and resolution of death with dignity concerns.

ACHE encourages all healthcare executives to play a significant role in addressing this issue:

• Executives should heighten awareness of ethical issues surrounding the right to choose treatment through information forums that promote open discussion among patients and their families, attorneys, clergy, journalists, physicians, and other healthcare professionals. By raising moral and ethical questions, healthcare executives will aid the public in understanding the growing impact of technology on death and dying.

• Healthcare executives should advocate the completion of advance directives, including living wills and durable powers of attorney for healthcare. Ideally, such documents should be prepared prior to hospitalization or medical crisis.

• These and similar legal mechanisms encourage people to consider under what circumstances they would not want certain life-prolonging treatments. Use of a power of attorney or laws that permit the appointment of a proxy have the added advantage of allowing individuals to designate a specific person who would make treatment choices

for them at any time they lack decision-making capacity. The ultimate objective of advance directives is to protect the rights of patients to influence clinical decisions affecting their care.

• Healthcare executives have a responsibility to ensure their organizations provide support for patients and their families as treatment decisions are reached. Patient autonomy (the right of an individual to influence decisions affecting his or her treatment) should remain at the core of this process.

• When there is disagreement on treatment for incompetent patients (even those patients who have valid advance directives or a durable power of attorney), the guidance of an ethics committee or similar resource may aid in resolution. Healthcare executives should develop clear guidelines to handle disputes and provide support to physicians and families responsible for making treatment choices.

• When developing and implementing guidelines, healthcare executives must encourage cooperation and understanding of ethical decision making among members of the governing body, executive management, physicians and other members of the healthcare team. Executives should work to develop methods of raising awareness and providing education regarding sensitivity to ethical dilemmas.

• If organizational policies limit end-of-life options for patients and families, healthcare executives have a responsibility to see that mechanisms are in place that provide disclosure of such limitations.

• Executives should support the development of resources and programs that promote pain control as a crucial modality in the management of patients at the end of life.

Healthcare executives must foster reasoned, compassionate decision making that considers the rights and values of patients and staff. While interpretation of these principles will vary by local custom and law, healthcare executives have a responsibility to ensure their organizations operate with respect for the inherent worth and human dignity of every individual.

Approved by the Board of Governors of the American College of Healthcare Executives on November 8, 2004.

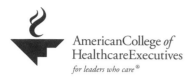 AmericanCollege *of*
HealthcareExecutives
for leaders who care ®

ETHICAL
POLICY STATEMENT

Ethical Decision Making for Healthcare Executives

August 1993
February 1997 (revised)
November 2002 (revised)
November 2007 (revised)

Statement of the Issue

Ethical decision making is required when the healthcare executive must balance the needs and interests of the individual, the organization and society. Those involved in this decision-making process must consider ethical principles such as justice, autonomy, beneficence and fairness as well as professional ethical standards and codes. Many factors have contributed to the growing concern in healthcare organizations with ethical issues, including issues of access and affordability, pressure to reduce costs, mergers and acquisitions, financial and other resource constraints, and advances in medical technology that complicate decision making near the end of life. Healthcare executives have a responsibility to address the growing number of complex ethical dilemmas they are facing, but they cannot and should not make such decisions alone or without a sound decision-making framework.

Healthcare organizations should have vehicles that may include ethics committees, ethics consultation services, processes for dealing with potential conflicts of interest or written policies and procedures to assist healthcare executives with the ethics decision-making process. With these organizational mechanisms, the sometimes conflicting interests of patients, families, caregivers, the organization, payors and the community can be appropriately weighed and balanced.

Policy Position

It is incumbent upon healthcare executives to lead in a manner that sets an ethical tone for their organizations. The American College of Healthcare Executives (ACHE) believes education in ethics is an important step in a healthcare executive's lifelong commitment to high ethical conduct, both personally and professionally. Further, ACHE supports the development of organizational mechanisms that enable healthcare executives

to appropriately and expeditiously address ethical dilemmas. Whereas physicians, nurses and other caregivers may primarily address ethical issues on a case-by-case basis, healthcare executives also have a responsibility to address those issues at broader organizational, community and societal levels. ACHE encourages its affiliates, as leaders in their organizations, to take an active role in the development and demonstration of ethical decision making.

To this end, healthcare executives should:

- Seek to create a culture that fosters ethical practices and ethical decision making throughout the organization.

- Communicate the organization's commitment to ethical decision making through its mission or value statements and its organizational code of ethics.

- Demonstrate through their professional behavior the importance of ethics to the organization.

- Offer educational programs to boards, staff, physicians and others on their organization's ethical standards of practice and on the more global issues of ethical decision making in today's healthcare environment. Further, healthcare executives should promote learning opportunities, such as those provided through professional societies or academic organizations, that will facilitate open discussion of ethical issues.

- Develop and use organizational mechanisms that reflect their organizations' mission and values and are flexible enough to deal with the spectrum of ethical concerns—clinical, organizational, business and management.

- Ensure that organizational mechanisms to address ethics issues are readily available, and include individuals who are competent to address ethical concerns and reflect diverse perspectives. An organization's ethics committee, for example, might include representatives

Ethical Decision Making for Healthcare Executives (cont.)

from groups such as physicians, nurses, managers, board members, social workers, attorneys, patient and/or community representatives, and clergy. All these groups are likely to bring unique and valuable perspectives to bear on discussions of ethical issues.

• ExecutivesEvaluate and continually refine organizational processes for addressing ethical issues.

Approved by the Board of Governors of the American College of Healthcare Executives on November 12, 2007.

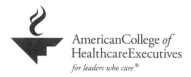
AmericanCollege *of*
HealthcareExecutives
for leaders who care®

ETHICAL
POLICY STATEMENT

Ethical Issues Related to a Reduction in Force

August 1995
November 2000 (revised)
November 2005 (revised)

Statement of the Issue

As the result of managed care, such as variable admissions, shorter lengths of stay, higher productivity, new technology, and other factors, the capacity of some healthcare organizations could significantly exceed demand. As a result, these organizations may be required to reduce their work force. Additionally, mergers and consolidations can result in further reductions and reassignments of staff. Financial pressures will continue to fuel this trend. However, patient care needs should not be compromised when determining staffing requirements.

Careful planning, diligent cost controls, effective resource management, and proper consultation can lessen the hardship and stress of a reduction in force. Formal policies and procedures should be developed well in advance of the need to implement them.

The decision to reduce staff necessitates consideration of the short-term and long-term impact on all employees—those leaving and those remaining. Decision makers should consider the potential ethical conflict between formally stated organizational values and their staff reduction actions.

Policy Position

The American College of Healthcare Executives recommends that specific steps be considered by healthcare executives when initiating a reduction in force process to support consistency between stated organizational values and those demonstrated before, during and after the process. Among these steps are the following:

• Recognize that cost reduction efforts must be appropriate—if they are too aggressive, the consequences for patients, staff and the organization can be as harmful as doing too little or proceeding too late;

• Consult with labor counsel;

• Provide timely, accurate, clear and consistent information—including the reasoning behind the decision—to stakeholders when staff reductions become necessary;

• Review the principles and ideals expressed in vision, mission and value statements, personnel policies, annual reports, employee orientation materials, and other documents to test congruence and conformance with reduction in force decisions;

• Support, if possible, through retraining and redeployment, employees whose positions have been eliminated. Also, consider outplacement assistance and appropriate severance policies, if possible; and

• Address the needs of remaining staff by demonstrating sensitivity to their potential feelings of loss, anger and survivor guilt. Also address their anxiety about the possibility of further reductions, uncertainty regarding changes in workload, work redesign, and similar concerns.

Healthcare organizations encounter the same set of challenging issues associated with reductions in force as do other employers. Reduction in force decisions should reflect an institution's ethics and value statements.

Approved by the Board of Governors of the American College of Healthcare Executives on November 7, 2005.

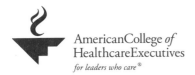

AmericanCollege *of*
HealthcareExecutives
for leaders who care ®

ETHICAL
POLICY STATEMENT

Ethical Issues Related to Staff Shortages

March 2002
November 2007 (revised)

Statement of the Issue

The effects of staff shortages are felt acutely by hospitals and other healthcare organizations. While less than a decade ago healthcare executives were struggling with how to reduce their organization's staff responsibly, today they face an equally daunting challenge. They must fulfill their responsibility to provide high-quality, affordable patient care in the face of work force shortages that may leave them with vacancies in many positions throughout their organization.

Alleviating work force shortages or adapting to them is a complex problem for which there are few easy solutions. Nevertheless, healthcare executives have an ethical responsibility to address any shortages that exist within their organizations in such a way that patient care is not compromised, existing staff are not unduly burdened and financial costs do not become excessive.

Policy Position

The American College of Healthcare Executives (ACHE) recommends that healthcare executives develop responsible action plans for delivering patient care in the face of staff shortages. To this end, ACHE recommends that such plans address the following:

- Attracting and retaining qualified staff by addressing issues important to today's work force, including strengthening the patient/clinician/executive partnership, treating each other with respect, promoting continuous quality improvement, and providing fair compensation, flexible scheduling and professional development;

- Maintaining workloads and expectations that strive to alleviate and prevent burnout;

- Creating systems for job assignments and backup coverage that ensure responsibilities are appropriately matched with qualifications;

- Being sensitive to the financial and nonfinancial consequences of utilizing temporary personnel to fill vacancies;

- Responding to potential disasters that would significantly impact staff availability over sustained periods, requiring multilevel backup capacity;

- Conducting employee opinion surveys and exit interviews, using results to identify steps to improve job satisfaction;

- Identifying ways to engage employees to help define and address issues adversely affecting recruitment and retention objectives;

- Maintaining a diverse and culturally competent work force;

- Analyzing departments or units with high turnover rates to determine whether management shortcomings, working conditions, and/or other factors may be contributing to staff morale problems; and

- Closing units or diverting patients if staff shortages become severe to ensure that patient care is not compromised and high-quality care is maintained.

Healthcare executives may find it beneficial to join forces with others in their service areas to address the problem of staff shortages. Collaboration to recruit qualified staff will prove to be a more effective long-term strategy than competition for the same resources. ACHE encourages healthcare executives to collaborate on the development of creative, sustainable strategies that will benefit their respective organizations as well as help ensure that high-quality, affordable healthcare remains available in their communities.

In addition, ACHE encourages healthcare executives to work to ensure the future supply of healthcare workers. Healthcare executives should collaborate with others to expose students to careers in healthcare, including both clinical and managerial careers.

Approved by the Board of Governors of the American College of Healthcare Executives on November 12, 2007.

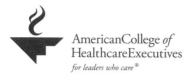

AmericanCollege *of*
HealthcareExecutives
for leaders who care®

ETHICAL
POLICY STATEMENT

Health Information
Confidentiality

February 1994
November 1997 (revised)
November 2004 (revised)

Statement of the Issue

Healthcare is among the most personal services rendered in our society; yet to deliver this care, scores of personnel must have access to intimate patient information. In order to receive appropriate care, patients must feel free to reveal personal information. In return, the healthcare provider must treat patient information confidentially.

However, maintaining confidentiality is becoming more difficult. Information systems technology allows instant retrieval of medical information, widening access to a greater number of people. Within healthcare organizations, personal information contained in medical records is reviewed not only by physicians and nurses, but also by professionals in many clinical and administrative support areas.

Healthcare executives must follow the laws governing use and release of information. Releases cannot be made without proper authorization except under limited circumstances. Healthcare executives must determine that patients or their legal representatives consented to the release of information and keep records of most disclosures for review upon patient request.

Some exceptions to patient confidentiality are necessary to promote public health, to protect children and spouses from abuse, and to comply with certain laws. Media representatives also seek access to health information, particularly when a patient is a public figure or when treatment involves legal or public health issues. Nevertheless, the rights of individual patients must be protected. Society's need for information rarely outweighs the right of patients to confidentiality.

Policy Position

The American College of Healthcare Executives believes all healthcare executives have a moral and professional obligation to protect the confidentiality of patients' med-

ical records. Additional legal restrictions imposed by the HIPAA Privacy and Security Rules must also be satisfied. As patient advocates, executives must obtain proper patient authorization to release information or follow carefully defined policies on the release of information without consent.

While the healthcare organization owns the health record, the information in that record remains the patient's personal property. Organizations must determine the appropriateness of all requests for patient information under applicable federal and state law and act accordingly.

In fulfilling their responsibilities, healthcare executives should seek to:

- Limit access to patient information to authorized individuals only. Non-treatment access should be limited to the minimum amount of information necessary.

- Ensure that institutional policies on confidentiality and release of information are consistent with regulations and laws.

- Educate healthcare personnel on confidentiality requirements and take steps to ensure all healthcare personnel are aware of and understand their responsibilities to keep patient information confidential, and impose sanctions for violations.

- Safeguard medical record files and computerized data with security and storage systems that protect against unauthorized access and ensure data integrity and availability.

- Provide for appropriate disaster recovery.

- Establish guidelines for masking patient identifiers in committee minutes and other working documents where the identity is not necessary.

Health Information Confidentiality (cont.)

- Ensure that policies concerning the right of patients to have access to their own medical records and an accounting of disclosures are clearly established and understood by appropriate staff.

- Create guidelines for securing necessary permissions for the release of medical information for research, education, utilization review and other purposes.

- Adopt a specialized process to further protect sensitive information such as psychiatric, HIV status or substance abuse treatment records.

- Identify special situations that require consultation with senior management prior to use or release of information.

- When appropriate, seek written agreements that detail the obligations of confidentiality and security for individuals and agencies who receive medical records information, including business associates (service providers).

- Follow all applicable policies and procedures regarding privacy of patient information even if information is in the public domain.

- Adopt procedures to address patient rights to request amendment of medical records and other rights under the HIPAA Privacy Rule.

- Educate patients about organizational policies on confidentiality, and use the notice of privacy practices as required by the HIPAA Privacy Rule.

- Participate in the public dialogue on confidentiality issues such as employer use of healthcare information and public health reporting.

The American College of Healthcare Executives urges all healthcare executives to maintain an appropriate balance between the patient's right to confidentiality and the need to release information in the public's interest in accordance with applicable state and federal law.

Approved by the Board of Governors of the American College of Healthcare Executives on November 8, 2004.

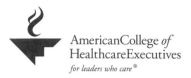

AmericanCollege *of*
HealthcareExecutives
for leaders who care®

ETHICAL
POLICY STATEMENT

Impaired Healthcare Executives

February 1991
March 1995 (revised)
November 2000 (revised)
November 2005 (revised)
November 2006 (revised)

Statement of the Issue

The American College of Healthcare Executives recognizes that impairment, defined broadly to include alcoholism, substance abuse, chemical dependency, mental/emotional instability or cognitive impairment, is a significant problem that crosses all societal boundaries.

Impairment occurs when the healthcare executive is unable to perform professional duties as expected. Impaired healthcare executives affect not only themselves and their families, but they also have a significant impact on their profession; their professional society; their organizations, colleagues, patients, clients and others served; their communities; and society as a whole. Impairment typically leads to misconduct in the form of incompetence and unsafe or unprofessional behavior, which also can lead to substantial costs associated with loss of productivity and errors in judgment.

The impaired healthcare executive can damage the public image of his or her organization of employment. Public confidence in the organization diminishes if it appears that the organization is not being managed with consistently high standards of professional and ethical practice. This lack of public confidence may cause the community to deem the organization unworthy of its support.

Society expects healthcare executives to practice the standards of good health that they advocate for the public. Impaired healthcare executives diminish the credibility of the profession and its ability to manage society's healthcare when they are not appropriately managing their own personal health.

Policy Position

The preamble of the American College of Healthcare Executives *Code of Ethics* states, "Healthcare executives have an obligation to act in ways that will merit the trust, confidence and respect of healthcare professionals and the general public. To do this, healthcare executives must lead lives that embody an exemplary system of values and ethics."

The American College of Healthcare Executives believes that all healthcare executives have an ethical and a professional obligation to:

• Maintain a personal health that is free from impairment.

• Refrain from all professional activities if impaired.

• Expeditiously seek treatment if impairment occurs.

• Urge impaired colleagues to expeditiously seek treatment and to refrain from all professional activities while impaired.

• Assist recovered colleagues when they resume their professional activities.

• Intervene and report the impairment to the appropriate person(s) should the colleague refuse to seek professional assistance and should the state of impairment persist.

• Support peers who identify healthcare executives in need of help.

• Recognize that individuals who have successfully received treatment for impairment and are no longer deemed impaired should be considered for employment opportunities for which they are qualified.

• Recommend or provide, within one's employing organization, confidential avenues for reporting impairment and either access or referral to treatment or assistance programs.

• Urge the community to provide information and resources for assistance and treatment of alcoholism, substance abuse, mental/emotional instability and cognitive impairment as needed and as appropriate.

• Raise the awareness of key stakeholders (such as employees, governing board members, etc.) on impairment issues and the resources available for assistance.

Approved by the Board of Governors of the American College of Healthcare Executives on November 6, 2006.

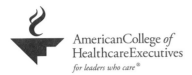

AmericanCollege *of*
HealthcareExecutives
for leaders who care®

ETHICAL
POLICY STATEMENT

Promise-Making, Keeping and Rescinding

March 2006

Statement of the Issue

In today's environment, healthcare executives are faced with making challenging and complex decisions that require balancing the current and future needs of the overall organization with various constituencies that serve and are served by the organization. Sometimes these decisions come about when healthcare executives are faced with making "promises" or revisiting previous promises made by executives. When this happens, new challenges can come about from the difficult task of weighing the needs of varied constituencies and the use of resources, not to mention the ethical responsibility to make such decisions.

Promises are verbal or written commitments made to another person or group of people. Promises can be formal written agreements, such as contracts, or informal agreements such as when a healthcare executive states to someone (or a group of people) an intention to do something. When the executive does the latter and recognizes that such a statement of intention will lead the person(s) to whom it is given to count on your following through, your statement of intention is a promise. Once made, adhering to a promise is a moral responsibility of the healthcare executive, even if made by one's predecessor.

Despite the moral responsibility that one ought to respect a promise, organizational circumstances may change sufficiently so that the promise should be reviewed, even though the promise may have become a long-standing tradition or expectation. This could be a situation regardless of whether the promise was made by the current healthcare executive or a prior executive in the same position.

However, because trust and honoring moral commitments are hallmarks of successful healthcare organizations, making, revising or rescinding a promise requires thoughtful consideration. A healthcare executive needs sufficient reasons for both making a promise and for

breaking a promise. In the latter case, the violation or breaking of a promise without adequate reason leads to harm, not only to the person(s) to whom the promise was made, but also to the executive and the image of the healthcare organization.

Policy Position

Making a Promise

The American College of Healthcare Executives (ACHE) firmly believes that healthcare executives have an ethical responsibility to use a systematic, deliberative and thoughtful approach to decision making when making a promise to a person or a group of people. To ensure such an approach, the following questions should be considered:

- What are the circumstances surrounding the promise? Why is the promise being considered? Why now?

- What are the facts regarding the promise? Is the promise legally binding? What does legal counsel suggest?

- What are the relevant ethical considerations regarding the promise? Is there an ethical rationale for justifying the promise?

- What are the options, such as maintaining the promise, rescinding the promise or altering the promise? Will future CEOs be able to uphold this promise? Are there circumstances under which this promise can or should be revisited? If so, what are they?

- What are the implications (benefits and harms) surrounding the above option(s)? How certain are you of those implications?

- What are the perspectives of the stakeholders affected by the promise?

Promise-Making, Keeping and Rescinding (cont.)

- Have you carefully reflected on the various options, including conducting a quantitative and qualitative analysis of each option and assessing both the short- and long-term ramifications of each option?

- After selecting a particular option, did you seek the appropriate approval, such as the board's?

- How is the promise going to be communicated and documented? Has this document been shared with the relevant stakeholders? Is it clear how future CEOs will know this promise exists?

Keeping or Rescinding a Promise

ACHE further believes that a similar systematic, deliberative and thoughtful approach to decision making be used when healthcare executives are faced with questions concerning the appropriateness of maintaining previous promises. In such a manner the healthcare executive can ensure that sound decisions are being made even in challenging and complex situations. The following aspects of the decision-making process can help foster a reasoned decision:

1. Making a Decision Regarding a Previous Promise

After clearly identifying and acknowledging the need to review whether a promise ought to be maintained, the following questions should be considered:

- What are the circumstances surrounding the promise? Why was the promise made? Why is it being questioned now?

- What are the facts regarding the promise? Is the promise legally obligated? What does legal counsel suggest?

- What are the relevant ethical considerations regarding maintaining, revising or rescinding the promise? Is there an ethical rationale for justifying the rescinding or revising of the promise?

- What are the options, such as maintaining the promise, rescinding the promise or altering the promise?

- What are the implications (benefits and harms) surrounding each option? How certain are you of those implications?

- What are the perspectives of the stakeholders affected by the promise?

- Have you carefully reflected on the various options, including conducting a quantitative and qualitative analysis of each option and assessing both the short- and long-term ramifications of each option?

- After selecting a particular option, did you seek the appropriate approval, such as the board's, giving the ethical grounding for the decision?

2. Implementing a Decision Regarding a Previous Promise

Decisions to rescind or revise an existing promise should be communicated in a timely manner to all key stakeholders, including the rationale for the action. When decisions are made to revise or rescind a promise, a clear communication plan is advised.

A comprehensive communication plan includes the following:

- Identifying the key audiences and messages.

- Choosing the appropriate spokesperson for the target audience.

- Obtaining the affected stakeholder perspectives and feedback, including being prepared to justify the decision and respond to all questions of concern.

- Considering the response if the decision was reported by the media.

During the communication process, if concerns or ramifications concerning the action arise that were not previously considered, executives should consider whether to review their decision regarding the promise.

Whether making a promise or reviewing a previous promise, the best decision outcome will be achieved when thoughtful, systematic reasoning and transparency serve as the primary guides for executive behavior.

Approved by the Board of Governors of the American College of Healthcare Executives on March 24, 2006.

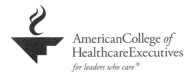

AmericanCollege *of*
HealthcareExecutives
for leaders who care®

PROFESSIONAL
POLICY STATEMENT

Board Certification in
Healthcare Management

November 1997
November 2002 (revised)
November 2007 (revised)

Statement of the Issue

By providing a credentialing program, a professional
society helps the field it serves by setting standards for
competence and excellence and assists the public by
providing a means by which to identify those who have
met this standard. Choosing to become credentialed in
healthcare management enables a professional to demonstrate his or her competence, leadership and commitment
to the profession. It also provides evidence of that individual's commitment to lifelong learning, management
excellence and ethical conduct.

The American College of Healthcare Executives (ACHE)
has a comprehensive, multifaceted credentialing program.
Healthcare executives who successfully meet the criteria
become board certified in healthcare management and are
recognized as ACHE Fellows. With this distinction,
Fellows earn the right to use the credential "FACHE"
(Fellow of the American College of Healthcare
Executives).

Policy Position

The American College of Healthcare Executives believes
that by participating in a voluntary credentialing program, healthcare executives are taking a meaningful and
visible step toward demonstrating their competence in
the field. Through their participation in such programs,
healthcare executives also are reaffirming their commitment to lifelong learning, management excellence and
ethical conduct.

The value of a credential is linked to the credibility of
the certifying organization and the rigor of the credentialing process itself. To this end, ACHE believes a
voluntary credentialing program that bestows certification in healthcare management should encompass
requirements addressing:

• Formal academic preparation beyond a bachelor's degree

• Position and responsibility

• Experience

Further, ACHE believes the program should require:

• Participation in continuing education

• Participation in healthcare and community affairs

• Commitment to the association as demonstrated
by tenure in ACHE

• Peer review

• Adherence to an ethical code of conduct

• Successful completion of a comprehensive exam
that measures knowledge and skills in healthcare
management

For a voluntary credentialing program to be a viable
indicator of an individual's competency, the program
must be designed using rigorous standards and periodically refined so that it remains a fair and predictable
indicator of professional competence in the changing
marketplace. To this end, the credentialing body should
adhere to the following steps as it relates to the development and refinement of its testing mechanism(s):

• Conduct periodic job analyses within the field to
ensure the testing mechanism is reflective of the
frequency and importance of job-related tasks performed by healthcare executives;

• Provide for periodic review of the testing mechanism
by a professional testing service or a psychometric
consultant;

• Establish a passing point for the test that is reflective
of professional competence, reasonable and accepted
in the psychometric community;

Board Certification in Healthcare Management (cont.)

• Administer each test according to established, consistent procedures;

• Follow prescribed security procedures that protect the integrity of the testing materials and the administration of the test.

Voluntary credentialing programs also should require individuals to periodically recertify—documenting their continuing education and other activities that are indicators of continued competency and their commitment to the profession. Finally, each year credentialed individuals should attest to uphold their professional Code of Ethics.

Approved by the Board of Governors of the American College of Healthcare Executives on November 12, 2007.

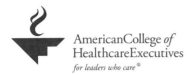

AmericanCollege *of*
HealthcareExecutives
for leaders who care ®

PROFESSIONAL
POLICY STATEMENT

Considering the Value of Older, Experienced Healthcare Executives

May 1992
May 1995 (revised)
December 1998 (revised)
March 2002 (revised)
November 2005 (revised)

Statement of the Issue

In recent decades, the world has witnessed unprecedented extensions in the longevity and well-being of citizens of developed nations. This prolongation of life is a remarkable achievement, but coping with the changes created by large numbers of long-lived people is forcing society and its institutions to make many adjustments.

Healthcare employers and employees must acknowledge the employment challenges presented by the new demographics. For employers, one challenge is overcoming unsubstantiated negative stereotypes of older, experienced employees concerning their attitudes, performance, physiological capacity, and ability to learn new techniques and skills. An opportunity for employers is to tap the extensive skills and experience of the older, experienced executive.

In 1967, the federal government enacted the Age Discrimination in Employment Act. Its purpose is protecting and promoting the employment opportunities of older workers and helping to find solutions to age-related employment problems. Healthcare organizations will engender more positive regard and support from their key stakeholders by striving to embrace the spirit and the letter of the law.

Policy Position

The American College of Healthcare Executives (ACHE) encourages healthcare executives and their organizations to employ individuals without regard to their age. While overt discrimination against employment of older, experienced healthcare executives is illegal and subject to sanction under federal law, even covert discrimination against the employment of older, experienced healthcare executives is incompatible with ACHE's *Code of Ethics*.

Executive employment decisions will become increasingly complex as organizations respond to demands for staff diversity and for changing leadership and management skills. To avoid actual and perceived discrimination against older, experienced healthcare executives, ACHE advocates the following to help create equitable employment opportunities.

ACHE encourages all healthcare executives and the organizations they represent to play a significant role in addressing this issue by actively pursuing the following:

- Employers should direct executive recruiters to identify and present candidates for senior-level positions irrespective of their age, and executive recruiters should suggest that their clients consider candidates for positions irrespective of their age.

- CEOs, trustees and recruitment and retention decision makers should avoid negative stereotypes of older, experienced workers and actively recruit seasoned executives for consideration, including those who are between positions.

- CEOs and trustees of healthcare organizations should establish human resources plans that provide for leadership succession and effective continuing education for older, experienced executives.

ACHE encourages older, experienced executives to actively pursue the following:

- Be flexible when seeking new positions by considering different organizational settings, geographic areas, levels of responsibility and compensations than they may have been accustomed to.

Considering the Value of Older, Experienced Healthcare Executives (cont.)

• Assume responsibility for continuously maintaining and improving their skills so they can contribute value to employing organizations in environments that continually change.

• Interact with colleagues and remain involved in professional associations.

Healthcare will continue to be regarded as a growing sector—one that not only offers the prospect of employment but also the opportunity to make important social contributions. Leaders in this field have an ethical responsibility to select and retain executives without regard to their chronological age.

Approved by the Board of Governors of the American College of Healthcare Executives on November 7, 2005.

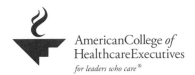
American College *of*
HealthcareExecutives
for leaders who care®

PROFESSIONAL
POLICY STATEMENT

Evaluating the Performance of the Hospital or Health System CEO

November 1993
December 1998 (revised)
November 2003 (revised)

Statement of the Issue

Board evaluation of the hospital or health system chief executive officer has long been an important way to ensure that performance expectations are mutually understood and that progress is being made toward their attainment. In an environment characterized by unprecedented change and uncertainty, the CEO's performance evaluation both assumes new significance and requires important changes to the nature and frequency of the CEO evaluation. The evaluation process should be viewed as an important tool for measuring leadership effectiveness.

Policy Position

The American College of Healthcare Executives believes hospitals and health systems should evaluate their chief executive officers using the following principles:

• Expectations of the CEO, expressed in terms of well-defined benchmark objectives, should be clearly identified well in advance of the evaluation to ensure that the evaluation will be a meaningful assessment of progress made on mutually understood goals.

• The evaluation should be a continuous, year-long process culminating in a formal, annual performance review that contains no surprises for either the evaluators or the CEO. Continuous evaluations are a way to provide meaningful feedback on many aspects of operations and clarify misunderstandings resulting from poor communication or lack of expertise in particular areas.

• The evaluation process should enhance the working relationship of and information-sharing between the CEO and the board, rather than be a one-directional process. The CEO should have an employment contract to further facilitate understanding of mutually understood expectations.

• The evaluation should link attainment of organizational objectives with the CEO's personal performance objectives. Two key organizational objectives should be considered in the CEO's performance evaluation: 1) the organization's contributions to community health and

2) organizational success. Professional role fulfillment—the CEO's personal performance goals—should be the third component of the evaluation. Among those items that should be included in the CEO's personal goals are 1) modeling ethical behavior and 2) participation in continuing education.

• Data, not subjective assessments, should be the mainstay of the CEO's performance evaluation. Hospitals and health systems should review data on how systems, e.g., efficiencies in patient admissions, accounts receivable, are working. In addition, because the CEO is ultimately accountable for the functioning of such systems and overall quality of care or service delivered, data about system effectiveness is among the determinants of the CEO's performance.

• The CEO's leadership of the organization to improve the community's health should also be evaluated. Examples of such contributions might include the extent of the organization's efforts to address issues such as prenatal care, smoking cessation, early detection of heart disease and diabetes as well as more global efforts to educate the community about important health issues.

• Board self-evaluations are an important enhancement to the evaluation process because they further build on the concept of mutually understood expectations. Consider conducting self-evaluations of the full board and of individual members.

• Although overall system performance is an important measure of CEO effectiveness, the CEO's salary increases must also be tied to individual performance as measured by the evaluation.

Reference

American College of Healthcare Executives, *Evaluating the Performance of the Hospital CEO, Third Edition* (Chicago: American College of Healthcare Executives, 2003).

Approved by the Board of Governors of the American College of Healthcare Executives on November 10, 2003.

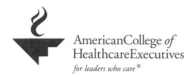
AmericanCollege *of*
HealthcareExecutives
for leaders who care®

PROFESSIONAL
POLICY STATEMENT

Increasing and Sustaining Racial/Ethnic Diversity in Healthcare Management

July 1990
May 1995 (revised)
December 1998 (revised)
March 2002 (revised)
November 2005 (revised)

Statement of the Issue

Racially/ethnically diverse employees represent a growing percentage of all healthcare employees, but they hold only a small percentage of top healthcare management positions.

This disparity persists despite recent successes in attracting racially/ethnically diverse students to graduate study in health administration. For example, by the 2000-2001 academic year, the proportion of racially/ethnically diverse individuals enrolled in and graduating from master's programs in health administration had nearly doubled compared to their representation in the 1992-1993 academic year. By 2003-2004, the proportion of racially/ethnically diverse individuals graduating from master's programs amounted to nearly 30 percent of the total. However, success in recruitment must be considered only a partial triumph as underrepresentation in healthcare management positions persists. Studies conducted jointly by the American College of Healthcare Executives (ACHE), the Institute for Diversity in Health Management, the National Association of Health Services Executives, the Association of Hispanic Healthcare Executives, and the Executive Leadership Development Program of the Indian Health Service show that proportionately fewer racially/ethnically diverse individuals attain high-level executive positions compared to whites. Racially/ethnically diverse women who do attain executive positions earn lower salaries, and they appear to be overrepresented in management positions in institutions serving a disproportionate share of the indigent population.

Our country's increasingly diverse communities result in a more diverse patient population. Studies suggest that diversity in healthcare management can enhance quality of care, quality of life in the workplace, community relations and the ability to affect community health status. Achieving diversity in senior management will involve a commitment to the awareness of diversity issues, hiring practices that attract diverse staff, development and mentoring in educational programs and organizations, and organization wide diversity training.

Policy Position

The American College of Healthcare Executives embraces diversity within the healthcare management field and recognizes that issue as both an ethical and business imperative. ACHE urges all healthcare executives, board members, educators and policymakers to actively strive to increase diversity within healthcare management ranks, especially in regard to race and ethnic background. ACHE actively strives to increase representation of racially/ethnically diverse individuals in healthcare management and works to create a supportive, collegial environment that encourages their membership and advancement within ACHE itself. ACHE, as a founding member, also is committed to collaborating with the Institute for Diversity in Health Management on these issues.

All stakeholders should renew and strengthen their commitment to redressing the imbalance in representation of racially/ethnically diverse individuals in leadership to enhance our profession now and in the future.

ACHE encourages all healthcare executives to play a significant role in addressing this issue by actively pursuing the following:

Recruitment

• Institute outreach mechanisms to attract promising racially/ethnically diverse candidates to healthcare management careers with special emphasis on increasing recruitment efforts at colleges and universities with predominately racially/ethnically diverse student enrollments.

• Advocate racial and ethnic diversity in the appointment of job search committee members and promote the provision of an ethnically diverse slate of candidates for senior management positions.

• Recruit racially/ethnically diverse individuals at every level, so as to increase current representation in management, but also to develop a pool of qualified candidates for the future.

Increasing and Sustaining Racial/Ethnic Diversity in Healthcare Management (cont.)

- Recruit candidates external to the healthcare field to broaden the pool of racially/ethnically diverse candidates.

- Direct executive recruiters to identify and present racially/ethnically diverse candidates for management positions.

Promotion

- At every opportunity advocate the goal of achieving full representation of racially/ethnically diverse individuals in healthcare management.

- Institute policies that (1) prevent discrimination on the basis of race/ethnicity, (2) increase diversity in the recruitment and hiring of candidates, and (3) create an environment that encourages retention and promotion of qualified racially/ethnically diverse employees. Ensure that policies are well known and understood and measure and reward changes resulting from these policies.

- Publicize career advancement opportunities, such as continuing education, professional development organizations, networking events and vacancies inside the organization, in a manner that appeals to everyone, especially racially/ethnically diverse individuals.

- Develop and disseminate specific criteria for advancement in management that would allow all individuals to have an equal opportunity for senior-level positions. Such criteria could be useful to racially/ethnically diverse individuals who wish to prepare themselves for senior-level positions.

- Conduct regular reviews of organizational compensation programs to ensure salaries are equitable and nondiscriminatory.

Support

- Work with organizations representing racially/ethnically diverse individuals within their communities to create sources for scholarships and fellowships.

- Advocate for governmental and private philanthropic programs that increase funding to underwrite advanced education, information dissemination and employment opportunities for racially/ethnically diverse individuals.

- Support organizations, such as the Institute for Diversity in Health Management, that champion racially/ethnically diverse executives through internships and other programming.

- Support and assist the development of mentoring programs within healthcare organizations specifically focused on developing long-term relationships between senior healthcare managers and racially/ethnically diverse candidates.

- Identify potential candidates to support and encourage retention and advancement of racially/ethnically diverse individuals.

- Provide diversity training at every level of the organization, including the board, to promote and encourage understanding.

- Urge racially/ethnically diverse healthcare executives who are not affiliates to join ACHE; extend invitations to events such as executive breakfasts, educational programs, clusters and Regent's Advisory Council meetings.

In addition, ACHE encourages racially/ethnically diverse healthcare executives to actively pursue the following:

- Earn an advanced degree in healthcare management or business.

- Seek positions in organizations in order to build their careers.

- Choose positions that offer new experiences and expand their skills sets and management abilities.

- Interact with colleagues and become involved in professional associations.

- Seek out mentors and serve as mentors to other professionals.

ACHE advocates a variety of approaches to improve the representation and equitable treatment of racial and ethnic diversity in healthcare management.

Approved by the Board of Governors of the American College of Healthcare Executives on November 7, 2005.

Data describing the demographic characteristics of individuals enrolled in and graduating from master's programs in health administration were obtained from studies conducted by the Association of University Programs in Health Administration.

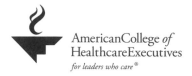
AmericanCollege *of*
HealthcareExecutives
for leaders who care ®

PROFESSIONAL
POLICY STATEMENT

Lifelong Learning and the Healthcare Executive

November 1994
November 1999 (revised)
November 2003 (revised)

Statement of the Issue

The need for healthcare executives to maintain their professional competency has never been greater. Changes in both the financing and delivery of care continue to occur at a rapid pace, and the expertise and skills that are needed to respond appropriately to the resultant challenges are not come by easily. At the same time, traditional career ladders are giving way to new opportunities that extend to all aspects of the healthcare continuum. Only through deliberate, ongoing career development can healthcare executives be assured they have the management and leadership skills they need to advance their careers and serve their organizations effectively.

Policy Position

The American College of Healthcare Executives (ACHE) believes that healthcare executives have a responsibility to foster their own professional development throughout their careers. Career development activities should include the following:

• Periodic self-assessment that involves taking stock of one's career in terms of professional strengths and weaknesses and current responsibilities. Self-assessments also should be used to focus on career aspirations and development of an action plan for achieving career goals.

• A commitment to regularly reading healthcare management periodicals, journals and books that provide insight into the trends, issues and challenges affecting the healthcare management field as well as a variety of media including Web-based or other resources offering broad-based business management information.

• Although ACHE requires an average of eight hours of external healthcare management continuing education annually for recertification as a Fellow, healthcare executives ideally should participate in both in-house education and external offerings that together provide a balance between healthcare management education and programming related to overall management effectiveness. To remain effective, healthcare executives must embrace and master new information and other emerging technologies that enhance professional performance. To this end, a minimum of 40 hours a year of continuing education is advisable.

• Active networking that includes both one-on-one interaction with peers and professional society and trade association involvement.

Approved by the Board of Governors of the American College of Healthcare Executives on November 10, 2003.

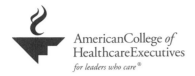

AmericanCollege *of*
HealthcareExecutives
for leaders who care ®

PROFESSIONAL
POLICY STATEMENT

Preventing and Addressing Harassment and Aggression in the Workplace

November 1996
November 1999 (revised)
November 2002 (revised)
November 2005 (reaffirmed)

Statement of the Issue

Healthcare executives have a professional responsibility to provide a work environment that protects staff from inappropriate behavior. To this end, healthcare executives have a responsibility to create an organizational culture that clearly conveys zero tolerance for harassment and aggression and to implement and enforce policies prohibiting them. Furthermore, healthcare executives must provide the necessary resources and mechanisms to safeguard against such behaviors.

Harassment and aggression in the workplace may cause physical and emotional repercussions. Besides the potential legal consequences of such activity, harassment and aggression can be linked to a loss of productivity, absenteeism, turnover, low morale, lack of trust, communication breakdowns, and long-term career and psychological damage.

Policy Position

The American College of Healthcare Executives believes that all healthcare executives have a professional and ethical responsibility to promote a workplace that is free from harassment on the basis of gender, sexual orientation, age, race, ethnicity, religion, national origin, disability, or any other personal characteristic, and to demonstrate zero tolerance for harassment and aggression. On behalf of their employing organizations, healthcare executives must further realize that they are responsible for implementing policy and monitoring compliance among their managers. To this end, healthcare executives should promote multifaceted programs in their organizations to prevent harassment and aggression, and employees should be encouraged to avoid or limit the harm from harassment and aggression. Sample program components include, but are not limited to, the following:

Clearly articulated policy against harassment and aggression. The policy should define "harassment" (preferably as defined by the Equal Employment Opportunity Commission—EEOC) and "aggression" and explicitly state that neither behavior is tolerated in the organization. The policy might include examples of prohibited conduct, delineate methods for making and investigating complaints, state that retaliation is prohibited and no reprisals will be taken against any employee filing a complaint under this policy, and provide that appropriate corrective action will be taken. The policy should be incorporated into the employee handbook as well as discussed in new employee orientation.

Employee training on harassment and aggression and their prevention. Training should be conducted by human resources staff or other individuals who have a technical and legal understanding of the issues, in addition to demonstrated ability to stimulate discussion about this sensitive topic. Training should be conducted with the goals of: raising awareness of harassment and aggression, clarifying misconceptions about what constitutes harassment and aggression, explaining the manager's role and responsibility in providing a safe and supportive work environment, and finally, sharing the specifics of the organization's policy prohibiting harassment and aggression.

Procedure for reporting allegations of harassment and aggression. The procedure should provide as much confidentiality as possible for both the complaining employee and the person accused of these behaviors. Employees should be protected from retaliation for filing a complaint or appearing as a witness in a harassment or aggression investigation. Further, if the procedure requires employees to make initial complaints to their supervisors, an alternate person should be designated to handle complaints when the supervisor is the alleged harasser or

Preventing and Addressing
Harassment and Aggression
in the Workplace (cont.)

aggressor. Supervisors should be required to report all complaints and be made aware of liability for failing to do so.

Procedure for expeditiously investigating complaints of harassment or aggression. According to EEOC guidelines, once an employee complains, employers should take "immediate and appropriate corrective action." The organization should, therefore, have a process in place for investigating complaints quickly, discreetly and completely. Investigations should be conducted by an objective party, and the results of the investigation should be reported to both the complaining employee and the person accused of harassment or aggression. Other staff should be informed on a "need to know" basis.

Standards for corrective action. Standards for corrective action are an essential part of any plan to prevent harassment or aggression. Disciplinary action should be proportionate to the severity of any behavior found; however, avoid providing specific punishments for specific actions. The policy, as it relates to corrective action, should be broad enough to give the freedom to exercise appropriate action. For example, the policy might state that such behaviors may result in discipline, up to and including discharge.

Legal counsel should review policies and procedures related to harassment and aggression because of the potential exposure to liability.

Approved by the Board of Governors of the American College of Healthcare Executives on November 7, 2005.

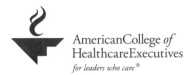
AmericanCollege *of*
HealthcareExecutives
for leaders who care ®

PROFESSIONAL
POLICY STATEMENT

Responsibility for Mentoring

November 1994
November 1999 (revised)
November 2004 (revised)

Statement of the Issue

The future of healthcare management rests in large measure with those entering the field as well as with mid-careerists who aspire to new and greater management opportunities. Although on-the-job experiences and continuing education will go a long way toward preparing tomorrow's leaders, the value of mentoring these individuals cannot be overstated. Mentorship is an important growth factor in the protégé's lifelong learning process. In turn, by sharing their wisdom, insights and experiences, mentors can give back to the profession and at the same time derive the personal satisfaction that comes from helping others realize their potential. For the organization, mentorship can lead to more satisfied employees and the generation of new ideas and programs.

Policy Position

The American College of Healthcare Executives (ACHE) believes that healthcare executives have a professional obligation to mentor both those entering the field as well as midcareerists preparing to lead the healthcare system of tomorrow.

Mentoring can take many forms, and the following options should be considered:

• Offer assistance recruiting, interviewing and working with qualified students interested in pursuing healthcare management careers.

• Volunteer to serve as a guest lecturer and use this opportunity to provide students with career planning guidance and insights gleaned from past experience.

• Help protégés develop clear expectations about their role so they will actively contribute to the mentoring relationship.

• Provide meaningful first-job opportunities to promising graduates and counsel them along the way.

• Encourage development of mentoring opportunities in culturally diverse, cross-generational and group settings as well as among individuals of different genders, races and ethnicities. Advocate for the value of mentoring for experienced executives from a variety of healthcare fields.

• Keep abreast of changes in mentoring philosophy and techniques. It will be key to ensuring your continued effectiveness as a mentor in an environment characterized by profound and rapid change.

• Seek out opportunities to contribute to local independent chapters of ACHE and members of the ACHE Higher Education Network.

• Promote mentoring opportunities and an organizational culture that promotes mentoring.

• Offer externships, internships, residencies and postgraduate fellowships.

Approved by the Board of Governors of the American College of Healthcare Executives on November 8, 2004.

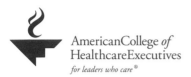

American College *of*
Healthcare Executives
for leaders who care®

PROFESSIONAL
POLICY STATEMENT

The Role of the Healthcare Executive in a Change in Organizational Ownership or Control: Consolidations, Mergers, Acquisitions, Affiliations, Divestitures, or Closures

November 1997
November 2000 (revised)
November 2005 (revised)

Statement of the Issue

Changes in organizational ownership or control present special challenges for healthcare executives. Executives must lead their organizations through the transition without self-serving motives. Perhaps most important is the challenge of community accountability—balancing the needs of the community for patient care and health improvement with the needs of the organization for adaptation.

Policy Position

The American College of Healthcare Executives (ACHE) believes that CEOs, their boards and members of their senior management teams should take a systematic approach to evaluating community health status and how the stakeholders might be affected by proposed changes to organization ownership or control. To this end, ACHE offers the following as a guide.

On an ongoing basis:

• Listen to the community and identify its future health improvement requirements. This assessment should include an evaluation of current health status, available healthcare resources, health improvement initiatives, and anticipated future needs.

• Ensure that a plan exists for providing care to the underserved in the community and for the continuation of other essential community services.

Before considering a change in ownership or control:

• Identify your organization's values and goals.

• Understand any legal limitations of your organization's certificate of incorporation, articles of organization, charter, or other binding documents that may restrict consideration of alternatives.

• Establish a code of conduct and specific criteria that the board, management team and other staff, and medical staff can use to evaluate proposals regarding change of ownership or control. Consider severance agreements for selected executives who will lead these studies to remove or lessen self-interest concerns related to loss of position and income.

• Conduct a study to assess various options for change that may be available to your organization and community. The study should examine your market and understand the changes that may affect your organization's ability to fulfill its vision and mission.

When considering specific proposals related to change of ownership or control:

• Assess the compatibility between your organization's values and philosophy and those of your potential partner.

• Identify financial incentives that may have an undue influence on the views of board members, executives and others involved in proposing and evaluating any change in ownership or control.

• Disclose all conflicts of interest, offers of future employment or future remuneration and other benefits related to the transaction.

The Role of the Healthcare Executive in a Change in Organizational Ownership or Control: Consolidations, Mergers, Acquisitions, Affiliations, Divestitures, or Closures (cont.)

- Evaluate proposals in terms of their likely impact on community healthcare and health status, organization mission and values, protection of the community's assets, and financial viability.

- Gain a thorough understanding of all the terms of the proposed transaction and of all collateral agreements.

- Develop and implement a communications plan that involves and informs all constituencies.

If the decision is made to proceed with a change of ownership or control:

- Obtain a valuation, by a party not involved in the transaction, of charitable assets being converted or restructured to ensure that reasonable value is received or used in structuring the transaction.

- In a nonprofit setting, prohibit private inurement or personal financial gain by individuals involved in the transaction.

- Ensure that control and administration of any foundation or charitable trust that would be created by the transaction be distinct from the restructured healthcare organization and that the foundation or trust continues to serve a healthcare-related charitable purpose in the community.

- Require that any foundation or trust created provide regular reports to the community on its efforts to improve community health status.

- Explain to the community the issues related to the change in ownership or control, the decision-making process and how the transaction will benefit the community.

- Provide an opportunity for public comment on the transaction, including stakeholders, before it becomes final.

- Make a public announcement at the earliest appropriate time.

- Inform the appropriate federal, state and local officials of the terms of the transaction in accordance with their requirements.

- Develop and implement a restructuring plan that provides for fair treatment of all employees.

In addition, ACHE affiliates also have a personal responsibility to:

- Abide by the standards set forth in the ACHE *Code of Ethics.*

- Place community and organizational interests above personal pride, ego or gain.

- Carry out the fiduciary responsibilities of their positions.

- Conduct all negotiations with honesty and integrity.

As consolidation and related activities continue in the healthcare field, organizations and their executives will be under increased scrutiny. Executives must demonstrate through their words and actions that their business decisions are guided by professional ethics and a commitment to improving community health status.

Adapted from the American Hospital Association's Guidelines for Hospital/Health System Leaders when Changing Ownership or Control, 1997.

Approved by the Board of Governors of the American College of Healthcare Executives on November 7, 2005.

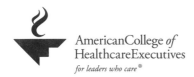

AmericanCollege *of*
HealthcareExecutives
for leaders who care ®

PUBLIC
POLICY STATEMENT

Access to Healthcare

May 1986
June 1986 (revised)
May 1994 (revised)
December 1998 (revised)
March 2002 (revised)
November 2005 (revised)

Statement of the Issue

At one time healthcare organizations could depend on income from public and private payors to underwrite a portion of the cost of care provided to the poor and un-insured. Although that source of income has eroded, the public expects healthcare organizations to maintain access to care regardless of the patient's ability to pay. Without question, meeting this expectation strains resources and puts some organizations in financial peril. In the absence of renewed support or other viable solutions, there will come a point where our commitment to ensuring access to all in need will be compromised.

The American College of Healthcare Executives (ACHE) urges society to guard against these threats to access. As leaders within the community, healthcare executives are well-positioned to actively participate in the effort to reach community consensus on how healthcare resources and needs should be balanced so that access to care is preserved.

Policy Position

The American College of Healthcare Executives believes no person should be denied necessary healthcare services because of inability to pay. Further, ACHE believes access to care is a shared responsibility of healthcare organizations, regardless of ownership, as well as government programs and agencies, community groups, and the private insurance market. To this end, ACHE urges healthcare executives to lead the effort within their organizations and on behalf of the communities their organizations serve to address issues related to funding services for the poor and underinsured. Consistent with ACHE's *Code of Ethics* and policy statement on "Ethical Decision Making for Healthcare Executives," there is a responsibility to consider broader community and societal implications as well as individual and organizational impact when addressing issues such as those affecting access.

Leadership responsibilities for healthcare executives include, but are not limited to:

• Developing and communicating access-to-care policies within their organizations and to the community.

• Managing their organizations efficiently to help under-write healthcare costs associated with uncompensated and undercompensated care.

• Collaborating with other healthcare providers in their community to develop shared approaches to ensure access to care.

• Encouraging and assisting trade and other professional associations to take proactive roles on access-to-care issues.

• Promoting shared leadership and funding responsibilities among government, healthcare organizations, employers, private insurers and consumers.

• Organizing grassroots advocacy efforts to secure needed funding from local, state and federal government bodies.

• Organizing or participating in local, state and regional task forces to resolve access problems.

• Spearheading discussions with key decision makers (e.g., legislators) and key stakeholders (e.g., public agencies) to identify community health priorities so that available resources can be allocated equitably and effectively.

An important role for healthcare executives has always been to translate social values into workable healthcare programs. In keeping with this role, healthcare executives have the opportunity to participate in public dialogue about new ways to finance and deliver healthcare so no one is denied care because of the inability to pay.

Approved by the Board of Governors of the American College of Healthcare Executives on November 7, 2005.

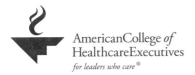
AmericanCollege *of*
HealthcareExecutives
for leaders who care®

PUBLIC
POLICY STATEMENT

Healthcare Executives' Responsibility to Their Communities

July 1989
May 1994
November 1997 (revised)
November 2000 (revised)
November 2003 (reaffirmed)
November 2006 (revised)

Statement of the Issue

A commitment to access to care regardless of the patient's ability to pay has long been a cornerstone of our healthcare system. It is also a commitment personally embraced by healthcare executives who lead healthcare organizations. But the healthcare executive's responsibility to the community does not end here—it encompasses commitment to improving community health status and addressing the societal issues that contribute to poor health as well as personally working for the betterment of the community-at-large. Taking a leadership role in serving the community is the responsibility of all healthcare executives regardless of occupational setting or ownership structure. Further, when providers, individuals and communities work toward common goals, the results can be significant: reduced healthcare costs, appropriate use of limited healthcare resources and, ultimately, a healthier community.

Policy Position

The American College of Healthcare Executives (ACHE) believes that all healthcare executives have a professional obligation to serve their communities through support of organizational initiatives and personal involvement in community and civic affairs. In addition, ACHE believes that healthcare executives should take a proactive role in individual and community health improvement efforts. ACHE recognizes that communities vary widely in demographics, resources, traditions and needs. Therefore, each community may identify different priorities and approaches.

Healthcare executives can lead or participate in community and organizational initiatives through the following actions:

• Work with other concerned organizations and individuals to develop effective measures of community health status. Collaborative efforts should lead to an accurate assessment of their community's health status, including the most prevalent health problems, causes of those problems, associated risk factors and available resources.

• Lead their organizations in collaborative efforts to address health concerns by working with public health and other government agencies, businesses, associations, educational groups, religious organizations, elected officials, financing entities, foundations and others. Diverse interests and resources could be applied to addressing community health concerns.

• Support the dissemination of accurate information about community health status, the services provided and programs available to prevent and treat illness and patients' responsibility for their own health.

• Participate in efforts to communicate organizational effectiveness in matching healthcare resources with community needs, improved clinical outcomes and community health status and their organizations' volunteerism roles.

• Incorporate community service responsibilities into policies and programs over which they have authority.

• Advocate and participate in their organizations' collaborative efforts with other community healthcare providers and social service agencies.

Healthcare Executives' Responsibility to Their Communities (cont.)

- Demonstrate that their organizations' commitment to the community is multifaceted and may include support of medical research, training of healthcare professionals, charity care and civic contributions as well as a host of other activities that contribute to the community's well-being.

- Offer health promotion and illness prevention programs to their employees, positively benefiting staff, as well as sending an important message to the community.

Healthcare executives can personally demonstrate their commitment to the community through the following actions:

- Embrace a healthy lifestyle. ACHE affiliates should model behavior they are advocating for their employees and the community-at-large. Appropriate behavior may include exercising regularly, taking steps to reduce stress and getting preventive checkups to address health problems before they become serious.

- Participate in local assessments of community need.

- Participate in regional, state and local task forces to resolve access to care and other community healthcare problems.

- Volunteer to meet on behalf of their organizations with the public, policymakers and other key stakeholders to define community healthcare priorities so that healthcare resources can be used equitably and effectively.

- Become involved in community service projects, civic organizations and public dialogue on healthcare policy issues affecting the community.

- Share models of successful healthy community projects with others to enhance efforts in other communities.

ACHE urges all healthcare executives to affirm their responsibility to their communities through their professional actions and personal contributions. To further strengthen its position on community responsibility, ACHE requires its affiliates to produce evidence of participation and leadership in healthcare and community/civic affairs to advance within ACHE.

In the current healthcare marketplace, the demand for health promotion and illness prevention activities will grow. By making a personal and professional commitment to improving the community's health status, healthcare executives will be taking an important step toward addressing this demand.

Approved by the Board of Governors of the American College of Healthcare Executives on November 6, 2006.

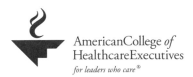

AmericanCollege *of*
HealthcareExecutives
for leaders who care®

PUBLIC
POLICY STATEMENT

Healthcare Executives' Role in Emergency Preparedness

November 2006

Statement of the Issue

Due to the complex nature of emergency preparedness, it is critical that healthcare executives ensure their organizations develop an all-hazards emergency operations plan relevant to their location and type of organization. The emergency operations plan should include a determination of which hazards are most probable and cover applicable responses to a natural disaster as well as potential CBRNE (chemical, biological, radiological, nuclear, explosive) events.

Hospitals and other healthcare delivery organizations must be prepared to care for those in need of medical services and, to the extent possible, protect staff and patients from being exposed to any further risk. The organization's emergency operations plan should recognize that a healthcare organization may be directly impacted by a disaster as well as be the recipient of victims. This is true for incidents of terrorism and natural occurrences such as hurricanes, tornados, floods, earthquakes or epidemics/pandemics.

It is vitally important that healthcare organizations monitor and update their emergency operations plans on an ongoing basis, maintaining a constant state of preparedness to ensure appropriate response and recovery within the shortest possible timeframes. Without proper planning, an incident involving the organization may result in either a temporary or permanent failure, thus disabling a crucial community resource. The emergency operations plan also should be fully integrated with that of other organizations and appropriate agencies at the local, state, regional and national levels. This is particularly important in situations such as a pandemic that may simultaneously impact large geographic areas for several months and disrupt national and international supply chains.

Policy Position

The American College of Healthcare Executives (ACHE) believes healthcare executives should actively participate in disaster planning and preparedness activities, striving to ensure that their emergency operations plan fits within overall community plans and represents a responsible approach to the risks an organization might face. Chief executive officers should lead efforts to ensure a comprehensive plan, including establishing board policy that delineates the organization's responsibilities and procedures to be followed. Healthcare executives also have a unique opportunity to help educate the community about infectious disease prevention and control efforts that may mitigate large-scale death during events such as a pandemic.

In developing a comprehensive emergency operations plan, ACHE encourages healthcare executives to pursue the following actions on an ongoing basis:

• Establish a process to understand and stay current regarding applicable national standards for emergency preparedness, including the National Response Plan and the National Bioterrorism Hospital Preparedness Program, as well as legal and ethical issues associated with emergency preparedness.

• Adopt an all-hazards framework to analyze the operational issues that would arise in relevant emergency situations.

• Coordinate and integrate organizational resources to address a full spectrum of actions (mitigation, preparedness, response and recovery), and ensure that the organization has the appropriate programs, trained and credentialed staff, supplies and equipment in place to quickly respond to events that their organization might face, which is identified by the organization's all-hazards analysis.

Healthcare Executives' Role in Emergency Preparedness

- Ensure active involvement in inter-agency planning efforts with all relevant organizations, including the development of an integrated communication plan, and community-wide exercises and drills to assess effectiveness and implement improvements.

- Develop policies and processes to ensure that all reasonable efforts are made to protect employees, patients and families while maintaining quality patient care to the best of the organization's ability during a crisis.

- Ensure that services are provided equitably and impartially based upon the vulnerability and needs of the individual and community affected by a disaster, including supporting the development of mental health response plans for patients, families, employees and their families.

- Adopt an incident command system and support the integration of a nationwide standardized approach to incident management and response (e.g., National Incident Management System).

As a critical component of a community's infrastructure, healthcare organizations should require proper planning for all-hazards events they may face. Healthcare executives should be active leaders in that planning and the creation of systems and processes to ensure that the emergency operating plan can be effectively and efficiently executed if ever needed.

Approved by the Board of Governors of the American College of Healthcare Executives on November 6, 2006.

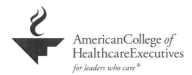

AmericanCollege *of*
HealthcareExecutives
for leaders who care®

PUBLIC
POLICY STATEMENT

Organ/Tissue/Blood/ Marrow Donation

November 1986
March 1993 (reaffirmed)
February 1997 (revised)
November 2000 (revised)
November 2003 (revised)
November 2006 (revised)

Statement of the Issue

Medical advances have provided a tremendous opportunity to save or improve lives through organ, tissue, blood, and marrow transplantation. Though tens of thousands of lives are saved each year through transplantation, thousands more continue to be tragically lost because need outpaces availability. Even when there is consent for organ donation, the actual number of organs utilized is suboptimal, with a failure to transplant nearly half of all organs available for transplant. Thus, waiting lists for these resources continue to grow at unprecedented levels.

Significant opportunities exist to increase both the percentage of eligible donors who become donors and the number of organs transplanted per donor. Donations and transplantation can be increased through:

• Specific hospital procedures that are developed in cooperation with affiliated organ and tissue procurement organizations to work with patients and families in maximizing donation rates.

• Best practices for increasing the donation conversion rate and the number of organs transplanted per donor, such as those developed by the Health Resources and Services Administration's (HRSA) Organ Donation and Transplantation Breakthrough Collaboratives.

• Heightened public and professional awareness of the problem and distribution of information related to potential solutions.

Though governments, medical professionals, hospitals, procurement organizations and insurance companies can provide resources that support donation, only individuals and their families have the ultimate power to offer the gift of life.

Policy Position

The American College of Healthcare Executives (ACHE) believes that all healthcare executives should work to increase the supply of available organs, tissues, blood, and marrow for transplantation. ACHE recognizes donation as a critical component of life-saving technology and end-of-life decision making and supports voluntary efforts to increase organ, tissue, blood, and marrow availability.

As business and community leaders, healthcare executives have the influence and credibility to motivate individuals and families to consider donation of organs, tissues, blood, and marrow. ACHE encourages its affiliates to actively pursue the following:

Establish Protocols and Information Programs

• Together with their affiliated organ and tissue procurement organization, establish effective and compassionate protocols for working with patients and their families. Families of dying patients should be provided with the option to donate. Many appreciate the opportunity to ease their personal loss with a selfless, giving act.

• Develop strong, ongoing public information and education programs that help people understand the process of organ and tissue donation and the importance of sharing with their families the decision they have reached. When individuals make their wishes known in advance, they ease the decision-making burden placed on their families during a difficult and vulnerable time. Usually it is the family that is asked for final consent for organ and tissue donation.

Organ/Tissue/Blood/Marrow Donation

- Develop strong, ongoing public information and education programs that help people understand the process of blood donation and how to become a potential marrow or peripheral blood stem cell donor.

Encourage Donation

- Encourage members of the medical community to develop protocols reflecting the best practices in the field to maximize organ, tissue, blood, and marrow donation, availability and transplantation.

- Consider serving as role models by publicizing their own personal decisions to sign donor cards, participate in blood drives or join the marrow registry. Healthcare executives can provide leadership in the resolution of this important social problem by encouraging their staff to follow their lead and in coordinating community efforts.

- Participate in national, state and local government and private-sector initiatives to promote organ, tissue, blood, and marrow donation.

The issue of organ, tissue, blood, and marrow donation and transplantation reaches beyond the limited availability of these precious resources in the face of growing demand, but one issue is clear: Transplantation cannot save lives and promote well-being unless caring individuals donate. ACHE encourages its affiliates to develop an environment that fosters this opportunity.

Note: Information on the Health Resources and Services Administration's (HRSA) Organ Donation and Transplantation Breakthrough Collaboratives can be found at: http://www.organdonor.gov/collaborative.htm

Approved by the Board of Governors of the American College of Healthcare Executives on November 6, 2006.

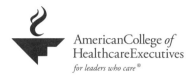

AmericanCollege *of*
HealthcareExecutives
for leaders who care ®

PUBLIC
POLICY STATEMENT

Strengthening Healthcare Employment Opportunities for Persons with Disabilities

May 1992
May 1995 (revised)
December 1998 (revised)
March 2002 (revised)
March 2006 (revised)

Statement of the Issue

Healthcare executives are well aware that diversity is one of the key ingredients to creating a strong, high-performing healthcare system. The diversity imperative also extends to the inclusion of persons with disabilities. Despite the passage of the Americans with Disabilities Act in 1990, disability, whether actual or perceived, presents an ongoing employment challenge in our society.

According to a 2003 U.S. Census Bureau survey, 6.3 percent of workers who did not reside in an institution had a disability. A 2005 survey of affiliates of the American College of Healthcare Executives (ACHE) showed a somewhat higher rate, with an estimated 7.6 percent of respondents being disabled, which is defined as having a condition that limits full participation in work and/or having specific conditions such as learning, emotional or mental disability or disease, a sensory impairment, physical handicap, pain or chronic fatigue syndrome.

Given the prevalence of disability among healthcare workers, as well as the nature of diversity as both an ethical and business imperative, healthcare executives should be vigilant in ensuring an inclusive environment, equitable workplace treatment and opportunities for persons with disabilities.

Policy Position

While overt discrimination against employment of persons with disabilities is illegal and subject to sanction under federal law, even covert discrimination against the employment of persons with disabilities is incompatible with the American College of Healthcare Executive's *Code of Ethics*. ACHE believes that healthcare executives should take the lead in their organizations to increase employment, advancement and leadership opportunities for persons with

disabilities. Additionally, healthcare executives should advocate on behalf of the employment of persons with disabilities in other organizations in their communities.

ACHE encourages all healthcare executives to pursue the following actions:

• Develop an organizational culture that encourages persons with disabilities to utilize their potential to contribute rather than discounting them on the basis of stereotypes or generalizations about their "limitations."

• Affirm that equal access to employment for persons with disabilities exists by recruiting governance leaders, executives, clinicians and support staff with auxiliary aids and services (such as Braille or large print, telecommunication devices for deaf persons and videotext displays); through using networks and recruiting firms committed to accommodating persons with disabilities; and by making auxiliary assistance available throughout the interview process.

• Reallocate or redistribute job responsibilities to accommodate individuals with disabilities and consider reallocating responsibilities to accommodate and retain an individual already on staff who acquires a disability.

• Determine appropriate accommodations using an informal, interactive problem-solving process involving the employer and the individual with a disability.

The American College of Healthcare Executives encourages its affiliates to take the lead in their organizations and their communities in creating working environments that enhance the opportunities of persons with disabilities to gain and maintain employment.

Approved by the Board of Governors of the American College of Healthcare Executives on November 6, 2006.

APPENDIX 3. IMPORTANT LISTS

Chairman Officers and Chief Executive Officers of ACHE
Honorary Charter Fellows, Charter Fellows, and Honorary Fellows
Recipients of Special ACHE Awards
Chapter Awards
Special Lectures

CHAIRMAN OFFICERS OF ACHE, 1933–2009

1933–1934	Charles A. Wordell	1965–1966	Boone Powell
1934–1935	Robert E. Neff	1966–1967	Peter B. Terenzio
1935–1936	Fred G. Carter, MD	1967–1968	Donald W. Cordes
1936–1937	Basil C. MacLean, MD	1968–1969	R. Zach Thomas Jr.
1937–1938	Howard E. Bishop	1969–1970	Arnold L. Swanson, MD
1938–1939	Robin C. Buerki, MD	1970–1971	Orville N. Booth
1939–1940	James A. Hamilton	1971–1972	Everett A. Johnson, PhD
1940–1941	Arthur C. Bachmeyer, MD	1972–1973	William N. Wallace
1941–1942	Lucius R. Wilson, MD	1973–1974	Gene Kidd
1942–1943	Joseph G. Norby	1974–1975	William S. Brines
1943–1944	Robert H. Bishop Jr., MD	1975–1976	James D. Harvey
1944–1946	Claude W. Munger, MD	1976–1977	Henry X. Jackson
1946–1947	Frank R. Bradley, MD	1977–1978	Norman D. Burkett
1947–1948	Edgar C. Hayhow, PhD	1978–1979	Ray Woodham
1948–1949	Jessie J. Turnbull	1979–1980	Chester L. Stocks
1949–1950	Wilmar M. Allen, MD	1980–1981	Donald R. Newkirk
1950–1951	Frank J. Walter	1981–1982	Charles T. Wood
1951–1952	Ernest I. Erickson	1982–1983	Earl G. Dresser
1952–1953	Fraser D. Mooney, MD	1983–1984	Alton E. Pickert
1953–1954	Merrill F. Steele, MD	1984–1985	Austin Ross
1954–1955	Albert C. Kerlikowske, MD	1985–1986	William E. Johnson Jr.
1955–1956	J. Dewey Lutes	1986–1987	D. Kirk Oglesby Jr.
1956–1957	Arthur J. Swanson	1987–1988	Francis J. Cronin
1957–1958	Frank S. Groner	1988–1989	David H. Jeppson
1958–1959	Anthony W. Eckert	1989–1990	H. W. Maysent
1959–1960	Ray E. Brown	1990–1991	James O. Hepner, PhD
1960–1961	Melvin L. Sutley	1991–1992	Paul S. Ellison
1961–1962	Tol Terrell	1992–1993	Robert R. Fanning Jr.
1962–1963	Frank C. Sutton, MD	1993–1994	Ronald G. Spaeth
1963–1964	Robert W. Bachmeyer	1994–1995	Col. William C. Head
1964–1965	Ronald D. Yaw	1995–1997	Garth A. H. Pierce

1997–1998	Larry L. Mathis	2003–2004	Larry S. Sanders
1998–1999	David W. Benfer	2004–2005	Richard A. Henault
1999–2000	Mark J. Howard	2005–2006	Samuel L. Odle
2000–2001	Michael C. Waters	2006–2007	William C. Schoenhard
2001–2002	Diane Peterson	2007–2008	Alyson Pitman Giles
2002–2003	Mark R. Neaman	2008–2009	Brig. Gen. David A. Rubenstein

CHIEF EXECUTIVE OFFICERS OF ACHE, 1933–2007

1933–1937	J. Dewey Lutes, *Director General*	1972–1978	Richard J. Stull, *President*
1937–1941	Gerhard Hartman, PhD, *Executive Secretary*	1979–1991	Stuart A. Wesbury Jr., PhD, *President*
1942–1965	Dean Conley, *Executive Director*	1991–	Thomas C. Dolan, PhD, *President*
1965–1971	Richard J. Stull, *Executive Vice President*		

HONORARY CHARTER FELLOWS

G. Harvey Agnew, MD
Otho F. Ball, MD
Richard P. Borden
Bert W. Caldwell, MD
Margaret M. Cummings
Matthew O. Foley
Maurice F. Griffin
Thomas Howell
E. H. Lewinski-Corwin, MD

Emma Lucas Louie
Malcolm T. MacEachern, MD
Christopher G. Parnell, MD
John M. Peters, MD
C. S. Pitcher
Rev. Alphonse M. Schwitalla
Daniel T. Test
W. H. Walsh, MD

CHARTER FELLOWS

Victor Anderson
E. Muriel Anscombe
Lawrence C. Austin
Arthur C. Bachmeyer, MD
Asa S. Bacon
W. D. Barker
Mabel Barr
Oliver H. Bartine
F. Oliver Bates
John G. Benson
Mabel Binner
Howard E. Bishop
B. W. Black, MD
E. M. Bluestone, MD
W. M. Breitinger

Burton A. Brown, MD
Robin C. Buerki, MD
L. H. Burlingham, MD
Arthur M. Calvin
Jessie M. Candlish
Muriel McKee Cariss
Fred G. Carter, MD
E. M. Collier
John G. Copeland
Allan Craig, MD
Clarence C. Cummings
Carolyn E. Davis
C. J. Decker
John C. Dinsmore
Joseph C. Doane, MD

Anna Lauman Driver
Maurice Dubin
Mark Eickenlaub
E. I. Erickson
Paul Fesler
Boris Fingerhood
J. B. Franklin
Rev. Herman Fritschel
Albert G. Hahn
Mrs. Albert Hahn
Guy M. Hanner
Harley A. Haynes, MD
A. K. Haywood, MD
Henry Hedden, MD
L.C. Vonder Heidt
S. R. D. Hewitt, MD
Howard E. Hodge
Clarence T. Johnson
Lake Johnson
Robert Jolly
Paul Keller, MD
E. E. King
Henry I. Klopp, MD
Mary R. Lewis, MD
Walter E. List, MD
Marie Louis
J. Dewey Lutes
Basil C. MacLean, MD
A. J. MacMaster
John R. Mannix
Elmer E. Matthews
Elizabeth McGregor
James McNee
Henry K. Mohler, MD
Donald Morrill, MD
Claude W. Munger, MD
Thomas T. Murray

Robert E. Neff
Robert A. Nettleton
Joseph G. Norby
James U. Norris
George O'Hanlon, MD
Russell H. Oppenheimer, MD
Charles E. Remy, MD
Georgia Rowan
Henry Rowland
Lewis Sexton, MD
George D. Sheats
Austin J. Shoneke
E. L. Slack
Donald C. Smelzer, MD
Clinton F. Smith
Herman Smith, MD
John M. Smith
Cecil T. Spry
Alfred G. Stasel
Merrill F. Steele, MD
George F. Stephens, MD
Mary V. Stephenson
Melvin L. Sutley
A. J. Swanson, MD
Jessie J. Turnbull
Bryce L. Twitty
Rev. Philip Vollmer
Fred M. Walker
Frank J. Walter
Peter D. Ward, MD
George W. Wilson
Lucius R. Wilson, MD
Robert B. Witham
C. S. Woods, MD
Charles A. Wordell
Carl P. Wright

HONORARY FELLOWS, 1933–2007

Hon. J. Chaiker Abbis ('85)
Robinson E. Adkins ('61)
G. Harvey Agnew, MD ('33)
Mother V. Allaire ('47)
Guillermo Almenara, MD ('44)
Stuart H. Altman ('97)
Odin W. Anderson, PhD ('67)
Maj. Gen. George E. Armstrong ('53)

Maj. Gen. Harry G. Armstrong ('53)
Arthur C. Bachmeyer, MD ('52)
Asa S. Bacon ('41)
Otho F. Ball, MD ('33)
Rt. Rev. Msgr. John W. Barrett ('49)
Karl D. Bays ('86)
Mme. L. De G. Beaubien ('39)
Stanley S. Bergen Jr., MD ('92)

Rev. Hector L. Bertrand ('70)

Ella Best ('58)

Jack C. Bills ('91)

Rev. John J. Bingham ('44)

Jan E. G. Blanpain, MD ('77)

F. J. L. Blasingame, MD ('60)

Frances P. Bolton ('44)

Vice Admiral Joel T. Boone ('55)

Richard P. Borden ('34)

Nelles V. Buchanan ('62)

LeRoy E. Burney, MD ('59)

Bert W. Caldwell, MD ('33)

G. D. W. Cameron, MD ('64)

Charles A. Cannon ('67)

Vice Admiral Richard H. Carmona, MD ('05)

Guy J. Clark ('54)

L. T. Coggeshall, MD ('65)

John A. D. Cooper, MD, PhD ('82)

Lawrence T. Cooper ('77)

Paul B. Cornely, MD ('73)

Nelson H. Cruickshank ('58)

Margaret M. Cummings ('34)

Robert M. Cunningham Jr. ('58)

Robert Cutler ('55)

Ward Darley, MD ('60)

Mrs. Maxwell Davidson ('79)

Graham L. Davis ('47)

Michael M. Davis ('35)

Michael DeBakey, MD ('90)

Mother Anna Dengel, MD ('62)

Marshall E. Dimock ('60)

Leland I. Doan ('55)

Avedis Donabedian, MD ('82)

William J. Driver ('68)

Leonard A. Duce, PhD ('72)

Merlin K. DuVal, MD ('80)

Bernard J. Echlin ('88)

C. Wesley Eisele, MD ('66)

William J. Ellis ('35)

Paul M. Ellwood Jr., MD ('87)

Haven Emerson, MD ('50)

Lester J. Evans, MD ('59)

Robert S. Ewing ('83)

James R. Felts Jr. ('78)

Zachary Fisher ('96)

Edmund Fitzgerald ('58)

Rev. John J. Flanagan ('58)

Matthew O. Foley ('33)

Marion B. Folsom ('66)

Mrs. W. W. Fondren ('63)

Thomas F. Frist Sr., MD ('89)

Rt. Rev. Msgr. John G. Fullerton ('57)

Mrs. S. Palmer Gaillard Jr. ('73)

John W. Gates ('81)

Lillian M. Gilbreth ('61)

Maurice Goldblatt ('58)

S. S. Goldwater, MD ('38)

Ignatio Gonzalez, MD ('46)

Annie Goodich ('48)

Hon. Willis D. Gradison Jr. ('90)

Harald M. Graning, MD ('71)

Rev. Msgr. Maurice F. Griffin ('33)

Gunnar Gundersen, MD ('59)

Mrs. Albert G. Hahn ('48)

Jack C. Haldeman, MD ('65)

Hon. Justice Emmett Hall ('80)

Paul R. Hawley, MD ('58)

Harley A. Haynes, MD ('48)

Emanuel Hayt ('58)

Lt. General Leonard D. Heaton ('60)

A. A. Heckman ('73)

Mrs. Clifford S. Heinz ('70)

Jane E. Henney, MD ('99)

Frederick T. Hill, MD ('62)

George W. Hill ('63)

Lister Hill ('54)

Vane M. Hoge, MD ('50)

Mrs. Chester A. Hoover ('59)

John F. Horty ('65)

Thomas Howell, MD ('33)

Sister John Gabriel (Ryan) ('35)

Lucius W. Johnson, MD ('57)

Robert W. Johnson ('62)

Richard M. Jones ('58)

William M. Kelley ('95)

Sidney R. Lamb ('36)

Eleanor C. Lambertsen, EdD ('71)

Peter B. Laubach, DBA ('84)

Charles S. Lauer ('94)

Lucien L. Leape, MD ('07)

Lucille P. Leone ('57)

Edward H. Lewinski-Corwin ('34)

Lucile Emma Lucas Louie ('34)

James E. Ludlam ('66)

Malcolm T. MacEachern, MD ('33)

Arthur Mag ('58)

Charles W. Mayo, MD ('54)

William G. (Billy) McCall ('88)

Ada Belle McCleery ('47)

John F. McCreary, MD ('69)

Foster G. McGaw ('62)
Msgr. Andrew J. McGowan ('93)
Rev. Donald A. McGowan ('51)
John Alexander McMahon ('74)
Fred A. McNamara ('52)
William S. McNary ('64)
Richard L. Meiling, MD ('80)
Karl P. Meister ('56)
William S. Middleton, MD ('57)
J. Roscoe Miller, MD ('51)
Emory W. Morris ('55)
Richard Moses ('79)
Maj. Gen. Oliver K. Niess ('61)
Maurice J. Norby ('58)
William A. O'Brien, MD ('43)
Rev. Joseph S. O'Connell ('39)
Basil O'Connor ('55)
Edward M. O'Herron Jr. ('76)
Dennis S. O'Leary, MD ('92)
Sister M. Olivia (Gowan) ('36)
Herluf V. Olsen, PhD ('58)
Christopher G. Parnall, MD ('34)
Thomas Parran, MD ('46)
Andrew Pattulo ('58)
Edmund D. Pellegrino, MD ('80)
Thomas L. Perkins ('66)
Earl Perloff ('70)
John M. Peters, MD ('34)
Marshall I. Pickens ('55)
W. Douglas Piercey, MD ('58)
Viola Pinanski ('64)
Charles S. Pitcher ('34)
Charles E. Prall, PhD ('59)
Rear Admiral Lemont Pugh ('53)
Richard L. Rand ('84)
W. S. Rankin, MD ('38)
Willard C. Rappleye, MD ('40)
Mary M. Roberts ('49)
Maj. Gen. Paul I. Robinson ('58)
David E. Rogers, MD ('87)
William L. Roper, MD ('02)
Hon. Joseph D. Ross, MD ('67)
Charles G. Roswell ('65)
F. Burns Roth ('58)

Howard A. R. Rusk, MD ('63)
John T. Ryan ('58)
James H. Sammons, MD ('86)
Leonard A. Scheele, MD ('53)
Rev. Alphonse M. Schwitalla ('34)
James Shannon, MD ('65)
Gen. Henry H. Shelton ('01)
Vergil N. Slee, MD ('69)
Raymond P. Sloan ('53)
Winford H. Smith, MD ('42)
Anne Ramsay Somers ('74)
Herman Miles Somers, PhD ('74)
Richard W. Soper ('37)
Henry J. Southmayd ('43)
Eric W. Springer, LLB ('78)
Nathan J. Stark, JD ('81)
Msgr. John C. Stauton ('72)
Sir Arthur G. Stephenson ('58)
Captain Joseph E. Stone ('47)
Jack I. Straus ('68)
Most Rev. Joseph Sullivan ('89)
James R. Tallon Jr. ('00)
William I. Taylor, MD ('66)
Lillian D. Terris, PhD ('78)
Luther L. Terry, MD ('64)
Daniel D. Test ('34)
Paul H. T. Thorlakson, MD ('72)
Thomas M. Tierney ('67)
Ambassador Randall L. Tobias ('06)
Rt. Rev. Msgr. Charles A. Towell ('54)
Col. Florence Turkington ('58)
Edward L. Turner, MD ('58)
Joseph F. Volker, DDS, PhD ('79)
William H. Walsh, MD ('34)
Clarence A. Warden Jr. ('64)
Frederic A. Washburn, MD ('40)
Malcolm Stuart McNeal Watts, MD ('75)
Lawrence L. Weed, MD ('75)
Lewis Weeks, PhD ('85)
Lloyd B. Wescott ('67)
Homer Wickenden ('58)
Kenneth Williamson ('58)
Richard E. YaDeau, MD ('76)
Morley A. R. Young, MD ('63)

GOLD MEDAL AWARD

The Gold Medal Award was established in 1964 to recognize exceptional individuals who exemplify the highest standards and values of the profession. It is awarded to Fellows of ACHE who have demonstrated outstanding leadership and fostered excellence in healthcare management. In 1991, the Board of Governors approved the merger of the Silver Medal Award with the Gold Medal Award, authorizing up to two Gold Medal recipients annually. The award is presented during ACHE's annual meeting banquet. On the special occasion of the inauguration of the award in 1964, four awards were granted.

1964	Robin C. Buerki, MD, CFACHE	1989	Austin Ross, LFACHE
	Pearl R. Fisher, FACHE	1990	David H. Hitt, LFACHE
	David Littauer, MD, FACHE	1991	Sister Irene Kraus, FACHE
	Tol Terrell, FACHE	1992	Horace M. Cardwell, FACHE
1965	Frank C. Sutton, MD, FACHE		John R. Griffith, FACHE
1966	Albert W. Snoke, MD, FACHE	1993	James W. Holsinger Jr., MD, FACHE
1967	Charles P. Cardwell Jr., FACHE		D. Kirk Oglesby Jr., LFACHE
1968	Frank S. Groner, FACHE	1994	John A. Russell, LFACHE
1969	Ray E. Brown, FACHE	1995	Reginald M. Ballantyne III, FACHE
1970	Boone Powell Sr., FACHE	1996	Scott S. Parker, LFACHE
1971	T. Stewart Hamilton, MD, FACHE	1997	Dan S. Wilford, LFACHE
1972	James D. Harvey, LFACHE	1998	Stephen M. Shortell, PhD, FACHE
1973	Ronald D. Yaw, FACHE	1999	Leo F. Greenawalt, FACHE
1974	George E. Cartmill Jr., LFACHE		Gail L. Warden, FACHE
1975	Donald W. Cordes, LFACHE	2000	Fred L. Brown, FACHE
1976	Peter E. Swerhone, LFACHE	2001	William C. Head, FACHE
1977	Donald C. Carner, LFACHE		James T. (Terry) Townsend, JD,
1978	R. Zach Thomas Jr., FACHE		FACHE, CAE
1979	William N. Wallace, FACHE	2002	C. Duane Dauner, FACHE
1980	Roy Rambeck, FACHE		Douglas D. Hawthorne, FACHE
1981	Pat N. Groner, LFACHE	2003	Patrick G. Hays, FACHE
1982	Ray Woodham, LFACHE	2004	Larry L. Mathis, LFACHE
1983	Stanley R. Nelson, LFACHE	2005	Ronald G. Spaeth, FACHE
1984	Bernard J. Lachner, FACHE	2006	Larry S. Sanders, FACHE
1985	Wade Mountz, LFACHE	2007	Jack O. Bovender Jr., FACHE
1986	H. Robert Cathcart, LFACHE		Diane Peterson, FACHE
1987	Samuel J. Tibbitts, FACHE	2008	Mark J. Howard, FACHE
1988	E. E. Gilbertson, LFACHE		Wayne Sorensen, PhD, FACHE

SILVER MEDAL AWARD

The Silver Medal Award was established in 1974 to recognize outstanding executives who are not in hospital or hospital system positions. The award served as the counterpart to the professional society's Gold Medal Award until 1991. At that time, the Board of Governors approved the merger of the Silver Medal Award with the Gold Medal Award, authorizing up to two Gold Medal recipients annually. The 1991 Silver Medal Award was the last given.

1974	Stanley W. Martin, LFACHE	1976	Matthew F. McNulty Jr., ScD, FACHE
1975	Gerhard Hartman, PhD, FACHE	1977	Richard J. Stull, FACHE

1978	Walter J. McNerney, FACHE	1985	David M. Kinzer
1979	O. Ray Hurst	1986	J. Alexander McMahon, HFACHE
1980	James O. Hepner, PhD, LFACHE	1987	Rear Adm. Lewis E. Angelo
1981	Donald L. Custis, MD	1988	Donald R. Newkirk, FACHE
1982	George Bugbee, FACHE	1989	Everett A. Johnson, PhD, FACHE
1983	Robert M. Cunningham Jr., HFACHE	1990	Bernard R. Tresnowski, LFACHE
1984	Richard L. Johnson, FACHE	1991	Stuart A. Wesbury Jr., PhD, FACHE

THE LIFETIME SERVICE AWARD

The Lifetime Service Award was created to recognize Life Fellows and Retired Fellows who have made significant contributions to ACHE.

2000	Paul S. Ellison, LFACHE	2006	Garth A. H. Pierce, LFACHE
2001	David H. Jeppson, LFACHE	2007	Donald S. Good, LFACHE
2002	Joseph H. Powell, LFACHE	2008	Francis J. Cronin Jr., LFACHE

ROBERT S. HUDGENS MEMORIAL AWARD

The Robert S. Hudgens Memorial Award for "Young Healthcare Executive of the Year" was established in 1969 as a tribute to Mr. Hudgens—ACHE's First Vice President (an elected office)—by the Alumni Association of the Graduate Program in Health Services Administration of the Medical College of Virginia, Virginia Commonwealth University. It is awarded to an exceptional healthcare executive who is under 40 years of age and serving as a chief executive officer or chief operating officer of a healthcare organization.

1969	Donald C. Wegmiller, FACHE	1990	Denise Williams
1970	Monroe Mitchell	1991	Michael J. Connelly, FACHE
1971	Nelson Lewis St. Clair Jr., FACHE	1992	Mark K. Wallace, FACHE
1972	Robert L. Montgomery, LFACHE	1993	Kevin E. Lofton
1973	Gail L. Warden, FACHE	1994	William F. Groneman, FACHE
1974	G. Edwin Howe, FACHE	1995	Stephen C. McCary, FACHE
1975	F. Kenneth Ackerman Jr., FACHE	1996	Kenneth A. Samet
1976	Paul B. Hofmann, DrPH, FACHE	1997	Sue G. Brody
1977	James L. Farley	1998	Lee H. Perlman, FACHE
1979	Lloyd L. Cannedy, PhD	1999	Rulon F. Stacey, PhD, FACHE
1980	Glen T. Randolph, FACHE	2000	Jon M. Foster, FACHE
1981	John T. Casey	2001	David A. Olson, FACHE
1982	Myles P. Lash	2002	Colleen L. Kannaday, FACHE
1983	Jan R. Jennings	2003	Anthony E. Munroe, EdD, FACHE
1984	David L. Bernd, FACHE	2004	James G. Springfield, FACHE
1985	David J. Fine, FACHE	2005	William E. Holmes
1986	Mark E. Celmer	2006	Danny L. Jones Jr., FACHE
1987	R. Timothy Stack, FACHE	2007	Lt. Col. Jessie L. Tucker III, PhD, FACHE
1988	Mark R. Neaman, FACHE		
1989	John B. Grotting	2008	David A. Stark, FACHE

EXECUTIVE OF THE YEAR AWARD

The Executive of the Year Award was introduced in 1961 and was presented annually at ACHE's Congress on Administration to an outstanding executive outside the hospital field. In 1975 the award was discontinued at the recommendation of the Committee on the Executive of the Year, action endorsed by the parent Committee on Awards and Testimonials and by the Board of Governors. All positions shown were those held at the time the award was bestowed.

1961   Clarence B. Randall
        Retired Chairman of the Board, Inland Steel Company

1962   George Romney
        President, American Motors Corporation

1963   Clark Kerr, PhD
        President, University of California

1964   John A. Barr
        Chairman of the Board, Montgomery Ward & Company

1965   General Robert W. Johnson
        Member, Board of Directors, Johnson & Johnson

1966   John W. Macy
        Chairman, U.S. Civil Service Commission

1967   Joseph L. Block
        Chief Executive Officer, Inland Steel Company

1968   Ray R. Eppert
        Chief Executive Officer, Burroughs Corporation

1969   George Champion
        Chairman of the Board, The Chase Manhattan Bank

1970   Robert G. Dunlop
        Chairman of the Board, Sun Oil Company

1971   Edwin J. Faulkner
        President, Woodman Accident and Life Company

1972   Walter K. Koch
        Attorney-at-Law, Holme Roberts & Owen

1973   Rev. Theodore M. Hesburgh
        President, University of Notre Dame

1974   Archie K. Davis
        Chairman of the Board, Wachovia Bank and Trust Company

DEAN CONLEY AWARD

The Dean Conley Award was established in 1958 to recognize outstanding articles on an administrative theme published in one of the major magazines or journals serving the healthcare management field. The award was named in tribute to Dean Conley, executive director of ACHE, serving from 1942 to 1965.

1958   "Principles of Administration"
        Wallace S. Sayre, PhD
        Hospitals

1960   "The Intellectual Development of the Operationalist"
        Rev. Robert J. Henle, SJ
        Hospital Progress

1961   "The Nature of Administration"
        Ray E. Brown, FACHE
        The Modern Hospital

1962   "The Administrator Must Be Adept at Adapting"
        Ray E. Brown, FACHE
        The Modern Hospital

1963   "Administrative Leadership in Hospital Research"
        Arnold L. Swanson, MD, LFACHE
        Canadian Hospital

1964   "The Top Management Triangle in the Voluntary Hospital"
        Paul J. Gordon, PhD
        Hospitals

1965   "Proliferation of Hospital Professions Is New Challenge to Management"
Donald W. Cordes, LFACHE
The Modern Hospital

1966   "Administration Is Not a Numbers Game"
Ray E. Brown, FACHE
The Modern Hospital

1967   "The Effective Hospital Administrator Leads Board and Community Thinking"
Robert B. Ferguson, FACHE
Hospital Administration in Canada

1968   "New Consensus Health Care for Everybody"
Harry Becker
The Modern Hospital

1969   "Promoting Quality Care Through Evaluating the Process of Patient Care"
Avedis Donabedian, MD, HFACHE
Medical Care

1970   "The Notion of Hospital Incentives"
Robert M. Sigmond, LFACHE
Hospital Progress

1971   "Hospital Costs and Payment: Suggestions for Stabilizing the Uneasy Balance"
Anne Ramsay Somers, HFACHE
Medical Care

1972   "Reaching the Unreachable"
H. Robert Cathcart, LFACHE
Hospitals

1973   "Beyond Responsibility: Toward Accountability"
Kenneth J. Williams, MD, LFACHE
Hospital Progress

1974   "Hospital Organization in the Post-Industrial Society"
Gordon L. Lippitt, PhD
Hospital Progress

1975   "Excessive Hospitalization Can Be Cut Back"
Peter Rogatz, MD, FACHE
Hospitals

1976   "The Promise of Multihospital Management
Montague Brown, DrPH, and William H. Money
Hospital Progress

1977   "Holding the CEO Accountable"
Harold Koontz, PhD
Hospital Progress

1978   "Reimbursement System Must Recognize Real Costs"
David H. Hitt, LFACHE
Hospitals

1979   "The Last Resort: Regulation by Law"
Thomas M. Tierney, HFACHE
Hospital Progress

1980   "The 1980's: Rise of HMO's and the Marketplace Competition"
Richard L. Johnson, LFACHE
Hospital Progress

1981   "Rethinking Health Policy for the Elderly: A Six-Point Program"
Anne Ramsey Somers, HFACHE
Inquiry

1982   "Predictions Too Rosy, Solutions Too Pat"
David M. Kinzer
Hospitals

1983   "Hospital Strategic Planning Must Be Rooted in Values and Ethics"
Joseph P. Peters, LFACHE, and Ronald C. Wacker
Hospitals

1984   "How to Create an Outstanding Hospital Culture"
Terrence E. Deal, PhD, Allan A. Kennedy, and Arthur H. Spiegel III
Hospital Forum

1985   "Death of a Paradigm: The Challenge of Competition"
Jeff C. Goldsmith, PhD
Health Affairs

1986   "Medical Staff of the Future: Replanting the Garden"
Stephen M. Shortell, PhD, FACHE
Frontiers of Health Services Management

1987   "How Companies Tackle Health Care Costs"
Regina E. Herzlinger and Jeffery Schwartz
Harvard Business Review

1988   "Where is Hospital Leadership Coming From"
David Kinzer
Frontiers of Health Services Management

1989   "The Uninsured: Response and
Responsibility"
Gail Wilensky, PhD, and Kala Ladenheim
Frontiers of Health Services Management

1990   "A Radical Prescription for Hospitals"
Jeff C. Goldsmith, PhD
Harvard Business Review

1991   "Improving Hospital Board Effectiveness:
An Update"
Anthony R. Kovner, PhD
Frontiers of Health Services Management

1992   "The Quest for Quality and Productivity in
Health Services"
Vinod K. Sahney, PhD, and Gail L.
Warden, FACHE
Frontiers of Health Services Management

1993   "Health Care Leadership in the Public
Interest"
Bruce C. Vladeck, PhD
Frontiers of Health Services Management

1994   "Managed Care: Past Evidence and
Potential Trends"
Robert H. Miller, PhD, and Harold S.
Luft, PhD
Frontiers of Health Services Management

1995   "The Architecture of Integration"
J. Daniel Beckham
Healthcare Forum Journal

1996   "The Illusive Logic of Integration"
Jeff C. Goldsmith, PhD
Healthcare Forum Journal

1997   "Managing the Transition to Integrated
Health Care Organizations"
John R. Griffith, FACHE
Frontiers of Health Services Management

1998   "The Emergence of Providers as Health
Insurers"
James J. Unland
Journal of Health Care Finance

1999   "Last Chance Therapies and Managed
Care: Pluralism, Fair Procedures, and
Legitimacy"
Norman Daniels, PhD, and James E.
Sabin, MD
Hastings Center Report

2000   "Challenges in Developing Physician
Leadership and Management"
Michael B. Guthrie, MD, FACPE
Frontiers of Health Services Management

2001   "Beyond Technology and Managed Care:
The Health System Considers Ten Future
Trends"
Wanda J. Jones
Frontiers of Health Services Management

2002   "Genomics: Implications for Health
Systems"
Chris Myers, Nicole Paulk, and Christine
Dudlak
Frontiers of Health Services Management

2003   "Why Integrated Health Networks Have
Failed"
Leonard Friedman, PhD, and Jim Goes,
PhD
Frontiers of Health Services Management

2004   "9/11: A Healthcare Provider's Response"
David J. Campbell, FACHE
Frontiers of Health Services Management

2005   "Prejudice and the Medical Profession"
Peter A. Clark, SJ, PhD
Health Progress

2006   "A Call for Board Leadership on Quality in
Hospitals"
Kanak S. Gautam, PhD
Quality Management in Health Care

2007   "Patient Safety: Mindful, Meaningful, and
Fulfilling"
Steven C. Winokur, MD, Kay Beauregard, RN
Frontiers of Health Services Management

2008   "Specialty-Service Lines: Salvos in the New
Medical Arms Race"
Robert A. Berenson, Thomas Bodenheimer,
and Hoangmai H. Pham
Health Affairs

EDGAR C. HAYHOW AWARD

The Edgar C. Hayhow Award was established in 1960 to recognize outstanding articles published in the journal *Hospital & Health Services Administration* (now the *Journal of Healthcare Management*). The award was named in tribute to Edgar C. Hayhow, Chairman of ACHE, 1947–1948, and the first practicing administrator to have earned a doctoral degree.

1960   "Motivation and Morale"
Oswald Hall, PhD

1961   "Problem-Oriented Administration"
Warren G. Bennis, PhD

1962   "The Qualities of an Administrator"
Ralph N. Traxler Jr., PhD

1963   "The Dynamics of Professionalism: The Case of Hospital Administration"
Harold L. Wilensky, PhD

1964   "The Spontaneous Development of Informal Organization"
E. Jackson Baur, PhD

1965   "The Impact of the Hospital on the Physician, the Patient and the Community"
George Rosen, MD, PhD

1966   "The Administrator and Policy Processes"
John W. Hennessey Jr., PhD

1967   "A Philosophical Dimension of Administration"
Leonard A. Duce, PhD

1968   "When Occupations Meet: Professions in Trouble"
Edward Gross, PhD

1969   "Applying Economic Concepts to Hospital Care"
Paul J. Feldstein, PhD

1970   "The Social Responsibility of General Hospitals"
Bright M. Dornblaser, FACHE

1971   "Professional Development Needs in Hospital Administration"
Louis E. Davis, PhD

1972   "Conflicting Economic Pressure in Health-Care"
James R. Jeffers, PhD

1973   "An Emerging Medical Staff Organization"
Everett A. Johnson, PhD, FACHE

1974   "Conflict of Interest: Ethical Dilemma"
Charles M. Ewell Jr., FACHE

1975   "The Crisis in Health Care System: A Contrary Opinion"
S. David Pomrinse, MD, FACHE

1976   "The Ashland Plan: An Ambulatory Care Outreach Alternative for a Community Hospital"
John N. Simpson, FACHE

1977   "Evaluation of Administrative and Organizational Effectiveness in Hospitals"
Charles M. Ewell Jr., PhD, FACHE

1978   "Old and New Thinking About Hospital Payments"
Everett A. Johnson, PhD, FACHE

1979   "Evaluating the Performance of the Chief Executive Officer"
James D. Harvey, LFACHE

1980   "The Management of Disruptive Conflicts"
Robert Veninga, PhD

1981   "What Motivates People to Work Effectively"
David Babnew, PhD, LFACHE

1982   "Administrative Linkages: Management Issues and Implications"
Austin Ross, LFACHE

1983   "Hospital Administration and Medicine at the Crossroads"
James W. Summers, PhD

1984   "Physician-Centered Marketing: A Practical Step to Hospital Survival"
Daniel A. Koger, PhD, and Frankie L. Perry, RN, MA, FACHE

1985 "Doing Good and Doing Well: Ethics, Professionalism and *Success*"
James W. Summers, PhD

1986 "Improving Hospital Productivity Under PPS: Managing Cost Reductions"
Stephen R. Eastaugh, PhD

1987 "In Search of Social Enterprise: A Fable"
David Starkweather, PhD, FACHE

1988 "Decision Points for Hospital-Based Health Promotion"
Eileen Malo and Laura E. Leviton, PhD

1989 "Voluntary Hospitals: Are Trustees the Solution?"
John R. Griffith, FACHE

1990 "The Keys to Successful Diversification: Lessons from Leading Hospital Systems"
Stephen Shortell, PhD, FACHE, Ellen Morrison, PhD, and Susan Hughes

1991 "Coping with Unbalanced Information about Decision-Making Influence for Nurses"
Robert H. Schwartz, PhD

1992 "The Power of Health Care Value-Adding Partnerships: Meeting Competition through Cooperation"
Stephen E. Foreman and Robert D. Roberts

1993 "Outcomes Measurement in Hospitals: Can the System Change the Organization?"
Jane C. Lindner, DBA

1994 "Total Quality Management in a Health Care Organization: How Are Employees Affected?"
Michael A. Counte, PhD; Gerald L. Glandon, PhD; Denise M. Oleske, PhD; and James P. Hill, JD

1995 "Creating Organized Delivery Systems: The Barriers and Facilitators"
Stephen M. Shortell, PhD, FACHE; Robin R. Gillies, PhD; David A. Anderson, CPA; John B. Mitchell, JD; and Karen Morgan Erickson

1996 "Continually Improving Governance"
Barbara Arrington, PhD, FACHE; Kanak Gautam, PhD; and William J. McCabe

1997 "The Role and Impact of Multiskilled Health Practitioners in the Health Services Industry"
Myron D. Fottler, PhD

1998 "Managing Clinical Integration in Integrated Delivery Systems: A Framework for Action"
David W. Young, DBA, and Diana Barrett, DBA

1999 "Rural Hospitals: Organizational Alignments for Managed Care Contracting"
Niccie L. McKay, PhD

2000 "The Emergency Department and Managed Care: A Synergistic Model"
Brent A. Fisher, FACHE

2001 "Strategic Cycling: Shaking Complacency in Healthcare Strategic Planning"
James W. Begun, PhD, and Kathleen B. Heatwole

2002 "Healing Models for Organizations: Description, Measurement, and Outcomes"
Kathy Malloch, PhD, RN

2003 "Measuring Comparative Hospital Performance"
John R. Griffith, FACHE, and Jeffrey A. Alexander, PhD

2004 "Healthcare Managers' Roles, Competencies, and Outputs in Organizational Performance Improvement"
William G. Wallick, PhD

2005 "Integrating Six Sigma with Total Quality Management: A Case Example for Measuring Medication Errors"
Lee Revere, PhD, and Ken Black, PhD

2006 "The Revolution in Hospital Management"
John R. Griffith, FACHE, and Kenneth R. White, PhD, FACHE

2007 "Self-Assessment of Cultural and Linguistic Competence in an Ambulatory Health System"
Martha A. Medrano, MD, MPH, Jean Setzer, PhD, Steven L. Enders, FACHE, Raymond Costello, PhD, Viola Benavente, RN

2008 "Return on Investment in Pay for Performance: A Diabetes Case Study"
Howard Beckman, MD, and Kathleen Curtin

JAMES A. HAMILTON AWARD

The James A. Hamilton Award for Book of the Year was established in 1958 to identify books of exceptional merit in the field of healthcare or general management. The award is underwritten by the Alumni Association of the Graduate Program in Health Services Research and Policy and Administration of the University of Minnesota, in tribute to its course founder and director, James A. Hamilton, Chairman of ACHE, 1939–1940.

1958   *Administrative Behavior*
Herbert A. Simon, PhD
The Macmillan Company

1959   *Personality and Organization*
Chris Argyris, PhD
Harper & Row

1960   *Managerial Psychology*
Harold Leavitt, PhD
University of Chicago Press

1961   *Men Who Manage*
Melville Dalton, PhD
John Wiley & Sons

1962   *The Human Side of Enterprise*
Douglas McGregor, PhD
McGraw-Hill Book Company

1963   *New Patterns of Management*
Rensis Likert, PhD
McGraw-Hill Book Company

1964   *The Community General Hospital*
Basil S. Georgopoulos, PhD, and Floyd C. Mann, PhD
The Macmillan Company

1965   *The Theory and Management of Systems*
Richard A. Johnson, PhD, Fremont E. Kast, PhD, and James E. Rosenzweig, PhD
McGraw-Hill Book Company

1966   *My Years With General Motors*
Alfred P. Sloan Jr.
Doubleday & Company

1967   *Men, Management and Morality: Toward a New Organizational Ethic*
Robert T. Golembiewski, PhD
McGraw-Hill Book Company

1968   *The Social Psychology of Organizations*
Daniel Katz, PhD, and Robert Kahn, PhD
John Wiley & Sons

1969   *Organization and Environment*
Paul R. Lawrence, PhD, and Jay W. Lorsch, PhD
Harvard University Press

1970   *The Exceptional Executive*
Harry Levinson, PhD
Harvard University Press

1971   *Ethos and Executive Values in Managerial Decision Making*
Clarence C. Walton, PhD
Prentice-Hall

1972   *Management Behavior, Performance and Effectiveness*
John P. Campbell, PhD, Marvin D. Dunnette, PhD, Edward E. Lawler III, PhD, and Karl E. Weick Jr., PhD
McGraw-Hill Book Company

1973   *Health Care in Transition: Directions for the Future*
Anne Ramsay Somers, HFACHE
Hospital Research and Education Trust

1974   *Organization Research on Health Institutions*
Basil S. Georgopoulos, PhD
ISR-The University of Michigan

1975   *Management: Tasks, Responsibilities, Practices*
Peter F. Drucker, PhD
Harper & Row Publishers

1976   *The Achieving Enterprise*
William F. Christopher
AMACOM

1977   *Management Control in Nonprofit Organizations*
Robert N. Anthony, PhD, and Regina E. Herzlinger, PhD
Richard D. Irwin

1978   *The Managerial Choice: To Be Efficient
and To Be Human*
Frederick I. Herzberg, PhD
Dow Jones-Irwin

1979   *Management Policy and Strategy*
George A. Steiner, PhD, and John B.
Miner, PhD
Macmillan Publishing Company

1980   *The New Managerial Grid*
Robert Blake, PhD, and Jane Mouton, PhD
Gulf Publishing Company

1981   *Leadership: What Effective Managers
Really Do...and How They Do It*
Leonard R. Sayles, PhD
McGraw-Hill Book Company

1982   *Managing in Turbulent Times*
Peter F. Drucker, PhD
Harper & Row

1983   *The Change Resisters: How They Prevent
Progress and What Managers Can Do
About Them*
George S. Odiorne
Prentice-Hall

1984   *The Social Transformation of American
Medicine*
Paul Starr, PhD
Basic Books

1985   *Managing Strategic Change in Hospitals:
Ten Success Stories*
Joseph P. Peters, LFACHE, and Simone
Tseng
American Hospital Publishing

1986   *CEO: Corporate Leadership in Action*
Harry Levinson, PhD, and Stuart
Rosenthal, MD
Basic Books

1987   *Corporate Pathfinders: Building Vision and
Values into Organizations*
Harold J. Leavitt
Dow Jones-Irwin

1988   *The Well-Managed Community Hospital*
John R. Griffith, FACHE
Health Administration Press

1989   *The Leadership Challenge*
James M. Kouzes and Barry Z. Posner, PhD
Jossey-Bass, Inc.

1990   *In Sickness and in Wealth: American
Hospitals in the Twentieth Century*
Rosemary Stevens, PhD
Basic Books, Inc.

1991   *What Kind of Life: The Limits of Medical
Progress*
Daniel Callahan, PhD
Simon and Schuster

1992   *Transforming Healthcare Organizations:
How to Achieve and Sustain
Organizational Excellence*
Ellen Gaucher and Richard J. Coffey, PhD
Jossey-Bass

1993   *Cornerstones of Leadership for Health
Services Executives*
Austin Ross, LFACHE
Health Administration Press

1994   *Improving Health Policy and
Management: Nine Critical Research
Issues for the 1990s*
Stephen M. Shortell, PhD, FACHE, and
Uwe E. Reinhardt, PhD
Health Administration Press

1995   *Managing the Whirlwind: Patterns and
Opportunities in a Changing World*
Michael H. Annison
Medical Group Management Association

1996   *Really Governing: How Health Systems and
Hospital Boards Can Make More of a
Difference*
Dennis D. Pointer, PhD, and Charles M.
Ewell Jr., PhD, FACHE
Delmar Publishers

1997   *Leading the Healthcare Revolution:
A Reengineering Mandate*
Gary D. Kissler, PhD
Health Administration Press

1998   *Market-Driven Health Care: Who Wins,
Who Loses in the Transformation of
America's Largest Service Industry*
Regina E. Herzlinger
Addison-Wesley Publishing Company, Inc.

1999   *Healthcare Strategic Planning: Approaches
for the 21st Century*
Alan M. Zuckerman, FACHE
Health Administration Press

2000   *Board Work: Governing Health Care Organizations*
Dennis D. Pointer, PhD, and James E. Orlikoff
Jossey-Bass

2001   *Leadership in Healthcare: Values at the Top*
Carson F. Dye, FACHE
Health Administration Press

2002   *Organizational Ethics in Health Care: Principles, Cases, and Practical Solutions*
Philip J. Boyle, PhD; Edwin R. DuBose, PhD; Stephen J. Ellingson, PhD; David E. Guinn, JD, PhD; and Rev. David B. McCurdy, DMin
AHA Press/Jossey-Bass

2003   *The Indispensable Health Care Manager: Success Strategies for a Changing Environment*
Wendy Leebov, EdD, and Gail Scott
Jossey-Bass

2004   *Putting Patients First: Designing and Practicing Patient-Centered Care*
Susan B. Frampton, PhD; Laura Gilpin; and Patrick A. Charmel, FACHE
Jossey-Bass

2005   *If Disney Ran Your Hospital: 9–1/2 Things You Would Do Differently*
Fred Lee
Second River Healthcare Press

2006   *Leading Your Healthcare Organization to Excellence: A Guide to Using the Baldrige Criteria.*
Patrice L. Spath
Health Administration Press

2007   *Redefining Health Care*
Michael E. Porter, Elizabeth Olmsted Teisberg
Harvard Business School Press

2008   *Leadership for Smooth Patient Flow*
Kirk Jensen, MD; Thom A. Meyer, MD; Shari J. Welch, MD; and Carol Hanaden, PhD
Health Administration Press

RICHARD J. STULL STUDENT ESSAY COMPETITION IN HEALTHCARE MANAGEMENT

This competition was introduced in 1989 and is open to students enrolled in those graduate and undergraduate health management programs in Canada and the United States that participate in the American College of Healthcare Executives higher education network. Listed are first-place winners in graduate and undergraduate programs for each year.

1989   "Confidentiality Issues for Health Care Administrators"
Sylvia A. Small
University of Texas–Medical Branch

"Legal Issues in Neonatal Intensive Care"
Barry M. Zajac
University of Michigan

1990   "Total Quality Management in Health Care"
Robert F. Casalou
University of Michigan

"Right to Refuse Medical Treatment"
Carol Lea Moody
University of Texas Medical Branch

1991   "Hospital Turf Battles: The Manager's Role"
Stephanie Lin Bloom, FACHE
The George Washington University

"The Significance of Transactional and Transformational Leadership Theory on the Hospital Manager"
Douglas B. Matey
University of New Hampshire

1992   "The Implications of Advance Directives on the Healthcare Institution"
Julie Pachmayer
Governors State University

"Organ Donation and Transplantation: The Need for a Multi-Pronged Approach for Equitable Allocation"
Mimi Modarress
University of Minnesota

1993   "Health Care Coalitions: An Emerging
       Force for Change"
       Karen Lowe Johnson
       Trinity University

       "Management Implications of Physician
       Practice Patterns—Strategies for Managers"
       Kristin O'Connor
       University of New Hampshire at Durham

1994   "Activity-Based Costing for Hospitals"
       Ralph H. Ramsey IV
       Texas Tech University

       "Reinventing Healthcare Delivery"
       Mark Bard
       James Madison University

1995   "Physician Practice Acquisitions: Valuation
       Issues and Concerns"
       Timothy B. Rimmer
       LaSalle University

       "Implementation Strategies of Patient
       Focused Care"
       Andreas L. Mang
       University of New Hampshire

1996   "Venturing into New Territory—Health
       Systems as Medicare Risk Contractors"
       Bradley A. Daniel, FACHE
       Virginia Commonwealth University

       "The Impact of Health Care Reform on
       HMO Administrators"
       Christopher R. Bolduc
       University of New Hampshire

1997   "Protecting the Public Interest: The Role of
       the State Attorney General in Regulating
       Hospital Conversions"
       Kara Marsche
       University of Michigan

       "Antitrust and Affiliations Among Health
       Care Providers: The Need for a Level
       Playing Field"
       Alison J. Heightchew
       James Madison University

1998   "A Cost-Savings Analysis of Prenatal
       Interventions"
       Susan L. Bonifield
       University of Memphis

       "Alternate Dispute Resolution: Methods to
       Address Workplace Conflict in Health
       Services Organizations"
       Jacqueline R. DeSouza
       James Madison University

1999   "Economic Credentialing: The Propriety of
       Managing Physician Costs Through
       Privileging"
       Brian A. Dahl
       University of Iowa

       "Hospital Customer Service in a Changing
       Health Care World: Does It Matter?"
       Julie E. Howard, DBA
       James Madison University

2000   "Disease Management: Old Wine in New
       Bottles?"
       Dawn R. Ritterband
       *Medical College of Virginia at Virginia
       Commonwealth University*

       "Mission and Organizational Performance
       in the Health Care Industry"
       Aimee B. Forehand
       James Madison University

2001   "Managing Strategic Outsourcing in the
       Healthcare Industry"
       Velma Roberts, PhD
       University of Alabama at Birmingham

       "The Adoption of Complementary and
       Alternative Medicine in Hospitals: A
       Framework for Decision-Making"
       Coleen F. Santa Ana
       James Madison University

2002   "Recruitment, Retention, and
       Management of Generation X with a
       Focus on Nursing Professionals"
       Judy A. Cordeniz, FACHE
       *Seton WorldWide, the online campus of
       Seton Hall University*

       "The Role of the Internet in Improving
       Health Care Quality"
       Kathryn E. Kerwin
       James Madison University

2003   "Robot-Assisted Surgery—The Future Is
       Here"
       Diana Gerhardus
       Trinity University

"Healthcare Reform Through Rationing"
Elizabeth J. Floyd
The University of Alabama, Tuscaloosa

2004   "Improving Care Interactions with
Racially and Ethnically Diverse Populations
in Healthcare Organizations: A Challenge
for Healthcare Management"
Duane E. Reynolds
The Ohio State University

"After 9–11: Elevating Bioterrorism
Preparedness in Hospitals"
Jenifer K. Murphy
James Madison University

2005   "The Plight of the Not-for-Profit: How
Current Controversies Are a Reflection of
the Historical, Regulatory, and Competitive
Environment of the Tax-Exempt Hospital"
R. Bramer Owens
Baylor University

"Addressing Variation in Hospital Quality:
Is Six Sigma the Answer?"
Tanisha D. Woodard
James Madison University

2006   "The Aging Nursing Workforce: How to
Retain Experienced Nurses"
Jeremye D. Cohen
Temple University

"The Importance of Middle Managers in
Healthcare Organizations"
Mari K. Embertson
Oregon State University

2007   "Hospital-Physician Informed Consent:
New Use of an Old Doctrine"
Edwin G. Ibay, JD
Virginia Commonwealth University

"Retail Medicine: The Cure for
Healthcare Disparities?"
Alicia Gallegos
Southern Illinois University

HEALTH MANAGEMENT RESEARCH AWARD

The Health Management Research Award was introduced in 1988 to enhance managerial effectiveness and career opportunities in health services administration. The award is supported through monies left to the Foundation of the American College of Healthcare Executives by Foster G. McGaw, founder of the American Hospital Supply Corporation. The award is granted only to affiliates of ACHE.

1988   "The Work of Middle Managers in Health
Care Organizations"
Linda Roemer, PhD

1989   "Discovering and Evaluating the Tactics
Used by Top Health Care Executives to
Carry Out Organizational Design"
Paul C. Nutt, PhD

1990   "Psychological Type, Health Care
Management, and the Myers-Briggs Type
Indicator: A Proposal for Research"
Stephen J. O'Connor, PhD, FACHE, and
Daniel J. Raab, FACHE

1991   "Diffusion and Adoption of Total Quality
Management"
Kit N. Simpson, DrPH, and Curtis
McLaughlin, DBA

1992   "Evaluating Hospital-Physician Integration
Strategies"
James B. Goes, PhD

1993   "Hospital Board Effectiveness: Board
Composition as a Predictor"
Carol Molinari, PhD

1994   "A Study of Administrative Costs and Intensity"
Samuel Levey, PhD, LFACHE

1995   "Performance Evaluation and Control of
Hospital CEOs: Implications for Corporate Strategy"
Gary J. Young, JD, PhD

1996   "How Marketing Oriented Are U.S. Hospitals in a Managed Care Environment?"
Patricia R. Loubeau, DrPH

1997   "Mentoring in Health Administration: The
Critical Link in Executive Development"
Anne Walsh, PhD, and Susan Borkowski,
PhD

1998	"Do Provider Incentive Withhold Arrangements Compensate Managed Care Plans for Agency Risk?" Patricia Driscoll, JD, and Rob Mauer, PhD	2003	"Succession Planning Practices and Outcomes in U.S. Hospitals: A Multilevel Analysis of Survey-Based Data" Andrew N. Garman, PsyD, and J. Larry Tyler, FACHE, FAAHC

1998　"Do Provider Incentive Withhold Arrangements Compensate Managed Care Plans for Agency Risk?"
Patricia Driscoll, JD, and Rob Mauer, PhD

1999　"Diversity Management Practices of Hospitals in Pennsylvania"
Janice L. Dreachslin, PhD; Robert Weech-Maldonado, PhD; Kathryn Dansky, PhD; and Gita De Souza, PhD

2000　"The Role of Internet Technologies in the Health Care Industry: Determinants and Outcomes of Adoption by Health Care Organizations"
E. Jose Proenca, PhD, and Michael George, FACHE

2001　"Building an Understanding of Qualities Needed for Health Administration Practice: A Cognitive Mapping Approach"
Richard M. Shewchuk, PhD; Stephen J. O'Connor, PhD, FACHE; and David J. Fine, MHA, FACHE

2002　"360 Feedback for Leadership Development in Health Administration"
Andrew N. Garman, PsyD, and J. Larry Tyler, FACHE, FAAHC

2003　"Succession Planning Practices and Outcomes in U.S. Hospitals: A Multilevel Analysis of Survey-Based Data"
Andrew N. Garman, PsyD, and J. Larry Tyler, FACHE, FAAHC

2004　"The Impact of Hospital CEO Turnover in U.S. Hospitals: A Web-Survey–Based Empirical Investigation"
Amir A. Khaliq, PhD; Steve Walston, PhD, FACHE; Steven E. Mattachione, JD, CPA, FHFMA; and David M. Thompson, PhD

2005　"Succession Planning Practices and Outcomes in U.S. Hospital Systems: A Survey of Current and Best Practices"
Andrew N. Garman, PsyD, and J. Larry Tyler, FACHE, FAAHC

2006　"Corporate Universities in Healthcare Organizations: Exploring the Evidence"
Ann Scheck McAlearney, ScD; David J. Reisman; Duane E. Reynolds; and Rebecca Schmake, PhD

2007　"The Incorporation of Non-Traditionally Educated Managers into Hospitals"
Amy K. Yarbrough, PhD, and Brian P. Baumgardner

STUART A. WESBURY Jr. POSTGRADUATE FELLOWSHIP

The Stuart A. Wesbury Jr. Postgraduate Fellowship was established in 1991 to further postgraduate education in healthcare and professional society management. The fellowship was named in honor of Stuart A. Wesbury Jr., PhD, FACHE, president of ACHE from 1979 to 1991. Student Associates of ACHE who have earned a graduate degree in health administration from a program accredited by the Commission on Accreditation of Healthcare Management Education are eligible. No Fellow was appointed in 1996.

1992	Ronald N. Feldman	2000	Gayle E. White
1993	Marie A. Rule	2001	Jana M. Meyer
1994	Trisha A. Seib	2002	Gloria I. San Miguel
1995	Chana L. Brady	2003	Lois R. Switzer
	Linda J. Walsh	2004	Ronald O'Shea Gamble
1997	D. Darren Opel	2005	Jonathan D. Wilbur
1998	Laura J. Cook	2006	Meryl J. George
1999	Frances C. Roesch, FACHE	2007	Reginald Cantave

AFFILIATED GROUP AWARD

The Affiliated Group Award was established in 1993 to recognize outstanding healthcare executive groups and women's executive networks affiliated with ACHE. The last award was given in 2004.

1993	The Metropolitan Health Administrators' Association New York, New York	1999	National Capital Healthcare Executives Washington, DC
1994	Association of Healthcare Executives of New Jersey	2000	Houston Chapter of the American College of Healthcare Executives Houston, Texas
1995	The Greater Philadelphia Health Assembly (renamed the Healthcare Leadership Network of the Delaware Valley) Philadelphia, Pennsylvania	2001	Health Care Executives of Southern California Ventura, California
1996	Health Care Administrators of Tidewater Tidewater, Virginia	2002	Georgia Association of Healthcare Executives Atlanta, Georgia
1997	Chicago Health Executives Forum Chicago, Illinois	2003	Healthcare Executives of Okinawa Okinawa, Japan
1998	Healthcare Executive Forum Buffalo, New York	2004	Michigan Healthcare Executives Group and Associates Detroit, Michigan

AWARD OF CHAPTER MERIT

This award is given to all fully chartered chapters that meet at least one of three performance standards needed to qualify for the Award for Chapter Excellence. The first awards were presented in 2007 based on the chapters' performance in 2006.

East Texas ACHE Forum
Eastern Pennsylvania Healthcare Executive
  Network
Health Care Executives of Southern
  California
Healthcare Leadership Network of
  Delaware Valley

Network of Overseas Healthcare Executives
North Dakota Healthcare Executives
  Forum
South Texas Chapter of the American
  College of Healthcare Executives
Triad Healthcare Executive Forum
Utah Healthcare Executives

ARTHUR C. BACHMEYER MEMORIAL ADDRESSES

This address is underwritten by alumni of the Graduate Program in Hospital Administration of The University of Chicago in tribute to their former director, Dr. Bachmeyer. There was no address in 1960, the year the site of the lecture was changed from ACHE's Annual Meeting to its educational program, the Congress on Healthcare Leadership. In 2005, the scheduled speaker was unable to give the address.

1949	"Mankind Is Your Concern" Stuart Chase *Economist, Author*	1950	"The Challenge of Liberty" William F. Russell, PhD *President, Teachers' College, Columbia University*

1951   "The Significance of Maturity"
James F. Bender, PhD
Director, National Institute of Human Relations

1952   "Education and Man's Quest for Freedom"
Clark G. Keubler, PhD
President, Ripon College

1953   "Principles of Effective Administration"
Paul S. Weaver, PhD
President, Lake Erie College

1954   "Perspective for Administration"
A. A. Suppan, PhD
Professor of Literature and Philosophy, Wisconsin State Teachers' College

1955   "The Administrator Reconsidered"
Robert M. Hutchins, PhD
President, Fund for the Republic

1956   "What it Means to Be an Administrator"
Marshall E. Dimock, PhD, HFACHE
Dean, Department of Government, New York University

1957   "A Practical Philosophy of Administration"
Elmore Petersen, PhD
Dean Emeritus School of Business, University of Colorado

1958   "Reflections on the Art of Administration"
Ordway Tead
Vice President, Harper & Brothers

1959   "The Challenge of Being an Administrator"
Ralph C. Davis, PhD
Professor of Management, Ohio State University

1961   "A Moral Philosophy for Management"
Benjamin M. Selekman, PhD
Kirstein Professor of Labor Relations, Harvard University

1962   "Ethics in Executive Action"
James C. Worthy
Partner, Cresap, McCormick and Paget

1963   "Statesmanship in Administration"
J. Martin Klotsche, PhD
Provost, University of Wisconsin-Milwaukee

1964   "Executives and Their Jobs Changing Organizational Structure"
Thomas L. Whisler, PhD
Professor of Industrial Relations, University of Chicago

1965   "Influences of Government on the Management Function"
Carl M. Frasure, PhD
Dean, College of Arts and Sciences, West Virginia University

1966   "New Trends in the Training of Administrators"
Henry A. Singer, PhD
Executive Director, Society for Advancement of Management

1967   "The Effective Executive"
Peter F. Drucker, PhD
Professor of Management, New York University

1968   "The Challenge of Communication"
Arthur Secord, PhD
Professor of Speech, Brooklyn College

1969   "Crisis in American Health Care"
Charles E. Odegaard, PhD
President, University of Washington

1970   "Universal Compulsory Health Insurance"
Odin W. Anderson, PhD, HFACHE
Associate Director, Center for Health Administration Studies, The University of Chicago

1971   "The Frontiers of Our Time"
Harold P. Plumier
Author, Lecturer, Consultant

1972   "Financial Prospects and Competition for Capital"
Henry Kaufman, PhD
Partner, Salomon Brothers

1973   "Training for Health Services Management"
Ray E. Brown, FACHE
Executive Vice President, Northwestern McGaw-Medical Center

1974   "Graduate Education Confronts the Market Place"
Robert H. Strotz, PhD
President, Northwestern University

1975   "National Health Insurance and the Hospital Administrator"
George Bugbee, FACHE
Director, Inter-Agency Institute for Federal Health Care Executives

1976   "Coercive vs. Representative Government
W. Allen Wallis
Chancellor, University of Rochester

1977   "Two Sides of the Same Coin: Voluntary Financing and Voluntary Management"
Walter J. McNerney, FACHE
President, Blue Cross Association

1978   "Spiritual Values in Hospital Administration"
Rev. Raymond C. Baumhart, SJ
President, Loyola University

1979   "Research Monitoring Systems"
J. Robert Clement
President, Trebor Health Associates, Inc.

1980   "Compensation for Health Service Executives"
John F. Sullivan
President, Sullivan & Shook

1981   "Self Renewal: A Divine Perspective for Hospitals and Managers"
Leland R. Kaiser, PhD
Director, Division of Health Administration, University of Colorado Medical Center

1982   "American Management: Losing Sight of 'Love of the Product'"
Thomas J. Peters, PhD
Principal, McKinsey & Company

1983   "What's Next?"
Peter B. Laubach, DBA, HFACHE
President, Center for Management Programs
Richard L. Rand, HFACHE
President, PermaHealth Enterprises

1984   "Administration and the Groves of Academe"
Hanna Holborn Gray, PhD
President, The University of Chicago

1985   "Healthcare and the Information Revolution"
Paul Starr, PhD
Professor, Harvard University

1986   "Risk Transfer and Other Management Alternatives"
John P. McLaughlin
Managing Director and Chairman, Health Care Industry Practice/Client Industry Committee, Marsh & McLennan, Inc.

1987   "Life Through an Elder's Eyes"
Patricia Moore
Gerontologist and Author, Moore & Associates

1988   "Breaking the Glass Ceiling: Can Women Reach the Top of the Corporate Ladder?"
Ann M. Morrison
Director, Center for Creative Leadership

1989   "Healthcare: The View from My Window"
Hon. Lynn M. Martin, FACHE
(R-Illinois) U.S. House of Representatives

1990   "Healthcare's Changing Corporate Culture"
Terrence Deal, PhD
Professor of Education and Human Development, Peabody College, Vanderbilt University

1991   "Access to Care"
Most Rev. Joseph M. Sullivan, HFACHE
Auxiliary Bishop, Diocese of Brooklyn

1992   "The Physician's Perspective on the Future of Healthcare Administration"
James Todd, MD
Executive Vice President, American Medical Association

1993   "Leadership Is an Art"
Charles S. Lauer, FACHE
Publisher, Modern Healthcare
Corporate Vice President, Crain Communications, Inc.

1994   "Communitarian Perspective on the Healthcare Crisis"
Amitai Etzioni, PhD
Professor, George Washington University

1995   "Healthcare Reform: Ten Percent Legislation and Ninety Percent Implementation"
William Kissick, MD, DrPH
Professor, University of Pennsylvania

1996   "The Future State of Healthcare"
J. Ian Morrison, PhD
Author, Lecturer, and Consultant

1997   "Accepting, Creating, and Thriving on Change"
Janet Lapp
President and Chief Executive Officer, CLD International

1998   "Thinking in the Future Tense"
Jennifer James, PhD
Cultural Anthropologist, Writer, Commentator, and Publisher

1999   "The Future of Medicare"
Bruce C. Vladeck, PhD
Director, Institute for Medicare Practice
Professor of Health Policy, The Mt. Sinai
School of Medicine, Senior Vice President for
Policy, The Mt. Sinai Medical Center

2000   "The Real Bottom Line"
Emily Friedman
Health Policy Analyst

2001   "Values and Health: Global Ethics for the
21st Century"
Rushworth M. Kidder
Founder and President, Institute for Global
Ethics

2002   "Aligning Purpose, Values, and
Management in the Healthcare Enterprise"
Reed V. Tuckson, MD
Senior Vice President of Consumer Health
and Medical Care Advancement,
UnitedHealth Group

2003   "Spirituality in the Workplace"
William A. Guillory, PhD
President and Chief Executive Officer,
Innovations Consulting International, Inc.

2004   "Leadership Lessons from the Jazz
Masters"
John Edward Hasse
Curator of American Music, Smithsonian
Institution's National Museum of
American History

2006   "From the Patient's Perspective"
Bertice Berry, PhD
Educator, Author, and Comedian

2007   "Access and the Business of Medicine:
The Path Ahead"
Risa Lavizzo-Mourey, MD
President and Chief Executive Officer,
Robert Wood Johnson Foundation

2008   "The Human Aspects of Quality
Improvement"
William F. Martin, PsyD
Associate Director, Human Resources,
DePaul University

MALCOLM T. MacEACHERN MEMORIAL LECTURES

An annual feature at ACHE's Congress on Healthcare Leadership since 1961, this lecture is underwritten by the Alumni Association of the Graduate Program in Hospital and Health Services Administration of Northwestern University in tribute to its former director, Dr. MacEachern.

1961   "The Inquiring Mind"
Cyril O. Houle, PhD
Professor of Education, The University of
Chicago

1962   "The Dynamics of Professionalization"
Harold L. Wilensky, PhD
Associate Professor of Sociology, University of
Michigan

1963   "Vision and Leadership in the Professions"
Eldridge T. McSwain, PhD
Dean, School of Education, Northwestern
University

1964   "The Administrator as Teacher"
Daniel R. Davies, PhD
Professor of Management, University of
Arizona

1965   "Graduate Education for Administration:
Some Recent Developments"
Leonard A. Duce, PhD
Dean, Graduate School, Trinity University

1966   "The Relevancy of Professional Education
for Management"
James H. Lorie, PhD
Professor of Business Administration,
Graduate School of Business,
The University of Chicago

1967   "Education Accreditation: Purposes and
Problems"
Frank G. Dickey, PhD
Chief Administrative Officer, National
Committee on Accrediting

1968   "The Adult Educated: A New Generation of Pioneers"
William L. Bowden, PhD
Chairman, Department of Adult Education, The University of Georgia

1969   "Educating for the Future"
Ralph Westfall, PhD
Associate Dean for Academic Affairs, School of Management Northwestern University

1970   "Education for Hospital Administration"
John A. Barr
Dean, Graduate School of Management, Northwestern University

1971   "The Dilemma of Hospitals—Is Public Utility Status the Answer?"
Fred P. Morrissey, PhD
Professor of Business Management, Graduate School of Business, The University of California

1972   "A Review of Some Major Administration Health Care Policies"
Scott Fleming
Deputy Assistant Secretary, Health and Scientific Affairs, HEW

1973   "The Challenge to Management of Today's Health Care World"
John Alexander McMahon, HFACHE
President, American Hospital Association

1974   "Leadership in Complex Institutions"
Warren G. Bennis, PhD
President, The University of Cincinnati

1975   "Implications of the Reports on the Commission on Education for Health Administration"
James P. Dixon, MD
President, Antioch College

1976   "Health Service Administration—Yesterday and Today"
James A. Hamilton, FACHE
Consultant

1977   "The Changing Nature of Society"
Howard F. Didsbury Jr.
Executive Director, World Future Society

1978   "The Manager as a Change Agent"
S. G. Huneryager, PhD
Professor of Management, University of Illinois Chicago

1979   "An Analysis of Governing Developments: Their Effects on the Business Community"
Richard R. Salzmann
Editor-in-Chief, Research Institute of America

1980   "Goals of Schools and Management: Positive Self-Image, Hope, and Love"
Zacharie J. Clements, PhD
Associate Professor of Education, University of Vermont, Burlington

1981   "Dealing with the Media During a Crisis"
Stephen C. Rare
Principal, Dynamic Innovations, Ltd.

1982   "Human Concern in Management"
Dan C. Baker

1983   "Health Care Ethics"
Joseph Cardinal Bernardin
Roman Catholic Archdiocese of Chicago

1984   "Healthcare: Past, Present and Future"
S. David Pomrinse, MD
President, Greater New York Hospital Association

1985   "Anti-Social Ethics"
Richard Lamm
Governor, State of Colorado

1986   "The Aging of America"
Ken Dychtwald, PhD
President, Age Wave

1987   "The New American Organization"
V. Clayton Sherman, EdD
President, Management House, Inc.

1988   "Healthcare—Also a Matter of Trust"
James E. Burke
Chairman and Chief Executive Officer, Johnson and Johnson

1989   "Assessing the Impact of DRGs on the American Healthcare System"
Stuart H. Altman, PhD
Dean, Heller School of Social Policy, Brandeis University

1990   "The Role of the Non-Profit Sector in Today's Healthcare"
George F. Moody
Chairman, American National Red Cross

1991   "Financing the Future of Healthcare"
Gail Wilensky, PhD
Administrator, Health Care Financing Administration

1992   "Managing Cultural Diversity"
Judy Rosener, PhD
Professor and Former Assistant Dean, Graduate School of Management, University of California

1993   "Delivering Primary Healthcare: Innovative Solutions in Urban Settings"
Ronald Anderson, MD
President and Chief Executive Officer, Parkland Memorial Hospital

1994   "Future Trends in Healthcare"
Richard T. Hoerl, PhD
President, Hoerl & Associates

1995   "Executive Renewal: A Human Approach to Productivity and Creativity"
Barbara Mackoff, PhD
Author and Management Psychologist

1996   "The Greater Social Responsibility of the Healthcare Executive"
Reed V. Tuckson, MD
Charles R. Drew University of Medicine and Science

1997   "The Evolving Healthcare Landscape: Managing the Transition"
Jacque J. Sokolov, MD
Chief Executive Officer, Advance Health Plans, Inc., and AHP Development Corp.

1998   "Predicting the Future of the U.S. Healthcare System"
Stuart A. Altman, PhD, HFACHE
Sol C. Chaikin Professor of National Health Policy, The Florence Heller Graduate School for Social Policy, Brandeis University

1999   "Leadership: Making a World of Difference"
Elaine Chao
Distinguished Fellow, The Heritage Foundation

2000   "Physician Collaboration: The Keys to Developing Productive Relationships"
Barbara C. LeTourneau, MD, FACPE
President, LeTourneau & Associates LLC

2001   "Teamwork Under Fire—Bringing Out the Best in Everyone During Times of Rapid Change"
Bonnie St. John Deane
Athlete, Author, Executive, and Motivator

2002   "Revisioning the Nursing Shortage: A Call to Caring and Healing the Healthcare System"
Janet F. Quinn, PhD, RN, FAAN
Associate Professor, University of Colorado School of Nursing

2003   "Corporate Culture for Uncertain Times"
Peg C. Neuhauser
Author and Consultant, PCN Associates

2004   "Convergence Health"
Lowell Catlett, PhD
Regent's Professor of Economics, Agriculture, and Genetic Engineering, New Mexico State University

2005   "The Art of Vision"
Erik Wahl
Founder, The Wahl Group

2006   "Evidence-Based Medicine: Key Concepts, Emerging Applications"
Paul H. Keckley, PhD
Executive Director, Vanderbilt Center for Evidence-Based Medicine

2007   "Managing Change: Understanding the Demographics of the Evolving Workforce"
Marilyn Moats Kennedy
President and Managing Partner

2008   "What it Takes to Lead Safety"
Donald Berwick, MD
President and Chief Executive Officer, Institute for Healthcare Improvement

PARKER B. FRANCIS FOUNDATION DISTINGUISHED LECTURES

Introduced in 1975 by ACHE in cooperation with the Puritan-Bennett Corporation of Kansas City, Missouri, in memory of Parker B. and Mary Francis, for the purpose of presenting outstanding executives from the worlds of commerce, education, and government to the health service field. No lecture was given in 1980.

1975   Peter G. Peterson
Chairman of the Board, Lehman Brothers, Inc.

1976   Gordon McLachlan
Former Secretary Nuffield Provincial Hospitals Trust

1977   Howard W. Hiatt, MD
Dean, Harvard School of Public Health

1978   Pierre A. Rinfret, PhD
President, Rinfret Associates, Inc.

1979   Richard S. Schweiker
United States Senator, State of Pennsylvania

1981   Herbert A. Simon, PhD
Professor of Computer Science & Psychology, Carnegie-Mellon University

1982   Peter Francese
Publisher, American Demographics

1983   Jane Bryant Quinn
Financial Analyst and Commentator

1984   William C. Freund, PhD
Senior Vice President and Chief Economist, New York Stock Exchange

1985   Lawrence R. Miller
Partner, L. M. Miller & Company

1986   Amitai Etzioni
Professor, George Washington University

1987   Nancy K. Austin
President, Nancy K. Austin, Inc.

1988   F. G. (Buck) Rogers
Former Senior Vice President-Marketing, IBM

1989   Lee Sherman Dreyfus
Former Governor, State of Wisconsin

1990   Rosemary A. Stevens, PhD
Professor and Chairman, Department of History and Sociology of Sciences, University of Pennsylvania

1991   Frances Hesselbein
President and Chief Executive Officer, Peter F. Drucker Foundation For Nonprofit Management

1992   Kevin Phillips
Author and Political Analyst

1993   Gloria Borger
Chief Congressional Correspondent, U.S. News & World Report

1994   Charles E. Cook Jr.
Columnist, Roll Call

1995   Jill Dougherty
White House Correspondent, CNN

1996   Eleanor Clift
Political Correspondent, Newsweek

1997   Steven V. Roberts
Political Analyst and Syndicated Columnist

1998   Fred Barnes
*McLaughlin Group Panelist
Executive Editor, The Weekly Standard*

1999   Bob Beckel
President, Bob Beckel and Associates

2000   Mara Liasson
White House Correspondent, National Public Radio

2001   Bill Press
Co-Host, "Crossfire," CNN

2002   Robert Novak
Syndicated Columnist

2003   Eleanor Clift
*Contributing Editor, Newsweek
McLaughlin Group Panelist*

2004   Robert Laszewski
President, Health Policy and Strategy Associates, Inc.

2005   Vice Admiral Richard H. Carmona, MD, MPH, FACS, HFACHE
United States Surgeon General

2006   Jeffrey C. Bauer, PhD
Senior Vice President, Superior Consultant Company

2007   Richard Umbdenstock, FACHE
President and Chief Executive Officer, American Hospital Association

2008   "New Frontiers in Safety and Quality in Healthcare"
Mark Chassin, MD
President, The Joint Commission

LEON I. GINTZIG COMMEMORATIVE LECTURES

An annual feature at ACHE's Congress on Healthcare Leadership since 1986, this lecture is underwritten by The George Washington University Alumni Association for Health Services Administration in tribute to the program's former professor and chairman, Dr. Gintzig.

1986   "Health, Healthcare Executives and their Communities"
Bruce C. Vladeck, PhD
President, United Hospital Fund

1987   "Leadership for Changing Times"
Gerald Greenwald
Chairman, Chrysler Motors Corporation

1988   "Marketing Warfare in Healthcare"
Jack Trout
President, Trout and Ries Advertising

1989   "Information Systems as a Strategic Asset"
Frank A. Metz Jr.
Senior Vice President, IBM

1990   "Reevaluating Healthcare Illusions"
Sen. John Kitzhaber, MD
President, Oregon State Senate

1991   "Creating the Future of Healthcare"
Leland R. Kaiser, PhD
President, Kaiser and Associates

1992   "Delivering Healthcare: Costs and Questions"
Richard Morrow, FACHE
Former Chairman and Chief Executive Officer, Amoco Corporation

1993   "Leadership and Moral Purpose"
Max De Pree
Chairman, Herman Miller, Inc.

1994   "Journey Toward Quality"
Amelia Trotter Tess
Managing Director, Ground Operations, Northland District, Federal Express Corporation

1995   "Positively Outrageous Customer Service"
T. Scott Gross
Author

1996   "Creating a Vision for Change: Knowing When to Act"
Karen Welke
Group Vice President, 3M Medical Products Group

1997   "Increasing Human Effectiveness: Managing the Rapids of Change"
Robert A. Moawad
Chairman and Chief Executive Officer, Edge Learning Institute

1998   "Relaxing at High Speed"
Jeff Davidson, CMC
Executive Director, Breathing Space Institute

1999   "Keeping Good People"
Roger E. Herman, CMC, CSP
Chief Executive Officer, The Herman Group

2000   "How Visionary Leaders Manage Change and Lead People"
Philip D. Steffen
Chief Executive Officer and Founder, Philip D. Steffen Associates, Inc., and Bottom Line Group, Inc.

2001   "Managing Change: Understanding the Demographics of the Evolving Workforce"
Marilyn Moats Kennedy
Founder and Managing Partner, Career Strategies

2002   "Thriving in Turbulent Times"
Alan Parisse
President, Parisse Group, Inc.

2003   "Positively Outrageous Service"
T. Scott Gross
T. Scott Gross & Company, Inc.

2004   "Inspiring Meaningful Change"
John Alston
Founder, American Institute for Stress Management

2005   "Managing the Unmanageable: Lessons from Harvard"
Mimi Donaldson
Author and Speaker

2006   "The Art of Innovation"
Thomas A. Kelley
General Manager, IDEO

2007   "Innovative Leadership: Building a High
Performance Culture"
Terry "Moose" Millard
*Former Southwest Airlines Pilot, Corporate
Culture Expert*

2008   "Stop Sabotaging Your Career: Eight
Proven Strategies to Succeed in Spite of
Yourself"
Lois Frankel, PhD
*President, Corporate Coaching
International*

INDEX OF NAMES

INDEX OF SUBJECTS